Novel PET Imaging Techniques in the Management of Hematological Malignancies

Editors

CRISTINA NANNI
PAOLO CASTELLUCCI
STEFANO FANTI
NEETA PANDIT-TASKAR

PET CLINICS

www.pet.theclinics.com

Consulting Editor
ABASS ALAVI

October 2024 • Volume 19 • Number 4

ELSEVIER

1600 John F. Kennedy Boulevard • Suite 1800 • Philadelphia, Pennsylvania, 19103-2899

http://www.pet.theclinics.com

PET CLINICS Volume 19, Number 4
October 2024 ISSN 1556-8598, ISBN-13: 978-0-443-24634-0

Editor: John Vassallo (j.vassallo@elsevier.com)
Developmental Editor: Varun Gopal

PET Clinics (ISSN 1556-8598) is published quarterly by Elsevier Inc., 360 Park Avenue South, New York, NY 10010-1710. Months of issue are January, April, July, and October. Periodicals postage paid at New York, NY, and additional mailing offices. Subscription prices per year are $288.00 (US individuals), $100.00 (US students), $304.00 (Canadian individuals), $100.00 (Canadian students), $306.00 (foreign individuals), and $140.00 (foreign students). For institutional access pricing please contact Customer Service via the contact information below. To receive student and resident rate, orders must be accompanied by name of affiliated institution, date of term, and the signature of program/residency coordinator on institution letterhead. Orders will be billed at individual rate until proof of status is received. Foreign air speed delivery is included in all Clinics subscription prices. All prices are subject to change without notice. Orders, claims, and journal inquiries: Please visit our Support Hub page https://service.elsevier.com for assistance.

Reprints. For copies of 100 or more of articles in this publication, please contact the Commercial Reprints Department, Elsevier Inc., 360 Park Avenue South, New York, NY 10010-1710. Tel.: 212-633-3874; Fax: 212-633-3820; E-mail: reprints@elsevier.com.

PET Clinics is covered in MEDLINE/PubMed (Index Medicus).

Contributors

CONSULTING EDITOR

ABASS ALAVI, MD, MD (Hon), PhD (Hon), DSc (Hon)
Professor of Radiology and Neurology, Director of Research Education, Division of
Nuclear Medicine, Department of Radiology, Hospital of the University of Pennsylvania, Perelman School of Medicine, University of Pennsylvania, Philadelphia, Pennsylvania, USA

EDITORS

CRISTINA NANNI, MD
Nuclear Medicine Physician, IRCCS Azienda Ospedaliero–Universitaria di Bologna, Bologna, Italy

PAOLO CASTELLUCCI, MD
Nuclear Medicine Physician, IRCCS Azienda Ospedaliero–Universitaria di Bologna, Bologna, Italy

STEFANO FANTI, MD
Nuclear Medicine Physician, IRCCS Azienda Ospedaliero–Universitaria di Bologna, Bologna, Italy

NEETA PANDIT-TASKAR, MD
Attending Radiologist, Molecular Imaging and Therapy Service, Department of Radiology; Member, Memorial Hospital, Memorial Sloan Kettering Cancer Center; Professor of Radiology, Weill Cornell Medical Center, New York, New York, USA

AUTHORS

ELISABETTA MARIA ABENAVOLI, MD
Researcher, Nuclear Medicine Unit, Careggi University Hospital, Florence, Italy

ABASS ALAVI, MD, MD (Hon), PhD (Hon), DSc (Hon)
Professor of Radiology and Neurology, Director of Research Education, Division of Nuclear Medicine, Department of Radiology, Hospital of the University of Pennsylvania, Perelman School of Medicine, University of Pennsylvania, Philadelphia, Pennsylvania, USA

LUDMILA SANTIAGO ALMEIDA, MD
Assistant Nuclear Physician, Division of Nuclear Medicine, University of Campinas (UNICAMP), Campinas, Brazil; Department of Diagnostic Imaging (Radiology) and Nuclear Medicine, University Hospital San Pedro and Centre for Biomedical Research of La Rioja, Logroño, La Rioja, Spain

SANDIP BASU, MBBS (Hons), DRM, DNB, MNAMS
Professor and Head of Radiation Medicine Centre (Medical), Radiation Medicine Centre (BARC), Tata Memorial Hospital Annexe, Parel, Mumbai, India; Homi Bhabha National Institute, Mumbai, India

FABRIZIO BERGESIO, PhD
Researcher, Medical Physics Division, Department of Medical Physics, Santa Croce e Carle Hospital, Cuneo, Italy

FRANCESCO BERTAGNA, MD
Professor, Nuclear Medicine, Department of Medicine and Surgery, Università degli Studi di Brescia and ASST Spedali Civili di Brescia, Brescia, Italy

VALENTINA BERTI, MD
Associate Professor, Nuclear Medicine Unit, Department of Experimental and Clinical

Biomedical Sciences "Mario Serio", University of Florence, Florence, Italy

DAVIDE BEZZI, MD
Physician, Nuclear Medicine Unit, AUSL Romagna, Italy

CHRISTOPHE BONNET, MD, PhD
Professor, Department of Hematology, University Hospital Liege, Liege, Belgium

RALPH A. BUNDSCHUH, MD
Deputy Head, Nuclear Medicine, Faculty of Medicine, University of Augsburg, Augsburg, Germany

ALESSIA CASTELLINO, MD
Hematologist, Department of Hematology, Santa Croce e Carle Hospital, Cuneo, Italy

ARRIGO CATTABRIGA, MD
Radiologist and PhD Student, Department of Radiology, IRCCS Azienda Ospedaliero-Universitaria di Bologna, Department of Medical and Surgery Sciences (DIMEC), University of Bologna, Bologna, Italy

STÉPHANE CHAUVIE, PhD
Chief, Department of Medical Physics, Santa Croce e Carle Hospital, Cuneo, Italy

RAINER CLAUS, MD
Attending Hematologist and Oncologist, Hematology and Oncology, Faculty of Medicine, University of Augsburg; Pathology, Faculty of Medicine, University of Augsburg, Augsburg, Germany

ADRIANO DE MAGGI, PhD
Researcher, Medical Physics Division, Department of Medical Physics, Santa Croce e Carle Hospital, Cuneo, Italy

SAMUEL DE SOUZA MEDINA, MD
Assistant Physician, Division of Hematology, Department of Internal Medicine, Faculty of Medical Sciences, Campinas University, Campinas, Brazil

ROBERTO C. DELGADO BOLTON, MD, PhD
Consultant, Department of Diagnostic Imaging (Radiology) and Nuclear Medicine, University Hospital San Pedro and Centre for Biomedical Research of La Rioja, Logroño, La Rioja, Spain; Servicio Cántabro de Salud, Santander, Spain

LAURENT DERCLE, MD, PhD
Associate Research Scientist, Department of Radiology, New York-Presbyterian Hospital, Columbia University Vagelos College of Physicians and Surgeons, New York, New York, USA

FRANCESCO DONDI, MD
Nuclear Medicine Physician, Department of Medicine and Surgery, Università degli Studi di Brescia and ASST Spedali Civili di Brescia, Brescia, Italy

REXHEP DURMO, MD
Research Assistant, Nuclear Medicine Division, Department of Radiology, Azienda USL IRCCS of Reggio Emilia, Reggio Emilia, Italy

JOHANNA S. ENKE, MD
Resident, Nuclear Medicine, Faculty of Medicine, University of Augsburg, Augsburg, Germany

NASEEM S. ESTEGHAMAT, MD, MS
Assistant Professor, Division of Malignant Hematology, Cellular Therapy and Transplantation, Department of Internal Medicine, University of California Davis, Sacramento, California, USA

ELBA ETCHEBEHERE, MD, PhD
Professor, Division of Hematology, Department of Internal Medicine, Faculty of Medical Sciences, Campinas University, Campinas, Brazil

PATRICK GLENNAN, BA
Research Fellow, Rutgers Robert Wood Johnson Medical School, Piscataway, New Jersey, USA

FELIPE GODINEZ, PhD
Assistant Professor and Graduate Advisor for the Biomedical Engineering Graduate Group, Department of Radiology, University of California Davis, UC Cavis Comprehensive Cancer Center, Sacramento, California, USA

VICTOR CABRAL HERINGER, MD
Nuclear Medicine Physician, Division of Nuclear Medicine, University of Campinas (UNICAMP), Campinas, Brazil

ROLAND HUSTINX, MD, PhD
Professor, Division of Nuclear Medicine and Oncological Imaging, Department of Medical

Physics, CHU of Liege, Quartier Hopital, GIGA-CRC In vivo Imaging, University of Liege, Liege, Belgium

DIKHRA KHAN, MD
Senior Resident, Diagnostic Nuclear Medicine Division, Nuclear Medicine, All India Institute of Medical Sciences, New Delhi, Delhi, India

RAKESH KUMAR, MD, PhD
Professor and Head, Diagnostic Nuclear Medicine Division, Nuclear Medicine, All India Institute of Medical Sciences, New Delhi, Delhi, India

CONSTANTIN LAPA, MD
Chair, Nuclear Medicine, Faculty of Medicine, University of Augsburg, Augsburg, Germany

FLAVIA LINGUANTI, MD
Nuclear Medicine Department, Ospedale San Donato, Arezzo, Italy; Nuclear Medicine Physician, Nuclear Medicine Unit, Department of Experimental and Clinical Biomedical Sciences "Mario Serio," University of Florence, Florence, Italy

EGESTA LOPCI, MD, PhD
Nuclear Medicine Physician, Nuclear Medicine Unit, IRCCS-Humanitas Research Hospital, Rozzano, Milano, Italy

CLEMENS MINGELS, MD
Post Doctoral Scholar, Department of Radiology, University of California Davis, Sacramento, California, USA; Department of Nuclear Medicine, Inselspital, Bern University Hospital, University of Bern, Bern, Switzerland

HANDE NALBANT, MD
Clinical Researcher, Department of Radiology, University of California Davis, Sacramento, California, USA

LORENZO NARDO, MD, PhD
Associate Professor, Division of Malignant Hematology, Cellular Therapy and Transplantation, Department of Internal Medicine, University of California Davis, Sacramento, California, USA

RAHUL V. PARGHANE, MBBS, MD
Professor and Nuclear Medicine Physician, Radiation Medicine Centre (BARC), Tata Memorial Hospital Annexe, Parel, Mumbai, India; Homi Bhabha National Institute, Mumbai, India

MONAELISABETH REVHEIM, MD, PhD, MHA
Chief Physician, The Intervention Center, Division for Technology and Innovation, Oslo University Hospital, Rikshospitalet, Professor, Institute of Clinical Medicine, Faculty of Medicine, University of Oslo, Oslo, Norway

ALICE ROSSI, MD
Radiologist, Radiology Unit, IRCCS Istituto Romagnolo per Lo Studio Dei Tumori (IRST) 'Dino Amadori,' Meldola, Italy

SAMBIT SAGAR, MD
Senior Resident, Diagnostic Nuclear Medicine Division, Nuclear Medicine, All India Institute of Medical Sciences, New Delhi, Delhi, India

HASAN SARI, PhD
Department of Nuclear Medicine, Inselspital, Bern University Hospital, University of Bern, Bern, Switzerland; Research Scientist, Siemens Healthineers International AG, Zurich, Switzerland

FATMA SEN, MD, MSc
Associate Clinical Professor, Department of Radiology, University of California Davis, Sacramento, California, USA

VANESSA SHEHU, BA
Research Technician, University of Pittsburgh School of Medicine, Pittsburgh, Pennsylvania, USA

SHASHI B. SINGH, MBBS
Postdoctoral Scholar, Molecular Imaging Program at Stanford (MIPS), Stanford University School of Medicine, The Richard M. Lucas Center for Imaging, Stanford, California, USA

KANANKULAM VELLIANGIRI SIVASANKAR, MD
Nuclear Medicine Physician, Diagnostic Nuclear Medicine Division, Nuclear Medicine, All India Institute of Medical Sciences, New Delhi, Delhi, India

BENJAMIN SPENCER, PhD
Assistant Professor, Department of Radiology,
University of California Davis, Sacramento,
California, USA

JOSEPH M. TUSCANO, MD
Professor, Division of Hematology
and Oncology, Department of Bone
Marrow Transplant, University of
California Davis, Sacramento, California,
USA

THOMAS J. WERNER, MSE
Clinical Research Assistant, Department of
Radiology, Hospital of the University of
Pennsylvania, Philadelphia, Pennsylvania, USA

NADIA WITHOFS, MD, PhD
Professor, Nuclear Medicine Physician,
Division of Nuclear Medicine and Oncological
Imaging, Department of Medical Physics, CHU
of Liege, Quartier Hopital, GIGA-CRC In Vivo
imaging, University of Liege, Liege, Belgium

Contents

The 2-deoxy-2-[^{18}F]fluoro-D-glucose positron emission tomography combined with computed tomography (PET/CT) has contributed to outcome improvement of patients with lymphoma. The use of [^{18}F]FDG PET/CT for staging and response assessment is successfully applied both in routine clinical practice and in clinical trials. The challenges lie in enhancing the outcomes of lymphoma patients, particularly those with advanced or refractory/relapsed disease, and to minimize the long-term toxicity associated with treatments, including radiation therapy. The objective of this review article is to present contemporary data on the use of [^{18}F]FDG PET/CT for treatment assessment of aggressive lymphomas.

While functional imaging with [^{18}F]Fluoro-deoxy-glucose positron emission tomography (PET)/computed tomography is a well-established imaging modality in most lymphoma entities, novel tracers addressing cell surface receptors, tumor biology, and the microenvironment are being developed. Especially, with the emergence of immuno-PET targeting surface markers of lymphoma cells, a new imaging modality of immunotherapies is evolving, which might especially aid in relapsed and refractory disease stages. This review highlights different new PET tracers in indolent and aggressive lymphoma subtypes and summarizes the current state of immuno-PET imaging in lymphoma.

In the1980s, radiolabeled cells helped understand the pathology of hemato-oncology. In the 1990s, preclinical trials evaluated radiolabeled immunotherapy with monoclonal antibodies (MoAbs) such as anti-CD20 agents labeled with Iodine-131 (Bexxar) or Yttrium-90 (Zevalin). Due to the safe and durable responses of radiolabeled MoAbs, the Food and Drug Administration approved these agents in the 2000s. Despite radioimmunotherapy's long journey, its application has recently decreased. This review will discuss the historical timeline of radioimmunotherapy, debate on advantages and difficulties, and explore trials. We will examine future directions of radioligand therapy in hemato-oncology, considering emerging molecules that may become the next theragnostic trend.

[^{18}F]fluoro-2-deoxy-D-glucose PET/computed tomography has been implemented in the management of patients with lymphoma, offering real-time metabolic information on lymphoma with the promise of more accurate staging, treatment response assessment, prognostication, and early detection of disease recurrence. The clinical management of lymphoproliferative disease has recently, rapidly evolved from initial chemotherapeutic to the use of immunotherapy, targeted agents, and to the use of chimeric antigen receptor T-cell therapies. The implementation of these new systems and imaging protocols together with new tracer development creates, in the field of lymphoproliferative disease, both opportunities and challenges that will be detailed in this comprehensive literature review.

The Food and Drug Administration and the European Medicines Agency have recently approved chimeric antigen receptor-engineered (CAR) T cells to treat several refractory/relapsed B-cell lymphomas. This comprehensive review aims to demonstrate the pivotal role that [^{18}F]-FDG PET/computed tomographic (CT) imaging can play to enhance the care of patients treated with CAR T-cell therapy. To this end, this review deciphers evidence showing the diagnostic, prognostic, predictive, and theragnostic value of [^{18}F]-FDG PET/CT-derived parameters.

Multiple myeloma (MM) is a hematologic malignancy characterized by the clonal proliferation of plasma cells within the bone marrow. Accurate staging and monitoring of disease progression are crucial for effective management. PET imaging has emerged as a powerful tool in the diagnosis and management of MM, with radiotracers like 18F-fluorodeoxyglucose and novel agents playing a pivotal role. This review explores the current state of PET imaging in multiple myeloma, focusing on its role in initial staging, response assessment, and prognosis prediction, with an emphasis on recent advancements.

According to international guidelines, patients with suspected myeloma should primarily undergo low-dose whole-body computed tomography (CT) for diagnostic purposes. To optimize sensitivity and specificity and enable treatment response assessment, whole-body MR (WB-MR) imaging should include diffusion-weighted imaging with apparent diffusion coefficient maps and T1-weighted Dixon sequences with bone marrow Fat Fraction Quantification. At baseline WB-MR imaging shows greater sensitivity for the detecting focal lesions and diffuse bone marrow infiltration pattern than 18F-fluorodeoxyglucose PET-CT, which is considered of choice for evaluating response to treatment and minimal residual disease and imaging of extramedullary disease.

The main finding that ^{18}F-FDG PET imaging can reveal in patients with leukemias is the presence of bone marrow (BM) infiltration in both acute or chronic forms. This ability can influence and guide the use of BM biopsy but also assess to therapy response. Additionally ^{18}F-FDG PET imaging has been reported as particularly useful for the diagnosis of leukemias in patients with non specific symptoms. In the case of acute leukemias it revealed also a role for the evaluation of extramedullary forms while in the case of chronic forms a role for the assessment of Richter transformation has been reported.

Hematological malignancies exhibit a widespread distribution, necessitating evaluation of disease activity over the entire body. In clinical practice, visual analysis and semiquantitative parameters are used to assess ^{18}F-FDGPET/CT imaging, which solely represents measurements of disease activity from limited area and may not adequately reflect global disease assessment. An efficient method for assessing the global disease burden of hematological malignancies is to employ PET/computed tomography based novel quantitative parameters. In this article, we explored novel quantitative parameters on PET/CT imaging for assessing global disease burden and the potential role of artificial intelligence (AI) to determine these parameters in evaluation of hematological malignancies.

Lymphoma represents a condition that holds promise for cure with existing treatment modalities; nonetheless, the primary clinical obstacle lies in advancing therapeutic outcomes by pinpointing high-risk individuals who are unlikely to respond favorably to standard therapy. In this article, the authors will delineate the significant strides achieved in the lymphoma field, with a particular emphasis on the 3 prevalent subtypes: Hodgkin lymphoma, diffuse large B-cell lymphomas, and follicular lymphoma.

The evolving field of chimeric antigen receptor (CAR) T-cell therapy, though promising, necessitates more comprehensive imaging methods to enhance therapeutic effectiveness and track cell trafficking in patients and ex vivo. This review examines the application of PET imaging in CAR T-cell trafficking and optimizing their therapeutic impact. The application of PET imaging using various radiotracers is promising in providing evaluation of CAR T-cell interaction within the host, thereby facilitating strategies for improved patient outcomes. As this technology progresses, further innovative strategies to streamline assessments of immunotherapeutic effectiveness are anticipated.

PET CLINICS

SERIES OF RELATED INTEREST

Advances in Clinical Radiology
Available at: Advancesinclinicalradiology.com
MRI Clinics of North America
Available at: MRI.theclinics.com
Neuroimaging Clinics of North America
Available at: Neuroimaging.theclinics.com
Radiologic Clinics of North America
Available at: Radiologic.theclinics.com

THE CLINICS ARE AVAILABLE ONLINE!
Access your subscription at:
www.theclinics.com

PROGRAM OBJECTIVE
The goal of the *PET Clinics* is to keep practicing radiologists and radiology residents up to date with current clinical practice in positron emission tomography by providing timely articles reviewing the state of the art in patient care.

TARGET AUDIENCE
Practicing radiologists, radiology residents, and other health care professionals who provide patient care utilizing radiologic findings.

LEARNING OBJECTIVES
Upon completion of this activity, participants will be able to:
1. Review existing treatment modalities for treating and understanding lymphoma.
2. Discuss the evolving field of CAR T-cell therapy and the application of positron emission tomography (PET) imaging in its evaluation.
3. Recognize using positron emission tomography (PET) imaging is a powerful tool in diagnosing and managing multiple myeloma.

ACCREDITATION
The Elsevier Office of Continuing Medical Education (EOCME) is accredited by the Accreditation Council for Continuing Medical Education (ACCME) to provide continuing medical education for physicians.

The EOCME designates this journal-based CME activity for a maximum of 11 *AMA PRA Category 1 Credit*(s)™. Physicians should claim only the credit commensurate with the extent of their participation in the activity.

All other health care professionals requesting continuing education credit for this enduring material will be issued a certificate of participation.

DISCLOSURE OF CONFLICTS OF INTEREST
The EOCME assesses conflict of interest with its instructors, faculty, planners, and other individuals who are in a position to control the content of CME activities. All relevant conflicts of interest that are identified are thoroughly vetted by EOCME for fair balance, scientific objectivity, and patient care recommendations. EOCME is committed to providing its learners with CME activities that promote improvements or quality in healthcare and not a specific proprietary business or a commercial interest.

The planning committee, staff, authors, and editors listed below have identified no financial relationships or relationships to products or devices they or their spouse/life partner have with commercial interest related to the content of this CME activity:
Elisabetta Maria Abenavoli, MD; Abass Alavi, MD, MD (Hon), PhD (Hon), DSc (Hon); Ludmila Santiago Almeida, MD; Sandip Basu, MBBS (Hons), DRM, Diplomate N.B., MNAMS; Fabrizio Bergesio, PhD; Francesco Bertagna, MD; Valentina Berti, MD; Davide Bezzi, MD; Roberto C. Delgado Bolton, MD, PhD; Christophe Bonnet, MD, PhD; Ralph A. Bundschuh, MD; Alessia Castellino, MD; Paolo Castellucci, MD; Arrigo Cattabriga, MD; Stéphane Chauvie, PhD; Rainer Claus, MD; Adriano De Maggi, PhD; Laurent Dercle, MD, PhD; Francesco Dondi, MD; Rexhep Durmo, MD; Johanna S. Enke, MD; Naseem S. Esteghamat, MD, MS; Elba Etchebehere, MD, PhD; Stefano Fanti, MD; Patrick Glennan, BA; Felipe Godinez, PhD; Varun Gopal; Victor Cabral Heringer, MD; Roland Hustinx, MD, PhD; Dikhra Khan, MD; Kothainayaki Kulanthaivelu; Rakesh Kumar, MD, PhD; Constantin Lapa, MD; Flavia Linguanti, MD; Michelle Littlejohn; Egesta Lopci, MD; Samuel de Souza Medina, MD; Clemens Mingels, MD; Hande Nalbant, MD; Cristina Nanni, MD; Rahul V. Parghane, MBBS, MD; Mona-Elisabeth Revheim, MD, PhD, MHA; Alice Rossi, MD; Sambit Sagar, MD; Vanessa Shehu; Shashi B. Singh, MD; KV Sivasankar, MD; Benjamin Spencer, PhD; Joseph M. Tuscano, MD; John Vassallo; Thomas J. Werner, MSE; Nadia Withofs, MD, PhD

The planning committee, staff, authors, and editors listed below have identified financial relationships or relationships to products or devices they or their spouse/life partner have with commercial interest related to the content of this CME activity:
Lorenzo Nardo, MD, PhD: *Researcher*: Novartis, Telix, Lantheus, GE Healthcare, Lilly, United Imaging

Neeta Pandit-Taskar, MD: *Consultant*: Actinium Pharmaceuticals, Inc., Innervate, Y-mAbs Therapeutics, Inc.; *Advisor*: Cellectar Biosciences, Inc., Telix Pharmaceuticals Limited; *Researcher*: Cellectar Biosciences, Inc., Clarity Pharmaceuticals, Fusion Pharma, ImaginAb, Innervate, Regeneron Pharmaceuticals Inc., Telix Pharmaceuticals Limited, Y-mAbs Therapeutics, Inc.

Hasan Sari, PhD: *Employee*: Siemens Healthcare AG

Fatma Sen, MD, MSc: *Researcher*: Biogen

UNAPPROVED/OFF-LABEL USE DISCLOSURE
The EOCME requires CME faculty to disclose to the participants:
1. When products or procedures being discussed are off-label, unlabelled, experimental, and/or investigational (not US Food and Drug Administration [FDA] approved); and

2. Any limitations on the information presented, such as data that are preliminary or that represent ongoing research, interim analyses, and/or unsupported opinions. Faculty may discuss information about pharmaceutical agents that is outside of FDA-approved labelling. This information is intended solely for CME and is not intended to promote off-label use of these medications. If you have any questions, contact the medical affairs department of the manufacturer for the most recent prescribing information.

TO ENROLL

To enroll in the *PET Clinics* Continuing Medical Education program, call customer service at 1-800-654-2452 or sign up online at http://www.theclinics.com/home/cme. The CME program is available to subscribers for an additional annual fee of USD 254.00.

METHOD OF PARTICIPATION

In order to claim credit, participants must complete the following:
1. Complete enrolment as indicated above.
2. Read the activity.
3. Complete the CME Test and Evaluation. Participants must achieve a score of 70% on the test. All CME Tests and Evaluations must be completed online.

CME INQUIRIES/SPECIAL NEEDS

For all CME inquiries or special needs, please contact elsevierCME@elsevier.com.

Preface

Novel PET Imaging Techniques in the Management of Hematologic Malignancies

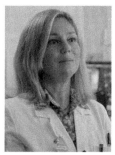

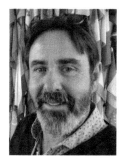

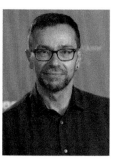

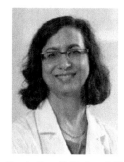

Cristina Nanni, MD   Paolo Castellucci, MD   Stefano Fanti, MD   Neeta Pandit-Taskar, MD

Editors

Hematology is probably the most relevant application field of PET since the widespread adoption of PET in the 1990s. Currently, the use of PET is indispensable in the natural history of almost all onco-hematologic diseases. With the advent of innovative therapies, such as CAR-T, the use of PET has gained further clinical diagnostic value. Significant innovations are also seen in the therapeutic and theranostic fields, and greater developments are anticipated in the future. Ultimately, the clinical applications of PET in onco-hematology likely represent the largest portion of the daily workload in most PET centers, and clinical hematologists have long relied on these molecular imaging techniques.

In the current issue, we have asked leading international experts in onco-hematology imaging and therapy to contribute their insights on the state-of-the-art applications of PET and therapeutic techniques in major hematologic diseases and to provide perspectives on potential future diagnostic and therapeutic applications in this field. Despite the necessarily limited space, we have endeavored to cover all relevant topics. Contributions have come from top experts in both established

application fields, which constitute the daily practice, such as in the article "[^{18}F]FDG PET Imaging for Therapy Assessment in Hodgkin and Non-Hodgkin Lymphomas" by the group led by Prof Roland Hustinx, and in new diagnostic possibilities in the article "New PET Tracers for Lymphoma." Therapeutic applications also have an important focus: the past and future of therapeutic applications in lymphomas have been brightly reported by a leading expert, such as Prof Elba Etchebehere, and collaborators. We have given ample space to current and future diagnostic applications in Multiple Myeloma, including a comparison of PET imaging with whole-body MR imaging. This issue would not be complete without mentioning the contribution of new PET machines with long axial fields of view, with an interesting article by Prof Nardo from the University of California, Davis, or the applications of PET in Chimeric Antigen Receptor T-Cell Trafficking, radiomics, or new quantitative PET methods in onco-hematology.

In conclusion, the use of PET and radioligand therapies in onco-hematology constitutes the present of our daily activities, but innovations in new theranostic radiopharmaceuticals and

PET Clin 19 (2024) xiii–xiv
https://doi.org/10.1016/j.cpet.2024.07.001
1556-8598/24/© 2024 Published by Elsevier Inc.

technological advancements ensure an increasingly bright future and an ever-greater significance of molecular imaging in onco-hematology.

We want to thank all the authors and collaborators for their spontaneous, free, and enthusiastic contributions to this project, which will undoubtedly be a valuable resource for both clinicians and imaging experts.

Cristina Nanni, MD
IRCCS Azienda Ospedaliero–
Universitaria di Bologna
Bologna, Italy

Paolo Castellucci, MD
IRCCS Azienda Ospedaliero–
Universitaria di Bologna
Bologna, Italy

Stefano Fanti, MD
IRCCS Azienda Ospedaliero–
Universitaria di Bologna
Bologna, Italy

Neeta Pandit-Taskar, MD
Molecular Imaging and Therapy Service
Department of Radiology
Memorial Hospital
Memorial Sloan Kettering Cancer Center
Weill Cornell Medical Center
New York, NY, USA

E-mail addresses:
cristina.nanni@aosp.bo.it (C. Nanni)
paolo.castellucci@aosp.bo.it (P. Castellucci)
stefano.fanti@aosp.bo.it (S. Fanti)
pandit-n@mskcc.org (N. Pandit-Taskar)

2-deoxy-2-[18F]FDG PET Imaging for Therapy Assessment in Hodgkin's and Non-Hodgkin Lymphomas

Nadia Withofs, MD, PhD[a,b,]*, Christophe Bonnet, MD, PhD[c],
Roland Hustinx, MD, PhD[a,b]

KEYWORDS

• PET • Lymphoma • Therapy • Assessment • Hodgkin • DLBCL • Adapted

KEY POINTS

• 2-deoxy-2-[18F]fluoro-D-glucose ([18F]FDG) PET response-adapted therapy has improved outcome of patients with Hodgkin lymphoma (HL). The standard treatment of HL is the combined modality therapy including both chemotherapy and involved site radiation therapy.
• PET response-adapted therapy in HL has contributed to the reduction of the long-term treatment-related toxicity.
• Circulating tumor DNA could complement [18F]FDG PET/CT scans, enhancing therapy outcome prediction in lymphoma. This is of particular interest in cases of positive interim and/or end-of-treatment PET scans within the context of immunotherapies.

INTRODUCTION

The estimated new cases of Hodgkin lymphoma (HL) and non-Hodgkin lymphoma (NHL) in the United States in 2022 are 8540 and 80,470, respectively, and the estimated deaths are 920 and 20,250, respectively.[1] NHL represents a varied spectrum of lymphoproliferative disorders originating in B lymphocytes, the diffuse large B-cell lymphoma (DLBCL) being the major subtype, T lymphocytes, or natural killer cells (NK/T-cell lymphomas are very rare).[2,3]

The 2-deoxy-2-[18F]fluoro-D-glucose ([18F]FDG) PET combined with computed tomography (PET/CT) has significantly contributed to improvement of patients' outcome. The Consensus of the International Conference on Malignant Lymphomas Imaging Working Group on the use of [18F]FDG PET/CT for staging and response assessment and the Lugano classification, including Lugano criteria adapted to immune-based therapy (LYRIC: the lymphoma response to immunomodulatory therapy criteria), are still successfully applied both in routine clinical practice and clinical trials.[4–8] A recent work within a panel of experts appointed by the European Association of Nuclear Medicine confirmed a consensus on most statements concerning the use of PET in NHL and HL.[9]

On the one hand, the challenges lie in enhancing the outcome of lymphoma patients, particularly those with advanced or refractory/relapsed disease. On the other hand, there is a need to prevent or minimize the long-term toxicity associated with treatments, including radiation therapy (RT).

The objective of this review article is to present contemporary data on the use of [18F]FDG PET/CT

[a] Division of Nuclear Medicine and Oncological Imaging, Department of Medical Physics, CHU of Liege, Quartier Hopital, Avenue de l'hopital 1, Liege, Belgium; [b] GIGA-Nuclear Medicine Lab, University of Liege, CHU - B34 Quartier Hôpital, Avenue de l'Hôpital 11, Liège, BELGIQUE; [c] Department of Hematology, CHU of Liege, Quartier Hôpital, Avenue de l'hôpital 1, 4000 Liege 1, Belgium
* Corresponding author. CHU of Liege, Quartier Hôpital, Avenue de l'hôpital, 1, 4000 Liege 1, Belgium.
E-mail address: nwithofs@chuliege.be

PET Clin 19 (2024) 447–462
https://doi.org/10.1016/j.cpet.2024.05.001

for treatment assessment of aggressive HL and NHL, including the potential future applications of semiquantitative and volumetric PET parameters.

HODGKIN LYMPHOMA

HL is an aggressive lymphoma of B-cell origin, with most patients diagnosed between the ages of 15 and 30 years, and with a secondary peak incidence occurring in adults aged 55 years and older.[10] The HL is subdivided into 2 main subtypes: the classic HL and nodular lymphocyte-predominant HL. The following discussion will focus on classic HL that is characterized by the presence of Hodgkin and Reed–Sternberg cells, constituting merely about 1% of the tumor mass. These cells, derived from germinal center B lymphocytes, are surrounded by a reactive inflammatory microenvironment. Treatment strategy depends on the stage of the disease according to Lugano modified Ann Arbor criteria, subdivided into early-stage and advanced-stage disease.[4] In early-stage HL, the disease is classified as favorable or unfavorable depending on baseline clinical risk factors such as patient age, the presence of B symptoms, the number of nodal sites or mediastinal–thoracic ratio (bulky disease), and erythrocyte sedimentation rate.[4] In advanced-stage HL, high-risk patients can be identified using the International Prognostic Score that includes 7 independent adverse prognostic factors (serum albumin <4 g/dL and hemoglobin <10.5 g/dL, male sex, age ≥45 years, stage IV disease, leukocytosis, and lymphocytopenia).[10,11]

The [18F]FDG PET is a strong prognostic biomarker in patients with HL.[12–22] Patients with negative [18F]FDG interim PET (iPET), performed after 2 cycles of chemotherapy, have an excellent overall outcome, whereas patients with positive iPET have a worse outcome in terms of progression-free survival (PFS) and overall survival (OS).[12–22]

The [18F]FDG PET/CT-adapted trials in HL outlined in **Table 1** contributed to the improvement of patient's outcome, with long-term remission rates exceeding 95% in early-stage HL.[12–19] These trials confirmed the survival benefit of early escalation in case of persistent positive disease at iPET while they helped prevent long-term treatment-related toxicity in patients demonstrating an early complete response at iPET by omitting unnecessary additional therapy. The Lugano classification for treatment assessment using [18F]FDG PET/CT is recommended to guide treatment choices.[4,7]

Early-Stage I–II Hodgkin Lymphoma

The primary treatment recommendation for early-stage IA–IIA favorable non-bulky disease is 2 cycles of ABVD (doxorubicin or trademark name Adriamycin, bleomycin, vinblastine, and dacarbazine) followed by restaging [18F]FDG iPET.[10,23] The standard treatment is the combined modality therapy (CMT) including both chemotherapy and involved site RT (ISRT).[10,14] The RAPID, EORTC/LYSA/FIL H10, and GHSG-HD16 trials tested the omission of ISRT from the standard CMT regimen in iPET responders (**Table 1**).[13,14,17–19]

The RAPID trial showed a modest improvement in the 3 year PFS rate with the addition of involved field RT (IFRT) in patients with non-bulky stage IA or IIA and negative PET [5-point Deauville scale (DS) score 1–2] scan after 3 cycles of ABVD, while the OS was similar.[19] Among the 32 patients with negative iPET scan who underwent second-line therapy, 31.8% (n = 7/22) in the group with no further therapy and 50.0% (n = 5/10) in the radiotherapy group received second-line high-dose chemotherapy followed by autologous stem-cell transplantation (ASCT) for recurrent HL.[19]

The EORTC/LYSA/FIL H10 trial did not demonstrate non-inferiority of ABVD only compared with CMT with 5 year PFS rates in favor of ABVD followed by INRT both in favorable group (hazard ratio [HR]: 15.8; 95% confidence interval [CI], 3.8–66.1) and unfavorable group (HR: 1.45; 95% CI, 0.8–2.5).[17,18] In the EORTC/LYSA/FIL H10 trial, the PET was performed after 2 cycles of ABVD and the mediastinal blood pool activity or surrounding activity was used as the reference background activity (corresponding to DS score 1–2).[17,18] In both RAPID and EORTC/LYSA/FIL H10 trials, omitting RT in iPET negative HL resulted in more relapses (11% vs 3% in H10 trial and 10% vs 4% in RAPID trial at 5 year median follow-up) mainly affecting originally involved areas.[24]

The long-term follow-up analysis of the GHSG HD16 trial concluded that RT cannot be omitted in patients with early-stage favorable HL after a negative iPET (DS score 1–2 after 2 cycles of ABVD); most relapses following treatment with ABVD alone occurred within the theoretic radiation field, underscoring the significant contribution of RT in achieving local tumor control and preventing relapses within the treatment area.[14] In the GHSG HD16 trial, patients with a positive iPET experienced a higher rate of recurrences, predominantly occurring outside the radiation field; therefore, enhancing response rates and PFS in these individuals might be attainable through chemotherapy intensification rather than intensifying or altering RT.[14] A meta-analysis published in 2016 demonstrated a significant reduction in PFS when RT is excluded through PET-adapted therapy. Hence, standard treatment for patients with early-stage HL remains CMT.[25]

Table 1
[^{18}F] fluoro-D-glucose PET/computed tomography-adapted trials in Hodgkin lymphoma

Trial, Year	Aim	iPET time-point	Negative PET Threshold	Number of Patients Enrolled. Disease Stage	Number (Percentage) of Patients with Negative iPET	5-y PFS Rates (if Not Otherwise Specified)	5-y OS Rates (if Not Otherwise Specified)
GHSG HD17,[12] 2021	• Investigate whether omitting consolidation RT was possible in iPET4 negative patients without substantially compromising 5-y PFS. • Investigate the prognostic effect of a positive iPET4 result in patients receiving combined-modality treatment.	After 2 cycles eBEACOPP +2 ABVD.	DS score 1–2	N = 1100. Stage IA, IB, or IIA unfavorable with at least one risk factor.[b]	Standard CMT arm: 318/486 (65.4%). PET4-guided treatment group: 333/493 (67.5%).	Standard CMT arm: 97.3% (95% CI, 94.5–98.7) PET4-guided treatment group: 95.1% (95% CI, 92.0–97.0) PET4-negativity allows omission of consolidation RT without a clinically relevant loss of efficacy (HR 0.523; 95% CI, 0.226–1.211).	In the per-protocol analysis population (n = 905): 98.8% (95% CI, 97.2–99.5) Intention-to-treat analysis population (n = 1096): 98.6% (95% CI, 97.3–99.3)
GHSG HD16,[13,14] 2019	Demonstrating non-inferiority when omitting consolidation RT in patients with a negative PET after 2 cycles of ABVD in terms of PFS as compared to CMT.	After 2 cycles of ABVD	DS score 1–2	N = 1150. Stage I–II favorable disease according to GHSG criteria.[b]	667/1007 centrally reviewed (66.2%) Note: 340/1007 (33.8%) positive iPET (n = 218 DS3; n = 122 DS4 and n = 0 DS5)	Standard CMT arm: 94.2%; 91.6%–96.9%. iPET-negative ABVD alone arm: 86.7% (82.5%–90.9%), significantly lower (HR 2.05; 95% CI: 1.20–3.51, P = .0072), with 5-y cumulative incidences of in-field recurrences significantly higher (10.4%; 6.7%–14.1%) than in the CMT group (2.0%; 0.4%–3.7%, P = .0002).	Not significantly different (P = .14) between CMT arm: 98.3% (96.9%–99.8%) and iPET-negative ABVD alone arm: 98.8% (97.4%–100%)

(continued on next page)

Table 1
(continued)

Trial, Year	Aim	iPET time-point	Negative PET Threshold	Number of Patients Enrolled. Disease Stage	Number (Percentage) of Patients with Negative iPET	5-y PFS Rates (if Not Otherwise Specified)	5-y OS Rates (if Not Otherwise Specified)
CALGB 50604,[16] 2018	Determine whether a population of patients with early-stage disease can be treated with short-course ABVD without RT on the basis of a negative interim PET/CT, thereby limiting the risks of treatment.	After 2 cycles of ABVD	DS score 1–3	N = 149. Stage I-II (no bulky disease)	135/149 (91%) The use of DS scores 1-3 rather than 1–2 to define negative iPET increased the iPET rate from 76% to 91%, thereby reducing the number of patients who would have received more toxic chemotherapy and RT.	3 y PFS rates significantly higher (HR, 3.84; 95% CI, 1.50–9.84; P = .011) in iPET-negative group (2 + 2 ABVD: 91% than in iPET-positive group (2 ABVD + 2 eBEACOPP + IFRT: 66%	NA
EORTC/LYSA/FIL H10,[17,18] 2017	Incorporate a randomized iPET response-adapted treatment strategy for both the iPET-negative and the iPET-positive patients with stage I and II HL to improve selection of patients who need reduced or more intensive treatments.	After 2 cycles of ABVD	Mediastinal blood pool activity or surrounding activity was used as the reference background activity (equivalent to DS score 1-2)	N = 754. Stage I-II favorable disease group (H10 F)	465 + 185 = 650/754 (86%)	*iPET-negative arm (4 ABVD):* 87.1% (82.1–90.8) vs 99.0% (95.9–99.7) in the standard CMT arm (3 ABVD + INRT; HR, 15.8; 95% CI, 3.8–66.1) *iPET-positive arm (2 ABVD + 2 eBEACOPP + INRT):* grouped with unfavorable patients (see below).	10 y OS rates: *iPET-negative arm:* 98.0% vs 100.0% in the standard CMT arm (HR, 2.80; 95% CI, 0.29–26.9; difference test P = .3522) *iPET-positive arm:* see below.
				N = 1196. Stage I-II unfavorable disease group (H10U)[a]	594 + 320 = 914/1196 (76%)	*iPET-negative arm (6 ABVD):* 89.6% (85.5–92.6) vs 92.1% (88.0–94.8) in the standard CMT arm (4 ABVD + INRT). *iPET-positive arm*	10 y OS rates: *iPET-negative arm:* 94.8% vs 94.3% in the standard CMT arm (HR, 0.84; 95% CI, 0.36–1.98; difference test

Study	Aim	Timing	DS score	Population	Randomization	Results
						(2 ABVD + 2 eBEACOPP + INRT): 90.6 (84.7–94.3) vs 77.4 (70.4–82.9) in the standard CMT arm (HR, 0.42; 95% CI, 0.23–0.74; P = .002). *P = .6908). iPET-positive arm:* 92.0% vs 90.4% in the standard CMT arm (HR, 0.92; 95% CI, 0.43–1.97; P = .8370)
RAPID,[19] 2015	To determine whether patients with clinical stage IA or stage IIA HL and negative PET findings after 3 cycles of ABVD require IFRT to delay or prevent disease progression.	After 3 cycles of ABVD	DS score 1–2	N = 602. Stage IA–IIA (non-bulky)	n = 426/602 (70.8%), of which 420 were randomized to either IFRT (n = 209) or observation (n = 211).	3 y PFS *IFRT arm:* 94.6% (95% CI, 91.5–97.7). *No IFRT arm:* 90.8% (95% CI, 86.9%–94.8%. No significant difference (P = .16). In the "per protocol" (as treated) analysis: 97.1% (95% CI, 94.7%–99.6%) vs 90.8% (95% CI, 86.8%–94.7%), favoring the use of CMT (P = .02). 3-y OS rates: *IFRT arm:* 97.1% (95% CI, 94.8%–99.4%). *No IFRT arm:* 99.0% (95% CI, 97.6%–100%) for patients who received no further treatment. No significant difference (P = .27)
RATHL,[20–22] 2016	To test: • Whether the omission of bleomycin from subsequent cycles in patients with negative iPET had any effect on control of the lymphoma or the toxic effects of therapy.	After 2 cycles of ABVD	DS score 1–3	N = 1119 Stage III, IV and II (500/119; 41,6%) with risk factors (B symptoms, bulky disease (>33% of the transthoracic diameter or >10 cm	937/1119 (84%), of which 933 were randomized.	3 y PFS rates: *6 ABVD group:* 85.7%; (95% CI, 82.1–88.6) *2 ABVD + 4 AVD group:* 84.4% (95% CI, 80.7–87.5) The 3 y PFS rates did not differ significantly and the omission of The 7 y OS did not differ significantly (HR, 0.84; 95% CI, 0.51–1.37): *6 ABVD group:* 93.2% (95% CI, 90.2–95.3). *2 ABVD + 4 AVD group:* 93.5% (95% CI, 90.5–95.5). *(continued on next page)*

Table 1
(continued)

Trial, Year	Aim	iPET time-point	Negative PET Threshold	Number of Patients Enrolled. Disease Stage	Number (Percentage) of Patients with Negative iPET	5-y PFS Rates (if Not Otherwise Specified)	5-y OS Rates (if Not Otherwise Specified)
	• Patients who had positive iPET findings underwent intensification with escalated BEACOPP or an accelerated version (BEACOPP-14).			elsewhere) or at least three involved sites.		bleomycin from the ABVD regimen led to a decrease in the incidence of pulmonary toxic effects when compared to continued ABVD. The potential value of added RT was not tested in the trial. *Positive-iPET group assigned to BEACOPP (n = 172):* Among 172 patients with positive iPET, the 7 y PFS was 65.9% (95% CI, 58.1–72.6).	Among 172 patients with positive iPET, the 7 y OS was 83.2% (95% CI, 76.2–88.3).

Abbreviations: ABVD, doxorubicin, bleomycin, vinblastine and dacarbazine; BEACOPP, bleomycin, etoposide, doxorubicin, cyclophosphamide, vincristine, procarbazine, and prednisone; BV, brentuximab vedotin; CI, confidence interval; CMT, combined modality therapy (chemotherapy and radiation therapy), DS, Deauville scale; eotPET, end-of-treatment positron emission tomography; GHSG, German Hodgkin study group; HR, hazard ratio; IFRT, involved field radiation therapy; INRT, involved node radiation therapy; IQR, interquartile range; iPET, interim positron emission tomography; PFS, progression-free survival; RT, radiation therapy; vs, versus.

[a] Unfavorable EORTC/LYSA criteria: ≥4 involved nodal areas, age of ≥50 y, bulky disease defined as a mediastinal/thoracic ratio ≥0.35, or elevated erythrocyte sedimentation rate of ≥50 mm/hour without B symptoms or 30 mm/hour or higher with B symptoms.

[b] GHSG unfavorable criteria: Clinical stages I or II, or nodular lymphocyte-predominant HL in Ann Arbor stages IB, IIA, or IIB, without any of the GHSG risk factors large mediastinal mass (≥ a third of the maximal thoracic diameter), extranodal lesions, elevated erythrocyte sedimentation rate (≥50 mm/h without B symptoms, ≥30 mm/h with B symptoms), or ≥3 involved nodal areas.

Data from Refs.[12–22]

The iPET after 2 cycles of ABVD is considered negative when DS score is 1 to 3.[26] Patients with early-stage I/II favorable disease and iPET DS score 1 to 3 can receive 2 additional cycles of ABVD combined with ISRT 30 Gy.[19] Patients with an iPET DS score 4 may continue with 2 additional cycles of ABVD with subsequent [18F]FDG PET restaging.[10] Patients with a DS score 5 at iPET restaging with a positive biopsy result (or if biopsy is not possible) are considered having a refractory disease, warranting an escalation in treatment.[10]

In patients with early-stage I/II unfavorable disease (B symptoms or bulky mediastinal disease or >10 cm adenopathy), treatment escalation with 2 cycles of BEACOPP (bleomycin etoposide doxorubicin [Adriamycin], cyclophosphamide vincristine [Oncovin], procarbazine prednisolone) is considered if iPET is positive (DS score 4–5) after 2 cycles of ABVD.[10] Indeed, the EORTC/LYSA/FIL H10 trial showed that escalation to BEACOPP followed by INRT in patients with unfavorable stage I–II HL and positive iPET was associated with an improvement in the 5 year PFS from 77.4% in the standard ABVD and INRT arm to 90.6% (HR: 0.42; 95% CI, 0.23–0.74; $P = .002$), with no increase in late adverse events.[17,18] However, in the 10 year follow-up, BEACOPP escalation was no longer associated with a statistically significant better outcome.[18] In the pre-PET era, the GHSG HD14 trial showed an improved 10 year PFS in patients with stage I–II unfavorable disease treated with 2 cycles of escalated-dose BEACOPP followed by 2 cycles of ABVD compared with patients treated with 4 cycles of ABVD, with both groups treated with IFRT.[27,28]

The GHSG HD17 trial then tested the non-inferiority of PET-guided treatment (2 BEACOPP +2 ABVD cycles followed by INRT only in PET4-positive patients) over standard CMT in terms of PFS in patients with early-stage unfavorable HL.[12] The 5 year PFS rate in the PET4-guided treatment group (95.1%; 95% CI, 92.0–97.0) was not inferior (HR: 0.523; 95% CI, 0.226–1.211) to the CMT group (97.3%; 95% CI, 94.5–98.7), suggesting that omission of consolidation RT can be considered without loss of efficacy in PET4-negative patients (see **Table 1**).[12] It means that with this approach, the majority of patients will achieve complete metabolic response (DS 1–3) and will avoid ISRT. In the GHSG HD17 trial, among patients with a DS score 4 who all received ISRT, the 5 year PFS rate was 81.6% (95% CI, 67.9–89.9).[12] Both approaches of H10 trial starting with 2 ABVD or HD17 starting with 2 BEACOPP can be considered and iPET guides the following treatment decision.[26]

The addition of brentuximab vedotin, a CD30-directed antibody–cytotoxic drug conjugate, to doxorubicin, vinblastine, and dacarbazine (BV-AVD) has been evaluated for first-line treatment of early-stage unfavorable HL in the BREACH trial.[15] It confirmed the hypothesis of a 10% increase in the PET-negative (DS score 1–3) rate after 2 cycles of BV-AVD (93 of 113 [82.3%] patients; 90% CI, 75.3%–88.0%) versus 2 cycles of ABVD (43 of 57 [75.4%] patients; 90% CI, 64.3%–84.5%).[15] Additionally, the BREACH trial showed that high total metabolic tumor volume (TMTV) was associated with a significantly shorter PFS (HR, 17.9; 95% CI, 2.2–145.5; $P = .001$); for patients with high TMTV, the 2 year PFS rate was 90.9% (95% CI, 74.4%–97.0%) and 70.7% (95% CI, 39.4%–87.9%) in the BV-AVD and ABVD arms, respectively.[15]

Advanced-Stage III–IV Hodgkin Lymphoma

In patients with advanced-stage III–IV HL, the preferred starting regimen is 2 cycles of ABVD or BV-AVD or escalated BEACOPP in selected patients.[10] At the end of treatment, radiotherapy may be considered following end-of-treatment (eot) PET to initially bulky or [18F]FDG PET-positive residual sites for consolidation.[10] In the case of ABVD, therapy is adapted based on [18F]FDG iPET scan results after 2 cycles. In case of complete metabolic response (DS score 1–3), 4 additional cycles of AVD are administered while escalated BEACOPP (3 cycles) is considered in case of positive iPET (DS score 4–5).[10] The subsequent PET restaging will help guide the following therapeutic decisions, and patients are classified as having refractory disease if PET results remain positive (DS score 4–5).[10]

The National Comprehensive Cancer Network (NCCN) guidelines have been refined based on findings from the PET for response adapted therapy in advanced Hodgkin Lymphoma (RATHL) trial, which evaluated iPET as a measure of early response to chemotherapy, tailoring treatment strategies for patients with advanced HL (see **Table 1**).[20,21] Treatment intensification (escalated-BEACOPP) adapted to early metabolic response assessed by iPET improved the long-term survival (>90%) of patients with advanced stage HL.[10,20,21,29–32]

In the GHSG HD18 and AHL2011 trials, the first-line therapy was 2 cycles escalated-BEACOPP and patients were assigned in different treatment groups based on the results of the iPET.[32–34] In the GHSG HD18 trial, patients with negative iPET (DS score <3) were randomly assigned to receive either additional cycles of escalated-BEACOPP (total 8 or 6 cycles) or 2 additional cycles (total 4 cycles); the 5 year PFS rate was 90.8% (95% CI, 87.9–93.7) in the 8 or 6 cycles (standard) group and 92.2% (95% CI, 89.4–95.0) in the 4 cycles group.[33] In the AHL2011 trial, patients with negative iPET scan switched to 2 cycles of ABVD.[32] The AHL2011 trial also showed that late responders (PET2-positive/PET4-negative patients) had a significantly lower 5 year PFS rates (75.4%; 95% CI, 62.5–84.4) than early responders (PET2-negative/PET4-negative patients [92.5; 95% CI, 90.1–94.3], $P = \cdot 0046$).[32] The meta-analysis of André and colleagues showed a slight OS benefit and PFS benefit of the frontline use of BEACOPP instead of ABVD.[34] The BEACOPP instead of ABVD increased secondary leukemia incidence but halved the requirement for ASCT.[34]

Unfortunately, a subset of patients experiences primary resistance or relapse following initial treatment. Hence, recent strategies have focused on targeting the tumor microenvironment, which constitutes the bulk of the tumor mass in classic HL. The ECHELON-1 trial showed a survival benefit of the addition of brentuximab vedotin (BV-AVD) compared to ABVD in patients with untreated stage III–IV HL, and treatment was not adapted based on iPET.[35–37] The 6 year OS benefit of BV-AVD over ABVD was present in both iPET-negative patients (94.9% vs 90.6%; HR, 0.54; 95% CI, 0.34–0.86) and iPET-positive patients (95% vs 77%; HR, 0.16; 95% CI, 0.04–0.72).[35] In the randomized SWOG S1826 trial, the addition of the checkpoint inhibitor nivolumab targeting programmed cell death 1 (PD-1) with AVD (N-AVD; 6 cycles) improved survival compared to BV-AVD in adult and pediatric patients with newly diagnosed advanced stage HL.[38] In this SWOG S1826 trial, patients received RT to residually metabolically active lesions on eotPET.[38] Lynch and colleagues tested concurrent pembrolizumab (anti-PD-1 monoclonal antibody), doxorubicin (Adriamycin), vinblastine, and dacarbazine (APVD) in 30 HL patients of whom 18/30 (60%) enrolled patients had advanced stage disease.[39] In this context of immunotherapy, they showed that the negativity rate of [18F]FDG PET/CT was low (57% after 2 cycles and 82% at the eot) with APVD.[39] By contrast, clearance of circulating tumor DNA (ctDNA) after 2 cycles of APVD and at the eot was associated with improved PFS, and none of the patients with positive PET and negative ctDNA (n = 4/30) at the eot have relapsed in the follow-up period.[39]

The EuroNet-PHL-C1 trial aimed to investigate whether RT could be omitted in children and adolescents with intermediate-stage and advanced-stage classic HL and adequate response to vincristine, etoposide, prednisone, and doxorubicin (OEPA), based on morphologic tumor-volume response with CT and [18F]FDG PET response.[40] Partial remission was defined as a reduction of at least 50% in tumor volume at any involved nodal site. Early-response assessment was not conducted according to the Lugano classification and DS score, but rather based on visual categories for PET negativity (category 1, no [18F]FDG uptake and category 2, slight uptake) and PET positivity (category 3, focal [18F]FDG uptake and category 4, strong [18F]FDG uptake), which corresponded, according to authors, to a visual DS score of 3 or higher as positive. In any case, the EuroNet-PHL-C1 has shown that RT can safely be avoided in patients who have an adequate response to intensified OEPA induction without compromising event-free or OS.

Refractory/Relapsed Hodgkin Lymphoma

Interestingly, the data of patients with positive iPET included in the GHSG HD18 trial were retrospectively analyzed and the pattern of suspected residual disease at iPET might be associated with the risk of treatment failure in advanced-stage HL.[41] Patients with greater than 2 iPET-positive lesions had a significantly higher risk of progression compared to patients with 1 to 2 iPET-positive lesions (HR: 2.17; 95% CI, 1.19–3.97; $P = .012$) and to patients with negative iPET receiving 6 to 8 cycles of chemotherapy (HR: 2.95; 95% CI, 1.62–5.37; $P<.001$).[33,41]

Nevertheless, restaging with [18F]FDG PET/CT after completion of treatment is recommended for all patients, and suspected refractory disease or relapse (DS score 4–5) should be confirmed with biopsy.[10] In case of positive biopsy, the patient should proceed to second-line therapy, with subsequent therapy decisions guided by the results of [18F]FDG PET/CT at restaging.[10] Patients should proceed to high-dose therapy followed by autologous stem cell transplantation if not contraindicated, with or without RT.[10]

DIFFUSE LARGE B-CELL LYMPHOMAS

The DLBCL is the major subtype of NHL (~30%), the others being chronic lymphocytic leukemia/small lymphocytic lymphoma (19%), follicular lymphoma (17%), marginal zone lymphoma (8%), mantle cell lymphoma (4%), and peripheral T-cell lymphoma, not otherwise specified (2%).[2] The indolent B-cell follicular lymphoma and marginal zone lymphoma hold the risk of histologic transformation to DLBCL that can be identified by [18F]FDG PET/CT in case of rapidly progressive or non-responding disease.[2] Risk factors for histologic transformation include elevated serum lactate dehydrogenase (LDH) levels, the presence of B symptoms, and high-risk International Prognostic Index (IPI) score at the time of diagnosis.[2] Primary mediastinal large B-cell lymphoma, a separate entity with a gene expression profile overlapping with HL, will not be discussed.[2]

DLBCL is a heterogeneous group, encompassing distinct clinical presentations, morphologic variants and molecular/genetic abnormalities, and ultimately outcomes. The DLBCL not otherwise specified represents the most common entity of large B-cell lymphomas and is subdivided into 2 subtypes based on morphologic and molecular features (gene expression profile): The activated B-cell-like subtype and the germinal center B-cell-like subtype, the latter being associated with a better outcome.[2,3] The IPI risk assessment and the revised-IPI rely on patient's ECOG performance status and age, Ann Arbor stage, number of extranodal sites, and serum LDH levels.[2,42] The presence of bulky disease ($\geq$7.5 cm) and, in advanced disease, the presence of *MYC* and *BCL2* (with or without *BCL6*) co-translocations (double-hit) are also incorporated in the risk assessment.[2,43] Chemoimmunotherapy with rituximab, cyclophosphamide, doxorubicin, vincristine, and prednisone (R-CHOP) is the first-line therapy of DLBCL.[2] The IFRT can be considered after 3 to 4 cycles of R-CHOP in patients with favorable stage I–II DLBCL in case of complete or partial response at iPET restaging, and in patients with advanced disease in case of bulky disease.[2,43] DLBCL is an aggressive lymphoma with long-term remission rate of about 60% to 70% and a 5 year OS varying from 33% to more than 90%, depending on risk factors at diagnosis.[2]

Therapy of DLBCL is guided by [^{18}F]FDG PET/CT response following Lugano classification, with DS score 1 to 3 defining PET complete metabolic response.[2,4,7,43] In the NCCN guidelines, the iPET is most commonly performed after 3 cycles of first-line therapy but it can be performed after 3 to 4 cycles in case of stage I–II with bulky disease or after 2 to 4 cycles in case of stage I–II with extensive mesenteric disease or stage III–IV disease. The eotPET is not required in case of limited stage I–II disease (bulky or not) with complete metabolic response (DS score 1–3) at iPET; these patients require only one additional cycle of R-CHOP and RT can be omitted.[2] The interpretation of a DS-4-5 at iPET depends on DLBCL stage: In stage I–II with extensive mesenteric disease or stage III–IV disease, therapy is continued in case of partial response with DS score 4 or 5, while in stage I–II (bulky or not), biopsy is required in case of partial response with DS score 4 or progressive disease (DS score 5) to confirm persistent (refractory) disease.[2] Due to the variable positive-predictive value of iPET (20%–74%), biopsy is strongly recommended prior to second-line treatment when iPET is positive.[43–45]

The retrospective analysis of the GOYA trial that enrolled patients randomly assigned to receive obinutuzumab (n = 706) or rituximab (n = 712) plus 6 or 8 cycles of CHOP demonstrated that a negative eotPET was an independent predictor of PFS and OS.[46] Two meta-analyses showed high negative predictive value of iPET for progression/2 year PFS (>80% except in 4 studies; 64%–95%), but wide variation in sensitivity (33%–87%), specificity (49%–94%), and positive predictive values (20%–74%).[44,45] Interim PET is a prognostic factor for PFS or event-free survival with iPET after 2 cycles (iPET2) and iPET4 (after 4 cycles) significantly discriminating good responders from poor responders, with the highest HRs for iPET4.[44,45]

Studies have been testing treatment strategies with the aim to reduce treatment-related toxicity. The LYSA/GOELAMS trial showed that RT can be omitted in patients with limited stage (non-bulky) DLBCL without impact on survival, preventing long-term toxicity.[47] The FLYER trial showed that in young patients with limited-stage (non-bulky) DLBCL with favorable prognosis (normal serum LDH levels, ECOG PS 0–1), 4 cycles R-CHOP (4 cycles + 2 rituximab) was not inferior to 6 cycles of R-CHOP in term of efficacy and was associated with reduced toxicity.[48] This was confirmed by the LYSA LNH 09-1b trial for a broader population (age 18–80 years, age-adjusted IPI = 0, bulky disease permitted).[49] The Intergroup National Clinical Trials Network Study S1001 assessed a PET-adapted treatment strategy in patients with non-bulky (<10 cm) stage I/II untreated DLBCL.[50] Patients who were iPET negative (DS score 1–3) after 3 cycles of R-CHOP (89%) received 1 additional cycle of R-CHOP, whereas patients who were iPET positive (11%; DS score 4–5) received ISRT followed by ibritumomab tiuxetan radioimmunotherapy, with similarly excellent long-term outcomes.[50] Interim PET-positive and PET-negative patients had similar outcomes, with PFS of 86% versus 89% and OS of 85% versus 91%, respectively.[50] In stage I–II DLBCL, RT remains recommended only for a small minority of patients with positive interim PET scan.[2]

To mitigate the burden of toxic therapies among older patients, the OPTIMAL >60 trial is assessing an iPET-adapted treatment strategy tailored for elderly patients with DLBCL.[51] Patients were randomized to receive 4 cycles of therapy, followed by either 2 additional cycles for patients with negative iPET or additional therapy cycles with ISRT for patients with positive iPET.[51] The first results demonstrated that the PET-based treatment strategy allowed sparing 2 cycles therapy in 82% of patients without compromising their outcome, and on the other hand, 2 additional therapy cycles plus ISRT appeared to compensate for the assumed worse prognosis of PET-positive patients.[51] Given the high negative predictive value of iPET in DLBCL, negative iPET can be a tool to refine treatment strategy, avoiding unnecessary therapy and related toxicity.[2] In contrast, the wide variation in the positive predictive value of [18F]FDG PET/CT scan at interim restaging can lead to false-positive results and potentially overtreatment.

DLBCL is associated with an aggressive clinical course with most relapses occurring in the first year after diagnosis. The IPI, revised-IPI, and NCCN-IPI scoring systems have been used to identify risk factors of relapse/progression from the diagnosis, stratifying patients into prognostic groups for OS; however, its precision is limited.[2,42] The baseline TMTV, surrogate marker of tumor burden, and the maximum distance between 2 lesions (Dmax) or between the bulkiest and the furthest lesion (Dmax$_{bulk}$), reflecting the spread of the disease, are known prognostic factors being explored together with the IPI to further improve patients risk stratification.[52–58] The TMTV delineation method using an standardized uptake value (SUV) threshold of 4.0 has shown to be robust and is now easy and quick to perform using academic and commercial software.[56,59] A benchmark standardized method, using the SUV threshold of 4.0 or greater and a minimum individual lesion volume of 3 cm^3, has been established and will be soon publicly available for users to check the reliability of their metabolic tumor volume (MTV) measurements performed locally and for software developers, and vendors.[56] Mikhaeel and colleagues have proposed a simple and robust prognostic index that predicts PFS for patients with individual DLBCL at baseline, which is named the International Metabolic Prognostic Index (IMPI).[57] The IMPI integrates age (as continuous variables), stage (I–IV) encompassing a measure of disease dissemination via the Ann Arbor stage, and MTV delineated using the SUV4.0 threshold.[57] The IMPI outperformed the IPI and exhibited superior capability in identifying a high-risk patient (examples of IMPI are depicted in Mikhaeel and colleagues[57]). The IMPI will aid in the identification of high-risk patients, which is particularly critical in DLBCL, where the curability rate is approximately 60%. Patients experiencing early progression or refractory disease often have a mere 6 month OS.[2] This highlights substantial gaps in addressing the needs of patients with DLBCL, prompting clinical studies focused on improving the prognosis for individuals at high risk. The IMPI might be a useful tool to select high-risk patients who might benefit from novel treatments such as bispecific monoclonal antibodies currently being tested into the first-line treatment in phase III trials.[60]

After treatment initiation, the change in the maximum standardized uptake value (ΔSUV_{max}=(-PET0 SUV$_{max}$-iPET SUV$_{max}$)/PET0 SUV$_{max}$ × 100%) is a quantitative measure being also explored to identify patients at risk of poor response.[45,53,61–64] The objective of measuring ΔSUV_{max} is to decrease the number of false positive cases determined by the visual DS score, thereby improving the identification of poor responders at iPET scanning compared to what the DS score 5 alone achieves.[45,53,61–64] An individual patient data meta-analysis including 1692 patients with de novo DLBCL from the PETRA database (Bologna, HOVON-84, IAEA, GSTT15, NCRI, Nordic-US Intergroup, PETAL, and SAKK 38/07 trials) aimed at determining the optimal timing and PET response criteria for iPET in DLBCL.[45] All PET scans were reviewed; DS score 5 was defined if the lesion SUV$_{max}$ exceeded 3 times the liver SUV$_{max}$, and a response was defined as a value of 66% or greater SUV$_{max}$ reduction between baseline and iPET scans after 1, 2, or 3 cycles, with a value of 70% or greater SUV$_{max}$ reduction after 4 cycles of therapy.[45] The IPI score and iPET scans (using DS score 4–5 or DS score 5 or ΔSUV_{max} to assign a PET-positive) were independent predictors of outcome.[45] PET criteria utilizing ΔSUV_{max} and DS score 5 positivity demonstrated a superior ability to differentiate between good and poor responders compared to the DS score 4 to 5 positivity, and performing iPET scans at later time points during therapy enhanced patient stratification.[45] Authors concluded that the optimal timing and response criteria depend on the clinical context: Patients with complete metabolic response at iPET2 may benefit from de-escalation, while patients with poor response at iPET4 using ΔSUV_{max} (<70%) may be included in randomized trials evaluating more aggressive treatment approaches.[45] In a post hoc analysis of the GAINED trial, authors have confirmed the superiority of ΔSUV_{max} (with cutoffs set at 66% for PET2 and 70% for PET4) over the Menton 2011 consensus, except in cases where the baseline SUV$_{max}$ is less than 10.0.[64] Additionally, they showed that patients with baseline SUV$_{max}$ less than 10.0 who were positive by ΔSUV_{max} at iPET2/iPET4 but PET-negative by Menton 2011 (n = 18) had a similar survival than patients with negative iPET2/iPET4, suggesting that ΔSUV_{max} yields false-positive results when the baseline SUV$_{max}$ is less than 10.0.[64] There are ongoing efforts to improve the interpretation criteria of [18F]FDG PET/CT in DLBCL; the incorporation of the ΔSUV_{max} at iPET4 might be a useful quantitative measure to further improve the prognostic impact of PET.

DLBCL exhibits heterogeneity in many aspects including clinical presentation, morphology, gene expression profile, and molecular subtypes, with distinct treatment response and prognosis. In patients from 2 HOVON trials, DLBCL patients with *MYC* gene rearrangements had significantly more positive eotPET scans (DS score 4–5) than patients with negative MYC (32.5 vs 15.7%, P = .004).[65] Genomic profiling is another research avenue for improving patients with DLBCL outcome.

For patients experiencing relapsed/refractory disease, if they meet the eligibility criteria, salvage high-dose chemotherapy followed by autologous stem cell transplant is the established second-line treatment.[2] Anti-CD19 antigenic receptor (CAR) T-cell therapies and T-cell-redirecting antibodies (CD20xCD3 bispecific monoclonal antibodies) have contributed to slightly improving the prognosis of patients with relapsed/refractory disease.[2] The [18F]FDG PET/CT scan conducted 1 month after CAR-T infusion serves as a predictive measure for CAR-T failure in large B-cell lymphoma.[66] Kuhnl and colleagues demonstrated that patients achieving a complete metabolic response (DS score 1–2) or exhibiting focal DS score 4 uptake in the RT field (behaving similarly to DS score 1–2 cases) had a 12 month PFS rate of 77.1%.[66] In contrast, patients with DS score 3 had a 12 month PFS rate of 63.5%, those with DS score 4 had a PFS rate of 43.5%, and patients with DS score 5 (considered indicative of treatment failure) had a PFS rate of 0%. The 12 month OS rates were 87.1%, 86.2%, 61.7%, and 38.1%, respectively.[66]

When performing [18F]FDG PET/CT in these patients treated with targeted immunotherapy, inflammation and flare-up phenomena are well-known immune-related pitfalls in the interpretation of the scans.[67–69]

DISCUSSION

The [18F]FDG PET scan performed early in the course of therapy has demonstrated robust prognostic value, serving as a valuable tool to guide treatment decisions.[2,10] The Lugano classification including the visual DS score has successfully contributed to the standardization of [18F]FDG PET/CT scan report both in clinical trials and in routine clinical practice.[4] Identifying nonresponder patients with PET enables the intensification of therapy, thereby enhancing the likelihood of efficacy, while unnecessary additional treatments can be avoided in PET responders, mitigating the risk of therapy-related toxicity, including in the long term.

The risk-adapted therapeutic strategies have contributed to enhancing the cure rate of patients with aggressive lymphomas, and consequently,

late treatment-related morbidity is increasingly taken into consideration in patient management, especially in HL affecting young individuals, for whom the long-term survival rate exceeds 90%.[70] The PET-adapted therapy in HL has contributed to the reduction of the long-term treatment-related toxicity. This approach contributes to reducing the risk of high-dose ionizing radiation, such as elevated risk of radiation-induced secondary malignancies (especially breast and lung cancer) and tissue reactions, for example, excess risk of cardiovascular and pulmonary disease.[34,71–73] The incorporation of [18F]FDG PET/CT in RT planning has enhanced the accuracy of determining disease extension at staging and the precision in delineating involved sites only, reducing the irradiated volume (and healthy tissue exposure), and thereby the subsequent toxicity risk associated with the treatment.[74] The RAPID, EORTC/LYSA/FIL H10, and GHSG-HD16 trials attempted to omit ISRT in patients with early-stage HL and negative iPET, but the recurrence rate was higher in patients not treated with RT, and therefore, CMT remains the standard treatment.[13,14,17–19] Escalated BEACOPP has improved survival of patients with advanced HL but with an increased risk of secondary malignancies and infertility.[20,29,31,32,75,76]

In the AHL2011 trial, Demeestere and colleagues have shown that de-escalated PET-driven treatment reduces the likelihood of infertility in advanced HL.[77] In the RATHL trial, the omission of bleomycin, part of the ABVD regimen, in the negative iPET (DS score 1–3) group led to the reduction of the incidence of pulmonary toxicity compared with continued ABVD, without impact on survival.[20] The non-inferiority of AVD compared with ABVD was recently confirmed in the long-term follow-up (median 7.3 years) results of the RATHL trial.[22] At long-term follow-up of RATHL trial, escalation with BEACOPP did not result in an increase in second malignancies.[22] For patients with advanced HL, the switch from BEACOPP to ABVD in early PET responders prevents the increased toxicity associated with BEACOPP while maintaining comparable survival outcomes.[32,76]

New biomarkers, including ctDNA and those related to [18F]FDG PET/CT imaging (TMTV), are being explored to further enhance therapy outcome prediction in HL.[78,79] Using machine learning techniques and analyses of ctDNA from liquid biopsy, researchers identified 2 classic HL subtypes with distinct outcome, as well as distinct transcriptional and immunologic profiles in patients from trials conducted in France, Belgium, Switzerland, and in the United States among which BREACH and AHL2011.[79] They also showed a significant correlation between the pretreatment ctDNA levels and the TMTV.[79] Patients with high pretreatment ctDNA levels had significantly shorter PFS ($P = 4.2 \; 10^{-6}$) and ctDNA was an independent prognostic factor (HR: 2.4; 95% CI, 1.5–3.7, $P = .0002$).[79] Positive ctDNA (minimal residual disease at cycle 3 day 1) was detected in 3 of 56 (5,3%) patients with negative iPET performed after 2 cycles and in 5 of 24 (20.8%) patients with positive iPET suggesting that iPET and ctDNA might be complementary for outcome prediction.[79]

The main challenge for DLBCL, the most frequent lymphoma subtype, is still improving outcome. At diagnosis, the prognostic index IMPI incorporating TMTV, age, and stage (I–IV) might further improve risk stratification and identify high-risk patients with DLBCL who might benefit from more intensive chemotherapy.[56,57] Interim [^{18}F]FDG PET/CT is not as robust as in HL to predict outcome of patients with DLBCL, with wide variation in positive predictive values.[44,45] The ΔSUV_{max} at iPET4 could complement the visual DS score and improve the prognostic impact of PET.[45,53,61–64] The LYSA group has begun compiling real-world data (Real World Data in Lymphoma and Survival in Adults) that could offer additional insights complementary to clinical trials, especially warranted in DLBCL.[80]

The use of artificial intelligence in lymphoma has been discussed in previous review articles.[81,82] The benefits will be manifold: the automated segmentation of tumor volumes, both metabolic and CT based, and the recognition of metabolic response will help accelerating the routine work flow in nuclear medicine while limiting interobserver variability. Harmonization across treatment centers should also accelerate research developments and clinical validation.

SUMMARY

Extended follow-up data validate the existing risk-adapted therapeutic approaches for HL. The [^{18}F]FDG PET response-adapted therapy contributed to both the improvement of patients' outcome and the reduction of the long-term treatment-related toxicity. The outcomes for patients with refractory/relapsed DLBCL are poor, and additional biomarkers such as TMTV integrated into the recently proposed IMPI at baseline and ctDNA could potentially contribute to improving patient outcomes.

CLINICS CARE POINTS

- The wide variation in the positive predictive value of [^{18}F]FDG PET/CT scan at interim restaging in DLBCL can lead to false-positive results and potentially overtreatment. Therefore, biopsy is strongly recommended prior to second-line treatment when iPET is positive.
- The proposed IMPI is a simple and robust prognostic index to predict PFS for individual patients with DLBCL at baseline. The IMPI integrates age (as continuous variables), stage (I–IV) encompassing a measure of disease dissemination via the Ann Arbor stage, and TMTV delineated using the SUV4.0 threshold.

DISCLOSURE

The authors have nothing to disclose. The authors declare that they have no commercial or financial conflict of interest.

REFERENCES

1. Siegel RL, Miller KD, Fuchs HE, et al. Cancer statistics, 2022. CA Cancer J Clin 2022;72(1):7–33.
2. NCCN Clinical Practice Guidelines in Oncology (NCCN Guidelines®) for B-Cell Lymphomas. Version 1.2024 — January 18, 2024. © National Comprehensive Cancer Network, Inc. 2024. All rights reserved. Accessed February 1, 2024. To view the most recent and complete version of the guideline, go online to NCCN.org.
3. Alaggio R, Amador C, Anagnostopoulos I, et al. The 5th edition of the World Health Organization classification of Haematolymphoid tumours: Lymphoid neoplasms. Leukemia 2022;36(7):1720–48.
4. Cheson BD, Fisher RI, Barrington SF, et al. Recommendations for initial evaluation, staging, and response assessment of Hodgkin and non-Hodgkin lymphoma: the Lugano classification. J Clin Oncol 2014;32(27):3059–68.
5. Barrington SF, Mikhaeel NG, Kostakoglu L, et al. Role of imaging in the staging and response assessment of lymphoma: consensus of the international Conference on malignant lymphomas imaging working group. J Clin Oncol 2014;32(27):3048–58.
6. Cheson BD, Ansell S, Schwartz L, et al. Refinement of the Lugano Classification lymphoma response criteria in the era of immunomodulatory therapy. Blood 2016;128(21):2489–96.
7. Ricard F, Cheson B, Barrington S, et al. Application of the Lugano classification for initial evaluation, staging, and response assessment of hodgkin and non-hodgkin lymphoma: the PRoLoG consensus initiative (Part 1-clinical). J Nucl Med 2023;64(1):102–8.
8. Ricard F, Barrington S, Korn R, et al. Application of the Lugano classification for initial evaluation, staging, and response assessment of hodgkin and

non-hodgkin lymphoma: the PRoLoG consensus initiative (Part 2-Technical). J Nucl Med 2023;64(2): 239–43.

9. Nanni C, Kobe C, Baessler B, et al. European Association of Nuclear Medicine (EANM) Focus 4 consensus recommendations: molecular imaging and therapy in haematological tumours. Lancet Haematol 2023;10(5):e367–81.

10. NCCN Clinical Practice Guidelines in Oncology (NCCN Guidelines®) for Hodgkin Lymphoma. Version 1.2024-October 12, 2023 © National Comprehensive Cancer Network, Inc. 2024. All rights reserved. Accessed February 1, 2024. To view the most recent and complete version of the guideline, go online to NCCN.org.

11. Hasenclever D, Diehl V. A prognostic score for advanced Hodgkin's disease. International prognostic factors Project on advanced Hodgkin's disease. N Engl J Med 1998;339(21):1506–14.

12. Borchmann P, Plutschow A, Kobe C, et al. PET-guided omission of radiotherapy in early-stage unfavourable Hodgkin lymphoma (GHSG HD17): a multicentre, open-label, randomised, phase 3 trial. Lancet Oncol 2021;22(2):223–34.

13. Fuchs M, Goergen H, Kobe C, et al. Positron emission tomography-guided treatment in early-stage favorable hodgkin lymphoma: final results of the international, randomized phase III HD16 Trial by the German Hodgkin Study Group. J Clin Oncol 2019; 37(31):2835–45.

14. Fuchs M, Jacob AS, Kaul H, et al. Follow-up of the GHSG HD16 trial of PET-guided treatment in early-stage favorable Hodgkin lymphoma. Leukemia 2024;38(1):160–7.

15. Fornecker LM, Lazarovici J, Aurer I, et al. Brentuximab vedotin plus AVD for first-line treatment of early-stage unfavorable hodgkin lymphoma (BREACH): a multicenter, open-label, randomized, phase II trial. J Clin Oncol 2023;41(2):327–35.

16. Straus DJ, Jung SH, Pitcher B, et al. Calgb 50604: risk-adapted treatment of nonbulky early-stage Hodgkin lymphoma based on interim PET. Blood 2018;132(10):1013–21.

17. Andre MPE, Girinsky T, Federico M, et al. Early positron emission tomography response-adapted treatment in stage I and II hodgkin lymphoma: final results of the randomized EORTC/LYSA/FIL H10 trial. J Clin Oncol 2017;35(16):1786–94.

18. Federico M, Fortpied C, Stepanishyna Y, et al. Long-term follow-up of the response-adapted Intergroup EORTC/LYSA/FIL H10 trial for Localized hodgkin lymphoma. J Clin Oncol 2024;42(1):19–25.

19. Radford J, Illidge T, Counsell N, et al. Results of a trial of PET-directed therapy for early-stage Hodgkin's lymphoma. N Engl J Med 2015;372(17):1598–607.

20. Johnson P, Federico M, Kirkwood A, et al. Adapted treatment guided by interim PET-CT scan in advanced Hodgkin's lymphoma. N Engl J Med 2016;374(25): 2419–29.

21. Barrington SF, Kirkwood AA, Franceschetto A, et al. PET-CT for staging and early response: results from the Response-Adapted Therapy in Advanced Hodgkin Lymphoma study. Blood 2016;127(12):1531–8.

22. Luminari S, Fossa A, Trotman J, et al. Long-term follow-up of the response-adjusted therapy for advanced hodgkin lymphoma trial. J Clin Oncol 2024;42(1):13–8.

23. Eichenauer DA, Aleman BMP, Andre M, et al. Hodgkin lymphoma: ESMO Clinical Practice Guidelines for diagnosis, treatment and follow-up. Ann Oncol 2018;29(Suppl 4):iv19–29.

24. Fiaccadori V, Neven A, Fortpied C, et al. Relapse patterns in early-PET negative, limited-stage Hodgkin lymphoma (HL) after ABVD with or without radiotherapy-a joint analysis of EORTC/LYSA/FIL H10 and NCRI RAPID trials. Br J Haematol 2023; 200(6):731–9.

25. Sickinger MT, von Tresckow B, Kobe C, et al. PET-adapted omission of radiotherapy in early stage Hodgkin lymphoma-a systematic review and meta-analysis. Crit Rev Oncol Hematol 2016;101:86–92.

26. Follows GA, Barrington SF, Bhuller KS, et al. Guideline for the first-line management of classical hodgkin lymphoma - a British Society for Haematology guideline. Br J Haematol 2022;197(5):558–72.

27. Gillessen S, Plutschow A, Fuchs M, et al. Intensified treatment of patients with early stage, unfavourable Hodgkin lymphoma: long-term follow-up of a randomised, international phase 3 trial of the German Hodgkin Study Group (GHSG HD14). Lancet Haematol 2021;8(4):e278–88.

28. von Tresckow B, Plutschow A, Fuchs M, et al. Dose-intensification in early unfavorable Hodgkin's lymphoma: final analysis of the German Hodgkin Study Group HD14 trial. J Clin Oncol 2012;30(9):907–13.

29. Stephens DM, Li H, Schoder H, et al. Five-year follow-up of SWOG S0816: limitations and values of a PET-adapted approach with stage III/IV Hodgkin lymphoma. Blood 2019;134(15):1238–46.

30. Press OW, Li H, Schoder H, et al. US Intergroup trial of response-adapted therapy for stage III to IV hodgkin lymphoma using early interim Fluorodeoxyglucose-positron emission tomography imaging: Southwest oncology group S0816. J Clin Oncol 2016;34(17): 2020–7.

31. Casasnovas RO, Bouabdallah R, Brice P, et al. Positron emission tomography-driven strategy in advanced hodgkin lymphoma: Prolonged follow-up of the AHL2011 phase III lymphoma study association study. J Clin Oncol 2022;40(10):1091–101.

32. Casasnovas RO, Bouabdallah R, Brice P, et al. PET-adapted treatment for newly diagnosed advanced Hodgkin lymphoma (AHL2011): a randomised, multicentre, non-inferiority, phase 3 study. Lancet Oncol 2019;20(2):202–15.

33. Borchmann P, Goergen H, Kobe C, et al. PET-guided treatment in patients with advanced-stage Hodgkin's lymphoma (HD[18]): final results of an open-label, international, randomised phase 3 trial by the German Hodgkin Study Group. Lancet 2017; 390(10114):2790–802.

34. Andre MPE, Carde P, Viviani S, et al. Long-term overall survival and toxicities of ABVD vs BEACOPP in advanced Hodgkin lymphoma: a pooled analysis of four randomized trials. Cancer Med 2020;9(18): 6565–75.

35. Ansell SM, Radford J, Connors JM, et al. Overall survival with brentuximab vedotin in stage III or IV Hodgkin's lymphoma. N Engl J Med 2022;387(4): 310–20.

36. Hutchings M, Radford J, Ansell SM, et al. Brentuximab vedotin plus doxorubicin, vinblastine, and dacarbazine in patients with advanced-stage, classical Hodgkin lymphoma: a prespecified subgroup analysis of high-risk patients from the ECHELON-1 study. Hematol Oncol 2021;39(2): 185–95.

37. Connors JM, Jurczak W, Straus DJ, et al. Brentuximab vedotin with chemotherapy for stage III or IV Hodgkin's lymphoma. N Engl J Med 2018;378(4): 331–44.

38. Herrera AF, LeBlanc ML, Castellino SM, et al. SWOG S1826, a randomized study of nivolumab(N)-AVD versus brentuximab vedotin(BV)-AVD in advanced stage (AS) classic Hodgkin lymphoma (HL). J Clin Oncol 2023;41(17_suppl):LBA4.

39. Lynch RC, Ujjani CS, Poh C, et al. Concurrent pembrolizumab with AVD for untreated classic Hodgkin lymphoma. Blood 2023;141(21):2576–86.

40. Mauz-Korholz C, Landman-Parker J, Balwierz W, et al. Response-adapted omission of radiotherapy and comparison of consolidation chemotherapy in children and adolescents with intermediate-stage and advanced-stage classical Hodgkin lymphoma (EuroNet-PHL-C1): a titration study with an open-label, embedded, multinational, non-inferiority, randomised controlled trial. Lancet Oncol 2022;23(1): 125–37.

41. Ferdinandus J, van Heek L, Roth K, et al. Patterns of PET-positive residual tissue at interim restaging and risk of treatment failure in advanced-stage Hodgkin's lymphoma: an analysis of the randomized phase III HD18 trial by the German Hodgkin Study Group. Eur J Nucl Med Mol Imaging 2024;51(2): 490–5.

42. Sehn LH, Berry B, Chhanabhai M, et al. The revised International Prognostic Index (R-IPI) is a better predictor of outcome than the standard IPI for patients with diffuse large B-cell lymphoma treated with R-CHOP. Blood 2007;109(5):1857–61.

43. Fox CP, Chaganti S, McIlroy G, et al. The management of newly diagnosed large B-cell lymphoma: a British Society for Haematology Guideline. Br J Haematol 2024. https://doi.org/10.1111/bjh.19273.

44. Burggraaff CN, de Jong A, Hoekstra OS, et al. Predictive value of interim positron emission tomography in diffuse large B-cell lymphoma: a systematic review and meta-analysis. Eur J Nucl Med Mol Imaging 2019;46(1):65–79.

45. Eertink JJ, Burggraaff CN, Heymans MW, et al. Optimal timing and criteria of interim PET in DLBCL: a comparative study of 1692 patients. Blood Adv 2021;5(9):2375–84.

46. Kostakoglu L, Martelli M, Sehn LH, et al. End-of-treatment PET/CT predicts PFS and OS in DLBCL after first-line treatment: results from GOYA. Blood Adv 2021;5(5):1283–90.

47. Lamy T, Damaj G, Soubeyran P, et al. R-CHOP 14 with or without radiotherapy in nonbulky limited-stage diffuse large B-cell lymphoma. Blood 2018; 131(2):174–81.

48. Poeschel V, Held G, Ziepert M, et al. Four versus six cycles of CHOP chemotherapy in combination with six applications of rituximab in patients with aggressive B-cell lymphoma with favourable prognosis (FLYER): a randomised, phase 3, non-inferiority trial. Lancet 2019;394(10216):2271–81.

49. Bologna S, Vander Borght T, Briere J, et al. Early positron emission tomography response-adapted treatment in Localized diffuse large B-cell lymphoma (Aaipi=0) : results of the phase 3 Lysa Lnh 09-1b trial. Hematol Oncol 2021;39(S2).

50. Persky DO, Li H, Stephens DM, et al. Positron emission tomography-directed therapy for patients with limited-stage diffuse large B-cell lymphoma: results of Intergroup National clinical trials Network study S1001. J Clin Oncol 2020;38(26):3003–11.

51. Pfreundschuh M, Murawski N, Christofyllakis K, et al. Excellent outcome of elderly patients with favourable-prognosis DLBCL treated with 4 cycles CHOP/Chlip-14 plus 8 applications of rituximab and a PET-based intensification strategy that includes involved-site radiotherapy (IS-RT): results of the first 120 patients of the OPTIMAL>60 trial of the Dshnhl. Blood 2017; 130(Supplement 1):1549.

52. Burggraaff CN, Eertink JJ, Lugtenburg PJ, et al. 18F-FDG PET improves baseline clinical predictors of response in diffuse large B-cell lymphoma: the HOVON-84 study. J Nucl Med 2022;63(7):1001–7.

53. Michaud L, Bantilan K, Mauguen A, et al. Prognostic value of 18F-FDG PET/CT in diffuse large B-cell lymphoma treated with a risk-adapted Immunochemotherapy regimen. J Nucl Med 2023;64(4): 536–41.

54. Cottereau AS, Meignan M, Nioche C, et al. Risk stratification in diffuse large B-cell lymphoma using lesion dissemination and metabolic tumor burden calculated from baseline PET/CT(dagger). Ann Oncol 2021;32(3):404–11.

55. Barrington SF, Meignan M. Time to prepare for risk adaptation in lymphoma by standardizing measurement of metabolic tumor burden. J Nucl Med 2019;60(8): 1096–102.

56. Barrington SF, Cottereau AS, Zijlstra JM. Is 18F-FDG metabolic tumor volume in lymphoma really happening? J Nucl Med 2024;65(4):510–1.

57. Mikhaeel NG, Heymans MW, Eertink JJ, et al. Proposed new Dynamic prognostic index for diffuse large B-cell lymphoma: international metabolic prognostic index. J Clin Oncol 2022;40(21): 2352–60.

58. Eertink JJ, Zwezerijnen GJC, Heymans MW, et al. Baseline PET radiomics outperforms the IPI risk score for prediction of outcome in diffuse large B-cell lymphoma. Blood 2023;141(25):3055–64.

59. Barrington SF, Zwezerijnen B, de Vet HCW, et al. Automated segmentation of baseline metabolic total tumor burden in diffuse large B-cell lymphoma: which method is most successful? A study on behalf of the PETRA consortium. J Nucl Med 2021;62(3): 332–7.

60. Hutchings M. The evolving therapy of DLBCL: bispecific antibodies. Hematol Oncol 2023;41(S1): 107–11.

61. Rekowski J, Huttmann A, Schmitz C, et al. Interim PET evaluation in diffuse large B-cell lymphoma using published recommendations: comparison of the Deauville 5-point scale and the DeltaSUV(max) method. J Nucl Med 2021;62(1):37–42.

62. Duarte S, Roque A, Saraiva T, et al. Interim FDG18-PET SUV(max) variation adds prognostic value to Deauville 5-point scale in the identification of patients with ultra-high-risk diffuse large B cell lymphoma. Clin Lymphoma Myeloma Leuk 2023;23(2): e107–16.

63. Allioux F, Gandhi D, Vilque JP, et al. End-of-treatment 18F-FDG PET/CT in diffuse large B cell lymphoma patients: DeltaSUV outperforms Deauville score. Leuk Lymphoma 2021;62(12):2890–8.

64. Itti E, Blanc-Durand P, Berriolo-Riedinger A, et al. Validation of the DeltaSUV(max) for interim PET interpretation in diffuse large B-cell lymphoma on the basis of the GAINED clinical trial. J Nucl Med 2023; 64(11):1706–11.

65. Eertink JJ, Arens AIJ, Huijbregts JE, et al. Aberrant patterns of PET response during treatment for DLBCL patients with MYC gene rearrangements. Eur J Nucl Med Mol Imaging 2022;49(3):943–52.

66. Kuhnl A, Roddie C, Kirkwood AA, et al. Early FDG-PET response predicts CAR-T failure in large B-cell lymphoma. Blood Adv 2022;6(1):321–6.

67. Danylesko I, Shouval R, Shem-Tov N, et al. Immune imitation of tumor progression after anti-CD19 chimeric antigen receptor T cells treatment in aggressive B-cell lymphoma. Bone Marrow Transplant 2021; 56(5):1134–43.

68. Cohen D, Luttwak E, Beyar-Katz O, et al. [18F]FDG PET-CT in patients with DLBCL treated with CAR-T cell therapy: a practical approach of reporting pre- and post-treatment studies. Eur J Nucl Med Mol Imaging 2022;49(3):953–62.

69. Adams HJA, Kwee TC. Proportion of false-positive lesions at interim and end-of-treatment FDG-PET in lymphoma as determined by histology: systematic review and meta-analysis. Eur J Radiol 2016; 85(11):1963–70.

70. Sasse S, Brockelmann PJ, Goergen H, et al. Long-term follow-up of contemporary treatment in early-stage hodgkin lymphoma: Updated analyses of the German hodgkin study group HD7, HD8, HD10, and HD11 trials. J Clin Oncol 2017;35(18): 1999–2007.

71. Oeffinger KC, Stratton KL, Hudson MM, et al. Impact of risk-adapted therapy for pediatric hodgkin lymphoma on risk of long-term morbidity: a report from the childhood cancer survivor study. J Clin Oncol 2021;39(20):2266–75.

72. Lo AC, Liu A, Liu Q, et al. Late cardiac toxic effects associated with treatment protocols for hodgkin lymphoma in children. JAMA Netw Open 2024;7(1): e2351062.

73. Giulino-Roth L, Pei Q, Buxton A, et al. Subsequent malignant neoplasms among children with Hodgkin lymphoma: a report from the Children's Oncology Group. Blood 2021;137(11):1449–56.

74. Wirth A, Mikhaeel NG, Aleman BMP, et al. Involved site radiation therapy in adult lymphomas: an overview of international lymphoma radiation oncology group guidelines. Int J Radiat Oncol Biol Phys 2020;107(5):909–33.

75. Sieniawski M, Reineke T, Nogova L, et al. Fertility in male patients with advanced Hodgkin lymphoma treated with BEACOPP: a report of the German Hodgkin Study Group (GHSG). Blood 2008;111(1): 71–6.

76. Merli F, Luminari S, Gobbi PG, et al. Long-term results of the HD2000 trial comparing ABVD versus BEACOPP versus COPP-EBV-CAD in untreated patients with advanced hodgkin lymphoma: a study by Fondazione Italiana Linfomi. J Clin Oncol 2016; 34(11):1175–81.

77. Demeestere I, Racape J, Dechene J, et al. Gonadal function recovery in patients with advanced hodgkin lymphoma treated with a PET-adapted regimen: prospective analysis of a randomized phase III trial (AHL2011). J Clin Oncol 2021;39(29):3251–60.

78. van Heek L, Stuka C, Kaul H, et al. Predictive value of baseline metabolic tumor volume in early-stage favorable Hodgkin Lymphoma - data from the prospective, multicenter phase III HD16 trial. BMC Cancer 2022;22(1):672.

79. Alig SK, Shahrokh Esfahani M, Garofalo A, et al. Distinct Hodgkin lymphoma subtypes defined

by noninvasive genomic profiling. Nature 2024; 625(7996):778–87.

80. Ghesquieres H, Cherblanc F, Belot A, et al. Challenges for quality and utilization of real-world data for diffuse large B-cell lymphoma in REALYSA, a LYSA cohort. Blood Adv 2024;8(2): 296–308.

81. Veziroglu EM, Farhadi F, Hasani N, et al. Role of artificial intelligence in PET/CT imaging for management of lymphoma. Semin Nucl Med 2023;53(3):426–48.

82. Hasani N, Paravastu SS, Farhadi F, et al. Artificial intelligence in lymphoma PET imaging: a scoping review (current trends and future directions). Pet Clin 2022;17(1):145–74.

New PET Tracers for Lymphoma

Johanna S. Enke, MD[a],*, Ralph A. Bundschuh, MD[a], Rainer Claus, MD[b,c], Constantin Lapa, MD[a]

KEYWORDS

- Lymphoma • Oncologic imaging • Molecular imaging • PET • CXCR4

KEY POINTS

- For most lymphoma entities, [^{18}F]FDG-PET/CT remains molecular imaging standard of reference for diagnosis and therapy evaluation.
- Receptor-directed vectors, such as tracers targeting chemokine receptors or surface proteins on tumor-associated cells in tumor microenvironment, have shown promising results in first clinical studies.
- With emerging immunotherapeutic approaches in lymphoma, immuno-PET/CT tracers could assist in therapeutic decision-making.

BACKGROUND

Functional imaging with 2-[fluorine 18]fluoro-2-deoxy-D-glucose (FDG) positron emission tomography (PET)/computed tomography (CT) plays a crucial role in lymphoma management as most entities present with high FDG-uptake.[1,2] Beyond historical categorization into Hodgkin's lymphoma (HL) and non-Hodgkin's lymphoma (NHL), lymphomas are also commonly classified as indolent or aggressive based on their biological and clinical behavior. Aggressive lymphomas are characterized by rapid proliferation and, hence, an increased FDG-avidity. In contrast, some indolent lymphomas, which partly show significantly less proliferative and metabolic activity, often are difficult to detect using FDG imaging.[2] Additionally, even though many potent treatment options for lymphomas exist, refractory or relapsed disease states are still difficult to treat. Therefore, there is a clinical need for molecular tracers beyond FDG not only to increase detection sensitivity but also to pave the way to novel targets for radionuclide-guided therapies. In this review, we discuss nuclear imaging of lymphomas using molecular tracers beyond FDG (Table 1).

NEW PET TRACERS IN INDOLENT LYMPHOMAS
Short Overview of Diseases/Molecular Background

Indolent lymphomas are a very heterogenous group of hematologic malignancies that can present with nodal, extranodal, and/or leukemic disease. Different subtypes are associated with a diverse tumor biology, often characterized by distinct molecular or genetic events. Follicular lymphoma (FL) is characterized by an overexpression of antiapoptotic BCL2 due to a t(14;18) translocation. Mantle cell lymphoma (MCL) can present as both a more indolent and a more aggressive disease and is often associated with a cyclin D1 overexpression based on a t(11;14) translocation. In hairy cell leukemia, almost every case harbors a distinct BRAF p.V600 E mutation, and in lymphoplasmocytic lymphoma (LPL or Morbus Waldenström) MYD88, L265 mutations are very common. Interestingly, a substantial part of LPLs shows mutations in the CXCR4 gene. Marginal zone lymphomas (MZLs; nodal, extranodal, or splenic), which are a rare and very heterogenous group,

[a] Nuclear Medicine, Faculty of Medicine, University of Augsburg, Stenglinstr. 2, 86156 Augsburg, Germany; [b] Hematology and Oncology, Faculty of Medicine, University of Augsburg, Stenglinstr. 2, 86156 Augsburg, Germany; [c] Pathology, Faculty of Medicine, University of Augsburg, Stenglinstr. 2, 86156 Augsburg, Germany
* Corresponding author.
E-mail address: Johanna.enke@uk-augsburg.de

PET Clin 19 (2024) 463–474
https://doi.org/10.1016/j.cpet.2024.05.002

Table 1
PET tracers in lymphoma imaging

Target	Tracer	Features
αvβ3-integrin receptor neoangiogenesis	Eg, [^{18}F]RGD-K5	Overexpressed by tumor-associated endothelial cells, assessment of tumor vascularity in lymphoma manifestations
CXCR4	[^{68}Ga]Ga-PentixaFor	Overexpressed by various indolent and aggressive lymphoma subtypes, theranostic option with [^{177}Lu]Lu-PentixaTher
Cellular proliferation	Eg, [^{18}F]FLT and [^{18}F]fludarabine	Thymidine/nucleoside analog, which is incorporated into DNA during cell proliferation. Uptake correlates with tumor aggressiveness and higher proliferation rates
FAP	[^{68}Ga]Ga-FAPI and [^{18}F]FAPI	Overexpressed by CAFs; targeting tumor microenvironment and fibrosis
cell death	[^{68}Ga]Ga-NOTA-duramycin	Targeting the membrane phosphatidylethanolamine molecule, which gets externalized to the cell surface during cell death
Immuno-PET imaging		
CD20	Eg, ^{89}Zr-zevalin, ^{89}Zr-rituximab, ^{89}Zr-obinutuzumab, and ^{89}Zr-ofatumumab	B-cell surface antigen, variably expressed in most B-cell lymphomas, target for CD20-directed immunotherapies
CD30	Eg, [^{89}Zr]Zr-DFO-AC-10	Physiologically expressed in B cells and T cells, expression in certain hematologic malignancies (eg, HL), target for CD30-directed immunotherapies
CD8	Eg, [^{89}Zr]Zr-Df-IAB22M2C and ^{89}ZED88082 A	Physiologically expressed on activated cytotoxic T cells, imaging of immune response after immune therapies. Expressed in T-cell lymphoma subtypes
PD(L)-1	Eg, ^{18}F-BMS-986192, ^{89}Zr-Df-nivolumab, and ^{89}Zr-pembrolizumab	Checkpoint inhibitor system expressed by immune cells and tumor cells

are mostly linked to infectious or autoimmune chronic inflammatory processes, for example, by Helicobacter pylori in the case of primary gastric MZL or by hepatitis C in the case of primary splenic MZL. The most prevalent indolent NHL is chronic lymphocytic leukemia (CLL) or small lymphocytic leukemia (SLL). Even though PET does not play a major role in CLL imaging, it becomes important during Richter transformation into an aggressive lymphoma subtype, usually diffuse-large B-cell lymphoma (DLBCL) and less frequently HL.

While most aggressive NHL and HL display intense FDG-tracer uptake,[3] FDG-avidity can vary between indolent lymphomas, ranging from positive cases in only 47% to 83% of CLL/SLL and 53% to 67% in patients with MZL up to 91% to 100% of patients with FL.[4] Thus, there is a clinical need for further tracers beyond FDG in lymphoma imaging, especially with emerging novel therapy options, such as immune and targeted therapies.

C-X-C Motif Chemokine Receptor 4

The C-X-C motif chemokine receptor 4 (CXCR4) is physiologically expressed by numerous hematological and immune cells and plays a crucial role in cell communication, proliferation, and migration. Overexpression of CXCR4 has been described for many cancer entities, including hematologic malignancies and been associated with a worse overall prognosis. CXCR4 receptor expression can be visualized using molecular imaging with [^{68}Ga]Ga-PentixaFor.[5,6]

In a study, which evaluated 690 patients with different tumor entities, patients with MCL were among the entities displaying the highest standardized uptake values (SUV).[7] While MCL displays FDG-avidity in most cases, sensitivity of [18F]FDG-PET/CT is especially limited in gastrointestinal and bone marrow involvement.[8,9] In a direct comparison of [68Ga]Ga-PentixaFor-PET/CT and [18F]FDG-PET/CT in MCL, the sensitivity was significantly higher in PentixaFor than in FDG (100% vs 75.2%). Furthermore, significantly higher SUVs and tumor-to-background ratios (TBRs) were observed for the CXCR4-directed imaging approach.[10]

While MZL displays inconsistent FDG-avidity,[4,11] CXCR4-directed imaging has proven to be an accurate imaging modality in staging and therapy response assessment. In 22 patients with newly diagnosed MZL, [68Ga]Ga-PentixaFor-PET/CT performed superior to conventional clinical staging (including CT, gastrointestinal endoscopy, and bone marrow biopsies).[12] Furthermore, CXCR4-directed imaging had a significant impact on staging and therapy decisions.[12] In direct comparison to [18F]FDG-PET/CT, [68Ga]Ga-PentixaFor identified more sites of disease, as 49.6% of MZL manifestations were only visible on CXCR4-directed imaging, while 2.7% were identified by [18F]FDG-PET/CT only.[13] In treatment response imaging, [68Ga]Ga-PentixaFor-PET/CT has also proven its general feasibility in the MZL subtype of gastric mucosa-associated lymphoid tissue (MALT) lymphoma: After H. pylori eradication, [68Ga]Ga-PentixaFor-PET/CT was used to evaluate residual disease.[14] CXCR4-directed imaging identified residual disease with a sensitivity of 95% and a specificity of 100% with gastric biopsies as reference standard, proving to be a potential tool in therapy response assessment.[14]

There are only limited data on CXCR4-directed imaging in further indolent lymphoma subtypes. Initial studies have demonstrated high [68Ga]Ga-PentixaFor uptake in patients with CLL.[7,15] Interestingly, Mayerhoefer and colleagues investigated the clinical hypothesis of a "compartment shift" in CLL from bone marrow and lymph nodes to peripheral blood after ibrutinib treatment initiation, where an increase of CLL blood cell count is frequently seen.[16,17] In this study [68Ga]Ga-PentixaFor-PET/MRI was performed prior to ibrutinib treatment and over the course of therapy. Within the first month of ibrutinib treatment, [68Ga]Ga-PentixaFor uptake decreased in bone marrow and lymph nodes, whereas increasing splenic CXCR4 uptake and an increasing leukocytosis could be noted.[16] In a small study of 17 patients

with Waldenström macroglobulinemia/LPL, [68Ga]Ga-PentixaFor demonstrated high sensitivity in detecting bone marrow involvement and extramedullary disease.[18]

Fibroblast Activation Protein

Since the development of fibroblast activation protein (FAP)-directed PET/CT tracers, FAP inhibitors (FAPI) as [68Ga]Ga-FAPI-PET/CT and [18F]FAPI-PET/CT have been evaluated in different cancer entities. FAP is highly expressed by cancer-associated fibroblasts (CAFs), which are regularly part of a strong desmoplastic stromal reaction surrounding cancer cells in different carcinomas, for example, breast, colon, or pancreatic cancer.[19–21] In contrast to carcinomas, the role of CAFs in lymphoma is not as clear and likely very heterogeneous depending on the lymphoma subtype and location. In FL, cocultivated CAFs had no effect on tumor cell viability, even though they displayed a protective mechanism hindering tumor cell apoptosis when exposed to cytotoxic treatment.[22] In imaging, there are only limited data on [18F]FAPI-PET/CT in hematologic neoplasms. In an initial study by Jin and colleagues, 73 patients with various lymphoma types underwent FAP-directed imaging.[23] While high SUVs were observed in some lymphoma subtypes, such as HL and primary mediastinal large B-cell lymphoma, indolent NHL displayed only mild-to-moderate [68Ga]Ga-FAPI uptake and weak FAP staining in immunohistochemistry (IHC), with the lowest SUV observed in MALT lymphoma.[23] In a direct comparison of FAP-directed imaging and [18F]FDG-PET/CT, [18F]FDG-PET/CT proved to be superior in terms of lesion detection to [68Ga]Ga-FAPI-PET/CT in 31 out of 41 indolent NHL cases.[24] Further research to evaluate the value of FAP-directed imaging in lymphoma is needed.

Further Tracers: Nucleoside-Based Imaging

[18F]deoxy-fluoro-thymidine ([18F]FLT), a nucleoside analog, is a marker for DNA-synthesis and cellular proliferation. By phosphorylation of [18F]FLT, which occurs during the S phase of the cell cycle,[25] intracellular trapping of [18F]FLT takes place.[26]. [18F]FLT-uptake has proven to correlate directly with tumor proliferation and Ki-67.[27] So far, most studies have been conducted in aggressive NHL with high proliferation indices. In contrast, indolent lymphomas exhibit only modest tracer uptake.[28] While this tracer might be useful in detecting progression/transformation into aggressive NHL subtypes, such as DLBCL,[28,29] no conclusion can be drawn at the moment.

NEW PET TRACERS IN HODGKINS DISEASE AND AGGRESSIVE NON-HODGKINS LYMPHOMA
Short Overview of Diseases/Molecular Background

Similar to indolent lymphomas, aggressive lymphomas also comprise a very heterogenous group of hematologic malignancies. The most common aggressive lymphoma is DLBCL, which itself is composed of different (gene-expression based) subtypes, such as activated B-cell and germinal center B-cell (GCB) DLBCL. Even though HL is considered a distinct entity (apart from NHLs) characterized by peculiar Reed-Sternberg cells in classic HL (and "popcorn" cells in nodular lymphocyte-predominant HL), HL shares common features with aggressive lymphomas and sometimes also shows rapid disease progression.

With a plethora of studies demonstrating its value, [18F]FDG PET/CT remains the standard-of-reference imaging modality in aggressive lymphomas as well as in HL. Nonetheless, recently developed tracers might hold other advantages.

C-X-C Motif Chemokine Receptor 4

So far, only a few studies on [68Ga]Ga-PentixaFor have included aggressive lymphoma subtypes.[30] In a small study by Pan and colleagues, 3 of 27 patients were diagnosed with DLBCL.[30] In all patients, lymphoma manifestations were CXCR4 positive but showed less uptake as compared to [18F]FDG imaging.[30]

In central nervous system lymphoma (CNSL), several studies have shown high [68Ga]Ga-PentixaFor uptake of intra-axial lesions[31,32] with excellent TBRs, as normal brain tissue does not express CXCR4 physiologically. In a pilot study by Herhaus and colleagues, lower CXCR4 expression was associated with a better response to methotrexate-based therapy.[32]

In T-cell lymphoma, there are currently only limited data on [68Ga]Ga-PentixaFor imaging: While T-cell lymphoma displayed good radiotracer uptake in a study conducted by Buck and colleagues,[7] others only reported PET-positivity in enteropathy-associated T-cell lymphoma (n = 3), with peripheral T-cell lymphoma, not otherwise specified (n = 1), and natural killer/T-cell lymphoma (NKTL) (n = 2) displaying no significant uptake of [68Ga]Ga-PentixaFor (**Fig. 1**).[30]

Beyond disease staging, CXCR4-directed imaging can be used for the identification of patients eligible for chemokine receptor-directed radioligand therapy (RLT).[33,34]

In T-cell lymphoma, CXCR4-directed RLT (using PentixaTher) with subsequent stem cell transplantation (SCT) has been evaluated in 4 patients. While 1 patient developed septicemia and died 16 days after therapy, the remaining 3 patients achieved encouraging objective responses.[35]

In DLBCL, Lapa and colleagues evaluated CXCR4-directed RLT in 6 patients with relapsed, advanced lymphoma as part of the conditioning regimen before allogenic SCT.[36] At follow-up 6 weeks after therapy, 2 partial (both in patients receiving combined radioimmunotherapy) and 2 mixed responses could be recorded; the remaining 2 patients had died due to infectious complications in therapy-induced aplasia.[36] A phase I/II trial (COLPRIT trial, Eudra-CT 2022-002989-33) will prospectively investigate the value of CXCR4-directed RLT in patients with advanced lymphoproliferative diseases.[33–36] Another phase I/II trial on PentixaTher in CNSL is currently recruiting (PTT101, NCT06132737).

Nucleoside-Based Imaging

As [18F]FLT-uptake is thought to be less affected by tumor-associated macrophage infiltration compared to [18F]FDG, persistent high [18F]FLT uptake after treatment initiation could serve as a negative prognostic factor in lymphoma.[29,37] In a prospective study with 66 patients with DLBCL, all lymphoma manifestations displayed increased tracer uptake.[29] Interestingly, at end of treatment (R-CHOP, rituximab, cyclophosphamide, doxorubicin, vincristine, prednisone), mean SUV were higher in patients who presented with progressive disease or partial response than in subjects with complete response.[29] At interim staging in patients with DLBCL, [18F]FLT-PET/CT had a higher positive predictive value in predicting residual disease than [18F]FDG-PET/CT.[37]

[18F]FLT usually accumulates in highly proliferative tissues, including the physiologic bone marrow. To improve sensitivity and specificity, [18F]fludarabine was developed as a new nucleoside-based tracer.[38–40]

In a preclinical murine study using CNSL and glioblastoma xenografts models, dynamic [18F]fludarabine-PET/CT demonstrated greater specificity for CNSL than [18F]FDG-PET/CT due to marked radiotracer retention in CNSL lesions in contrast to rapid clearance from glioblastoma lesions.[41]

In an initial clinical study of 5 patients with DLBCL and 5 patients with CLL, increased [18F]fludarabine uptake in nodal and extranodal DLBCL, manifestations considered abnormal in CT or [18F]FDG PET, was observed.[42] Noteworthy, diverging [18F]FDG and [18F]fludarabine uptake was noted in some

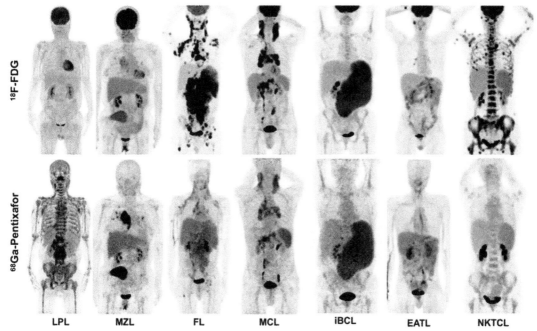

Fig. 1. Direct comparison by Pan and colleagues of [^{18}F]FDG and [^{68}Ga]Ga-PentixaFor-PET/CT in different lymphoma entities with superior TBR in LPL, where bone marrow involvement could be detected, and MZL.[30] One patient with NK/T-cell lymphoma (NKTCL) was negative in CXCR4-imaging. EATL, enteropathy-associated T-cell lymphoma; FL, follicular lymphoma; iBCL, indolent B cell lymphoma; MCL, mantle cell lymphoma. (*Figure from* Pan Q, Luo Y, Zhang Y, Chang L, Li J, Cao X, et al. Preliminary evidence of imaging of chemokine receptor-4-targeted PET/CT with [^{68}Ga]pentixafor in non-Hodgkin lymphoma: comparison to [^{18}F]FDG. EJNMMI Res. 2020;10(1):1-8. https://doi.org/10.1186/S13550-020-00681-7 creative commons licence CC BY 4.0.)

cases: One testicular lymphoma manifestation showed no uptake in [^{18}F]fludarabine. In contrast, mediastinal lymph nodes, which never displayed [^{18}F]fludarabine-uptake remained [^{18}F]FDG-avid after the completion of therapy in another patient, who is still in complete remission 2 years after end of treatment.[42]

[^{18}F]Fluorine-Arginine-Glycine-Aspartic

The transmembrane glycoprotein $\alpha v\beta3$-integrin plays an important role in neoangiogenesis, endothelial growth, and cell migration. Thus, by targeting this specific marker with molecular imaging tracers, for example, [^{18}F]fluorine-arginine-glycine-aspartic ([^{18}F]RGD-K5), more information on the tumor environment and a potential target for new antiangiogenic treatment strategies could be gained.[43–45] So far, [^{18}F]RGD-K5 has been mainly used in solid tumor entities, such as head and neck cancer and lung cancer.[46,47] In lymphoma imaging, Tonnelet and colleagues evaluated [^{18}F]RGD-K5 in a cohort of 18 patients with HL and NHL at baseline and after 2 cycles of chemotherapy.[48] High initial RGD-uptake was present in patients with HL (n = 5) and one gray-zone lymphoma, while other NHL only showed modest to no uptake (**Fig. 2**).[48] After

2 cycles of chemotherapy, nonresponders presented with significantly higher SUV parameters than therapy responders.[48]

Fibroblast Activation Protein

In aggressive lymphoma subtypes like DLBCL, stromal cells and their corresponding gene expression signatures are associated with longer overall survival,[49–51] while stromal gene expression is associated with a worse overall prognosis in solid cancers.[52] In FAP-directed imaging, aggressive lymphomas displayed higher quantitative parameters (like SUV and TBR) as compared to indolent subtypes.[23] In a pilot study, HL, DLBCL, and Burkitt's lymphoma had the highest FAP-uptake.[23] However, imaging with [^{18}F]FDG-PET/CT still proved to be superior in most aggressive lymphoma subtypes.[24] Nonetheless, with emerging therapy options targeting the tumor microenvironment and stromal response, FAP-directed imaging might offer valuable pretherapeutic insights on tumor microenvironment and prognosis. In a recent case report, Lu and colleagues reported on a patient suffering from stage IV DLBCL, with no FAP-uptake in lymphoma manifestations, maybe indicating a subgroup of DLBCL with poorer outcome.[53]

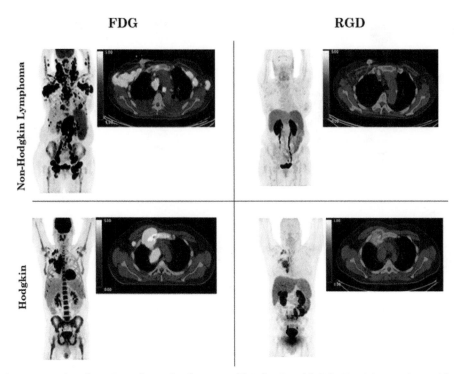

Fig. 2. Direct comparison from Tonnelet and colleagues of [18F]FDG and [18F]RGD-K5 in a patient with NHL and a patient with HL. While HL showed mild-to-moderate uptake of RGD, NHL showed no tracer uptake.[48] (*Figure from* Tonnelet D, Bohn MDP, Becker S, Decazes P, Camus V, Thureau S, et al. Angiogenesis imaging study using interim [18F] RGD-K5 PET/CT in patients with lymphoma undergoing chemotherapy: preliminary evidence. EJNMMI Res. 2021;11(1). https://doi.org/10.1186/S13550-021-00776-9 licensed under the creative commons license CC-BY 4.0.)

Further Tracers

[68Ga]Ga-triazacyclononane-triacetic acid (NOTA)-duramycin is a novel marker for early apoptosis, targeting the membrane phosphatidylethanolamine molecule, which gets externalized to the cell surface during cell death.[54] In an initial report, Gill and colleagues evaluated 10 patients with lymphoma after anthracycline-based chemotherapy for response and anthracycline-induced cardiotoxicity.[55] With high blood pool activity 4 hours after tracer injection, the assessment of abnormal cardiac uptake was not possible, whereas an increased tracer uptake of lymphoma manifestations after chemotherapy could be noted.[55] Further studies are needed to validate those findings.

NEW IMMUNO-TRACERS IN LYMPHOMA IMAGING

In recent years, the characterization of the tumor microenvironment, immune response to cancer, and associated therapeutic agents have been in the focus of extensive research. With rapidly emerging immunotherapeutic agents, for example, checkpoint inhibitors and chimeric antigen receptor (CAR) T-cell therapies, current surveillance methods are confronted with new challenges, such as pseudoprogression and immune-related adverse effects.[56–58] To provide information on the functional/molecular status of the immune system, new PET tracers have recently emerged, visualizing key components such as surface markers of immune cells, cytokines, and immune checkpoints. By labeling tumor-targeting vectors (such as monoclonal antibodies, nanobodies, and bispecific antibodies) with radionuclides, highly specific and sensitive PET tracers are being developed.

Not surprisingly, immuno-PET tracers are of great interest in hematological malignancies, as such tracers could potentially help to quantify molecular interactions and simulate subsequent targeted therapies. So far, there are only limited data available on the clinical use of immuno-PET in lymphoma imaging.[59,60]

CD20 Expression

CD20, a surface antigen, which is overexpressed in most B-cell lymphomas, plays a pivotal role in lymphoma diagnosis and treatment. By targeting CD20 with monoclonal antibodies, such as rituximab, or more recently with CD20-directed bispecific antibodies, patient outcomes could be significantly improved. While CD20-targeted therapies have shown remarkable efficacy, some patients experience relapse or develop resistance—sometimes associated with downregulation of CD20 as an evasion mechanism.[61] Immuno-PET targeting CD20 could aid in the visualization and assessment of eligibility for different treatment strategies. So far, a variety of CD20 targeting antibodies have been developed and labeled for immuno-PET, such as rituximab, obinutuzumab, and ibritumomab tiuxetan.[59] The first in-human use of [89]Zr-zevalin, an [89]Zr-labeled CD20 antibody, was performed by Perk and colleagues in a patient with NHL, who had undergone [^{18}F] FDG-PET 2 weeks before.[62] All tumor manifestations were visible in [89]Zr-zevalin-PET/CT.[62] Lymphoma uptake of [89]Zr-rituximab correlated with CD20-expression as confirmed by IHC in a study by Jauw and colleagues (**Fig. 3**), with one patient displaying [89]Zr-rituximab-positive lymphoma manifestations even though no CD20 expression was observed in IHC.[63] [89]Zr-rituximab-PET/CT was evaluated in 5 heavily pretreated patients with relapsed/recurrent lymphoma (4 FL, 1 HL) prior to RLT.[64] In direct comparison, [89]Zr-obinutuzumab and [89]Zr-ofatumumab displayed better tumor localization capabilities prior to radioimmunotherapy than labeled rituximab.[65]

CD30 Expression

The cell surface receptor CD30 is physiologically expressed by activated B and T cells and is part of the tumor necrosis factor receptor superfamily.[66,67] Among other B-cell and T-cell lymphomas, expression of CD30 is particularly seen in certain hematopoietic malignancies, especially in Reed–Sternberg cells in HL. With the development of anti-CD30-guided therapies, such as brentuximab vedotin as antibody–drug conjugate, CD30 has become an interesting target for immunotherapy.[67] Similar to other cell surface receptors, downregulation of receptor expression due to therapy regimen is frequently observed,[68] leading to the clinical need for noninvasive CD30-directed imaging. Brentuximab vedotin, labeled with [89]Zr and [124]I, has been investigated in mice with [89]Zr providing superior images[69]; tracer accumulation of [89]Zr-labeled brentuximab vedotin has been observed in CD30-positive lymphoma manifestations.[69] Rylova and colleagues used [89]Zr-deferoxamine (DFO)-labeled CD30-specific AC-10 antibodies ([[89]Zr]Zr-DFO-AC-10), which showed promising preclinical results in mice with high tumor-to-background contrast.[70] However, so far, no in-human study has been conducted.

CD8 Expression

CD8 is primarily expressed in T-cell lymphomas, such as cutaneous T-cell lymphoma, peripheral

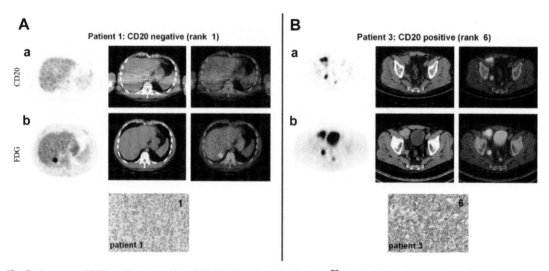

Fig. 3. Immuno-PET imaging targeting CD20 in DLBCL patients with [89]Zr-rituximab. (*A*) DLBCL patient with hepatic lymphoma manifestation, as shown by FDG-PET/CT (b) and no CD20 expression in CD20-directed PET/CT (a) and confirmed by IHC (Score 0, A1) (*B*) Intensive CD20-expression of all lymphoma manifestations as shown by [89]Zr-rituximab-PET/CT (a) and IHC (Score 3+, B6) of an inguinal lymph node, as shown by FDG-PET/CT (b). (*Modified from* Jauw YWS, Zijlstra JM, De Jong D, Vugts DJ, Zweegman S, Hoekstra OS, et al. Performance of 89Zr-Labeled-Rituximab-PET as an Imaging Biomarker to Assess CD20 Targeting: A Pilot Study in Patients with Relapsed/Refractory Diffuse Large B Cell Lymphoma. PLoS One. 2017;12(1). https://doi.org/10.1371/JOURNAL.PONE.0169828 licensed under the creative commons license CC BY 4.0.)

T-cell lymphoma, not otherwise specified and anaplastic T-cell lymphoma. Furthermore, cytotoxic CD8-positive T cells are an important part of the immune response to cancer. The presence of cytotoxic T cells, particularly within the tumor microenvironment, is often considered a predictive biomarker for response to immunotherapies such as immune checkpoint inhibitors.[66] High levels of tumor-infiltrating cytotoxic T cells have been frequently associated with better treatment outcomes in different cancer types.[71] Immuno-PET targeting CD8-positive cells could assess the presence and activity of cytotoxic T-cells within a tumor, providing insights into (early) immune/therapy response and supporting early treatment decisions. So far, no study has been conducted in patients with lymphoma, but CD8-targeted PET/CT with [[89]Zr]Zr-Df-IAB22M2C and [89]ZED88082 A has been evaluated in solid cancers.[72,73] In a study by Ruijter and colleagues, tracer uptake correlated to immunohistochemically confirmed CD8 expression. Higher tracer uptake was noted in lesions with stromal/inflamed rather than in desert immunophenotypes and higher SUV correlated with longer overall survival.[72] Noteworthy, heterogeneity in CD8+ T-cell distribution and pharmacodynamics was noted within and among patients.[72] Further studies are needed to evaluate the role of CD8-directed PET/CT imaging in treatment assessment in different cancer entities including lymphoma.

Further Tracers: CD19, Programmed-cell Death Protein (Ligand) 1

CD19 is physiologically expressed during B-cell differentiation and, therefore, expressed by most B cell lymphoma subtypes. However, there are only very limited data on PET or single photon emission computed tomography targeting CD19-positive cells available.[74–76] With the advent of CD19-targeted CAR T cells in the treatment of relapsed/refractory B-cell lymphoma,[77] CD19-directed PET tracers might be of great clinical interest.

In recent years, immunotherapies targeting the programmed-cell death protein (ligand)1 (PD-1/PD-L1) immune checkpoint axis have shown remarkable results in many types of cancers, including hematological malignancies, which underlines the importance of PD-1 and PD-L1 in immune escape mechanisms.[78] In relapsed/refractory lymphoma, the highest response rates could be achieved in classic HL.[79,80] Radiolabeled tracers targeting PD-1 or PD-L1 (eg, ^{18}F-BMS-986192, [89]Zr-Df-nivolumab, and [89]Zr-pembrolizumab) have been developed offering noninvasive information on PD-(L)1 expression status.[81–84] In lymphoma, an initial study with [89]Zr-labeled PD-1 immunoglobulin G in mice bearing T-cell lymphoma revealed high tracer uptake of PD-1-positive lesions. Since checkpoint inhibitors could become increasingly important in lymphoma therapy,[85] the role of PD-1-targeted PET/CT in lymphoma warrants further research.

SUMMARY

While [^{18}F]FDG-PET/CT is the most established tracer in molecular imaging and has proven its value in various types of lymphoma and clinical settings, its specificity is limited. Furthermore, FDG-avidity, especially in indolent lymphoma subtypes can vary. In recent years, novel, potentially more specific tracers for molecular imaging of lymphoma were developed. These imaging agents target specific molecular pathways, or key components of the tumor microenvironment provide further insights into the complex biology of lymphoma.

Tracers directed at immune checkpoints such as PD-1 and PD-L1, as well as markers of immune cell activity like CD8, offer great potential for assessing therapy response and predicting outcomes in patients with lymphoma undergoing immunotherapy. Moreover, the exploration of novel immuno-targets such as CD20 and CD30 could offer guidance in treatment decisions.

Most of these new PET tracers have shown encouraging preliminary results and could eventually assist in diagnostic and therapeutic decision-making improving patient outcomes. However, further research is urgently needed to translate these findings into clinical practice in lymphoma management.

CLINICS CARE POINTS

- In patients with FDG-avid lymphomas, [^{18}F] FDG-PET/CT remains the imaging modality of choice for staging, therapy response evaluation and end of treatment assessment.

- In indolent lymphomas (including marginal zone lymphoma), CXCR4-directed PET/CT might prove a valuable imaging tool that warrants further investigation in future trials.

- CXCR4-directed radiopharmaceutical therapy requires a close collaboration between nuclear medicine and hematology.

DISCLOSURE

The authors have no relevant conflicts of interest relating to the topic.

REFERENCES

1. Swerdlow SH, Campo E, Harris NL, et al, editors. WHO classification of tumours of haematopoietic and lymphoid tissues. 4th edition. Lyon: International Agency for Research on Cancer; 2017.

2. Weiler-Sagie M, Bushelev O, Epelbaum R, et al. 18F-FDG avidity in lymphoma readdressed: a study of 766 patients. J Nucl Med 2010;51(1):25–30.

3. Bruzzi JF, Macapinlac H, Tsimberidou AM, et al. Detection of Richter's transformation of chronic lymphocytic leukemia by PET/CT. J Nucl Med 2006; 47(8).

4. Barrington SF, Mikhaeel NG, Kostakoglu L, et al. Role of imaging in the staging and response assessment of lymphoma: consensus of the international conference on malignant lymphomas imaging working group. J Clin Oncol 2014;32(27):3048–58.

5. Buck AK, Stolzenburg A, Hänscheid H, et al. Chemokine receptor – directed imaging and therapy. Methods 2017;130:63–71.

6. Kircher M, Herhaus P, Schottelius M, et al. CXCR4-directed theranostics in oncology and inflammation. Ann Nucl Med 2018;32(8):503–11.

7. Buck AK, Haug A, Dreher N, et al. Imaging of C-X-C motif chemokine receptor 4 expression in 690 patients with solid or hematologic neoplasms using 68Ga-pentixafor PET. J Nucl Med 2022;63(11): 1687–92.

8. Albano D, Treglia G, Gazzilli M, et al. 18F-FDG PET or PET/CT in mantle cell lymphoma. Clin Lymphoma, Myeloma & Leukemia 2020;20(7):422–30.

9. Bailly C, Carlier T, Touzeau C, et al. Interest of FDG-PET in the management of mantle cell lymphoma. Front Med 2019;6(APR). https://doi.org/10.3389/FMED.2019.00070.

10. Mayerhoefer ME, Raderer M, Lamm W, et al. CXCR4 PET imaging of mantle cell lymphoma using [68Ga] Pentixafor: comparison with [18F]FDG-PET. Theranostics 2021;11(2):567–78.

11. Hoffmann M, Kletter K, Becherer A, et al. 18F-fluorodeoxyglucose positron emission tomography (18F-FDG-PET) for staging and follow-up of marginal zone B-cell lymphoma. Oncology 2003;64(4):336–40.

12. Duell J, Krummenast F, Schirbel A, et al. Improved primary staging of marginal-zone lymphoma by addition of CXCR4-directed PET/CT. J Nucl Med 2021;62(10):1415–21.

13. Kosmala A, Duell J, Schneid S, et al. Chemokine receptor–targeted PET/CT provides superior diagnostic performance in newly diagnosed marginal zone lymphoma patients: a head-to-head comparison with [18F]FDG. Eur J Nucl Med Mol Imag 2023;51(3):749–55.

14. Mayerhoefer ME, Raderer M, Lamm W, et al. CXCR4 PET/MRI for follow-up of gastric mucosa–associated lymphoid tissue lymphoma after first-line Helicobacter pylori eradication. Blood 2022; 139(2):240–4.

15. Mayerhoefer ME, Jaeger U, Staber P, et al. Ga-pentixafor PET/MRI for CXCR4 imaging of chronic lymphocytic leukemia: preliminary results. Invest Radiol 2018;53(7). https://doi.org/10.1097/RLI.0000000000 000469.

16. Mayerhoefer ME, Haug A, Jäger U, et al. In human visualization of ibrutinib-induced CLL compartment shift. Cancer Immunol Res 2020;8(8). https://doi.org/10.1158/2326-6066.CIR-19-0880.

17. Mayerhoefer ME, Haug A, Jaeger U, et al. In human visualization of ibrutinib-induced CLL compartment shift. Blood 2019;134(Supplement_1). https://doi.org/10.1182/blood-2019-131469.

18. Luo Y, Cao X, Pan Q, et al. 68Ga-Pentixafor PET/CT for imaging of chemokine receptor 4 expression in Waldenström macroglobulinemia/lymphoplasmacytic lymphoma: comparison to 18F-FDG PET/CT. J Nucl Med 2019;60(12):1724–9.

19. Loktev A, Lindner T, Mier W, et al. A tumor-imaging method targeting cancer-associated fibroblasts. J Nucl Med 2018;59(9):1423–9.

20. Hamson EJ, Keane FM, Tholen S, et al. Understanding fibroblast activation protein (FAP): substrates, activities, expression and targeting for cancer therapy. Proteonomics Clin Appl 2014;8(5–6):454–63.

21. Kratochwil C, Flechsig P, Lindner T, et al. 68Ga-FAPI PET/CT: tracer uptake in 28 different kinds of cancer. J Nucl Med 2019;60(6):801–5.

22. Staiger AM, Duppel J, Dengler MA, et al. An analysis of the role of follicular lymphoma-associated fibroblasts to promote tumor cell viability following drug-induced apoptosis. Leuk Lymphoma 2017;58(8): 1922–30.

23. Jin X, Wei M, Wang S, et al. Detecting fibroblast activation proteins in lymphoma using 68Ga-FAPI PET/CT. J Nucl Med 2022;63:212–7.

24. Chen X, Wang S, Lai Y, et al. Fibroblast activation protein and glycolysis in lymphoma diagnosis: comparison of 68Ga-FAPI PET/CT and 18 F-FDG PET/CT. J Nucl Med 2023;00:1–7.

25. Barthel H, Cleij MC, Collingridge DR, et al. 3-Deoxy-3-[18F]fluorothymidine as a new marker for monitoring tumor response to antiproliferative therapy in vivo with positron emission tomography 1. Cancer Res 2003;63:3791–8.

26. Rasey JS, Grierson JR, Wiens LW, et al. Validation of FLT uptake as a measure of thymidine kinase-1 activity in A549 carcinoma cells. J Nucl Med 2002; 43:1210–7.

27. Barthel H, Perumal M, Latigo J, et al. The uptake of 3′-deoxy-3′-[18F]fluorothymidine into L5178Y tumours in vivo is dependent on thymidine kinase 1 protein levels. Eur J Nucl Med Mol Imag 2005; 32(3):257–63.

28. Buck AK, Bommer M, Stilgenbauer S, et al. Molecular imaging of proliferation in malignant lymphoma. Cancer Res 2006;66(22):11055–61.

29. Herrmann K, Buck AK, Schuster T, et al. Predictive value of initial 18F-FLT uptake in patients with aggressive non-hodgkin lymphoma receiving R-CHOP treatment. J Nucl Med 2011;52(5):690–6.

30. Pan Q, Luo Y, Zhang Y, et al. Preliminary evidence of imaging of chemokine receptor-4-targeted PET/CT with [68Ga]pentixafor in non-Hodgkin lymphoma: comparison to [18F]FDG. EJNMMI Res 2020;10(1):1–8.

31. Starzer AM, Berghoff AS, Traub-Weidinger T, et al. Assessment of central nervous system lymphoma based on CXCR4 expression in vivo using 68Ga-pentixafor PET/MRI. Clin Nucl Med 2021;46(1):16–20.

32. Herhaus P, Lipkova J, Lammer F, et al. CXCR4-Targeted PET imaging of central nervous system B-cell lymphoma. J Nucl Med 2020;61(12):1765–71.

33. Herrmann K, Schottelius M, Lapa C, et al. First-in-Human experience of CXCR4-directed endoradiotherapy with 177Lu- and 90Y-labeled pentixather in advanced-stage multiple myeloma with extensive intra- and extramedullary disease. J Nucl Med 2016;57(2):248–51.

34. Schottelius M, Osl T, Poschenrieder A, et al. [177Lu] pentixather: comprehensive preclinical characterization of a first CXCR4-directed endoradiotherapeutic agent. Theranostics 2017;7(9):2362.

35. Buck AK, Grigoleit GU, Kraus S, et al. C-X-C motif chemokine receptor 4–targeted radioligand therapy in patients with advanced T-cell lymphoma. J Nucl Med 2023;64(1). https://doi.org/10.2967/jnumed.122.264207.

36. Lapa C, Hänscheid H, Kircher M, et al. Feasibility of CXCR4-directed radioligand therapy in advanced Diffuse large B-cell lymphoma. J Nucl Med 2019;60(1):60–4.

37. Minamimoto R, Fayad L, Advani R, et al. Diffuse large B-cell lymphoma: prospective multicenter comparison of early interim FLT PET/CT versus FDG PET/CT with IHP, EORTC, deauville, and PERCIST criteria for early therapeutic monitoring. Radiology 2016;280(1):220–9.

38. Scordo M, Flynn JR, Gonen M, et al. Identifying an optimal fludarabine exposure for improved outcomes after axi-cel therapy for aggressive B-cell non-Hodgkin lymphoma. Blood adv 2023;7(18):5579–85.

39. Samaniego F, McLaughlin P, Neelapu SS, et al. Initial report of a phase II study with R-FND followed by ibritumomab tiuxetan radioimmunotherapy and rituximab maintenance in patients with untreated high-risk follicular lymphoma. Leuk Lymphoma 2021;62(1):58–67.

40. Guillouet S, Patin D, Tirel O, et al. Fully automated radiosynthesis of 2-[18F]fludarabine for PET imaging of low-grade lymphoma. Mol Imag Biol 2014;16(1):28–35.

41. Hovhannisyan N, Fillesoye F, Guillouet S, et al. [18F] Fludarabine-PET as a promising tool for differentiating CNS lymphoma and glioblastoma: comparative analysis with [18F]FDG in human xenograft models. Theranostics 2018;8(16):4563–73.

42. Chantepie S, Hovhannisyan N, Guillouet S, et al. 18F-Fludarabine PET for lymphoma imaging: first-in-humans study on DLBCL and CLL patients. J Nucl Med 2018;59(9):1380–5.

43. Liu J, Yuan S, Wang L, et al. Diagnostic and predictive value of using RGD PET/CT in patients with cancer: a systematic review and meta-analysis. BioMed Res Int 2019;2019. https://doi.org/10.1155/2019/8534761.

44. Li L, Chen X, Yu J, et al. Preliminary clinical application of RGD-containing peptides as PET radiotracers for imaging tumors. Front Oncol 2022;12:1.

45. Gu Y, Dong B, He X, et al. The challenges and opportunities of αvβ3-based therapeutics in cancer: from bench to clinical trials. Pharmacol Res 2023;189:106694.

46. Chen SH, Wang HM, Lin CY, et al. RGD-K5 PET/CT in patients with advanced head and neck cancer treated with concurrent chemoradiotherapy: results from a pilot study. Eur J Nucl Med Mol Imag 2016;43(9):1621–9.

47. Beer AJ, Lorenzen S, Metz S, et al. Comparison of integrin alphaVbeta3 expression and glucose metabolism in primary and metastatic lesions in cancer patients: a PET study using 18F-galacto-RGD and 18F-FDG. J Nucl Med 2008;49(1):22–9.

48. Tonnelet D, Bohn MDP, Becker S, et al. Angiogenesis imaging study using interim [18F] RGD-K5 PET/CT in patients with lymphoma undergoing chemotherapy: preliminary evidence. EJNMMI Res 2021;11(1). https://doi.org/10.1186/S13550-021-00776-9.

49. Raffaghello L, Vacca A, Pistoia V, et al. Cancer associated fibroblasts in hematological malignancies. Oncotarget 2015;6(5):2603.

50. Ciavarella S, Vegliante MC, Fabbri M, et al. Dissection of DLBCL microenvironment provides a gene expression-based predictor of survival applicable to formalin-fixed paraffin-embedded tissue. Ann Oncol 2018;29(12):2363–70.

51. Menéndez V, Solórzano JL, García-Cosío M, et al. Immune and stromal transcriptional patterns that influence the outcome of classic Hodgkin lymphoma. Sci Rep 2024;14(1):710.

52. Haro M, Orsulic S. A paradoxical correlation of cancer-associated fibroblasts with survival outcomes in B-cell lymphomas and carcinomas. Front Cell Dev Biol 2018;6(98). https://doi.org/10.3389/FCELL.2018.00098.

53. Lu L, Bin J. Complete absence of FAPI uptake in a patient with aggressive Diffuse large B-cell

lymphoma involving multiple nodal and extranodal sites. Clin Nucl Med 2023;48(12):E591–2.

54. Kaur G, Shukla J, Sood A, et al. Potential role of 68Ga-NOTA-Duramycin PET/CT imaging for early response evaluation in a lymphoma patient: a case report. Clin Nucl Med 2023;48(1):E19–21.

55. Gill G, Krishnaraju V, Pandey S, et al. 68Ga-duramycin PET/CT imaging of anthracycline-induced cell death in patients with lymphoma. J Nucl Med 2023;64(supplement 1):P1198.

56. Frelaut M, Le Tourneau C, Borcoman E. Hyperprogression under immunotherapy. Int J Mol Sci 2019; 20(11). https://doi.org/10.3390/ijms20112674.

57. Sortais C, Cordeil S, Bourbon E, et al. Flare-up phenomenon or pseudoprogression after CAR T-cell infusion in non-Hodgkin aggressive lymphomas. Leuk Lymphoma 2023;64(3). https://doi.org/10.1080/10428194.2022.2161304.

58. Lee AJ, Kim KW, Cho YC, et al. Incidence of immune-mediated pseudoprogression of lymphoma treated with immune checkpoint inhibitors: systematic review and meta-analysis. J Clin Med 2021; 10(11). https://doi.org/10.3390/jcm10112257.

59. Dun Y, Huang G, Liu J, et al. ImmunoPET imaging of hematological malignancies: from preclinical promise to clinical reality. Drug Discov Today 2022;27(4): 1196–203.

60. Triumbari EKA, Morland D, Laudicella R, et al. Clinical applications of immuno-PET in lymphoma: a systematic review. Cancers 2022;14(14):3488.

61. Hiraga J, Tomita A, Sugimoto T, et al. Down-regulation of CD20 expression in B-cell lymphoma cells after treatment with rituximab-containing combination chemotherapies: its prevalence and clinical significance. Blood 2009;113(20):4885–93.

62. Perk LR, Visser OJ, Stigter-Van Walsum M, et al. Preparation and evaluation of (89)Zr-Zevalin for monitoring of (90)Y-Zevalin biodistribution with positron emission tomography. Eur J Nucl Med Mol Imag 2006;33(11):1337–45.

63. Jauw YWS, Zijlstra JM, De Jong D, et al. Performance of 89Zr-Labeled-Rituximab-PET as an imaging biomarker to assess CD20 targeting: a pilot study in patients with relapsed/refractory Diffuse large B cell lymphoma. PLoS One 2017;12(1). https://doi.org/10.1371/JOURNAL.PONE.0169828.

64. Muylle K, Flamen P, Vugts DJ, et al. Tumour targeting and radiation dose of radioimmunotherapy with (90) Y-rituximab in CD20+ B-cell lymphoma as predicted by (89)Zr-rituximab immuno-PET: impact of preloading with unlabelled rituximab. Eur J Nucl Med Mol Imag 2015;42(8):1304–14.

65. Yoon JT, Longtine MS, Marquez-Nostra BV, et al. Evaluation of next-generation anti-CD20 antibodies labeled with 89Zr in human lymphoma xenografts. J Nucl Med 2018;59(8):1219–24.

66. Raskov H, Orhan A, Christensen JP, et al. Cytotoxic CD8+ T cells in cancer and cancer immunotherapy. Br J Cancer 2020;124(2):359–67.

67. Wang D, Zeng C, Xu B, et al. Anti-CD30 chimeric antigen receptor T cell therapy for relapsed/refractory CD30+ lymphoma patients. Blood Cancer J 2020; 10(8):1–4.

68. Chen R, Hou J, Newman E, et al. CD30 downregulation, MMAE resistance, and MDR1 upregulation are all associated with resistance to brentuximab vedotin. Mol Cancer Therapeut 2015;14(6):1384.

69. Moss A, Gudas J, Albertson T, et al. Abstract 104: preclinical microPET/CT imaging of 89Zr-Df-SGN-35 in mice bearing xenografted CD30 expressing and non-expressing tumors. Cancer Res 2014; 74(19_Supplement):104.

70. Rylova SN, Del Pozzo L, Klingeberg C, et al. Immuno-PET imaging of CD30-positive lymphoma using 89Zr-Desferrioxamine-Labeled CD30-specific AC-10 antibody. J Nucl Med 2016;57(1):96–102.

71. Li F, Li C, Cai X, et al. The association between CD8+ tumor-infiltrating lymphocytes and the clinical outcome of cancer immunotherapy: a systematic review and meta-analysis. EClinicalMedicine 2021;41: 101134.

72. Kist de Ruijter L, van de Donk PP, Hooiveld-Noeken JS, et al. Whole-body CD8+ T cell visualization before and during cancer immunotherapy: a phase 1/2 trial. Nat Med 2022;28(12):2601–10.

73. Farwell MD, Gamache RF, Babazada H, et al. CD8-Targeted PET imaging of tumor-infiltrating T cells in patients with cancer: a phase I first-in-humans study of 89Zr-Df-IAB22M2C, a radiolabeled anti-CD8 minibody. J Nucl Med 2022;63(5):720–6.

74. Simonetta F, Alam IS, Lohmeyer JK, et al. Molecular imaging of chimeric antigen receptor T cells by ICOS-ImmunoPET. Clin Cancer Res 2021;27(4). https://doi.org/10.1158/1078-0432.CCR-20-2770.

75. Simonetta F, Alam IS, Lohmeyer JK, et al. Molecular imaging of chimeric antigen receptor T cells by ICOS-immunopet. Blood 2020;136(Supplement 1). https://doi.org/10.1182/blood-2020-136331.

76. Vervoordeldonk SF, Heikens J, Goedemans WT, et al. 99mTc-CD19 monoclonal antibody is not useful for imaging of B cell non-Hodgkin's lymphoma. Cancer Immunol Immunother 1996;42(5). https://doi.org/10.1007/s002620050285.

77. Sterner RC, Sterner RM. CAR-T cell therapy: current limitations and potential strategies. Blood Cancer J 2021;11(4). https://doi.org/10.1038/s41408-021-00459-7.

78. Xu-Monette ZY, Zhou J, Young KH. PD-1 expression and clinical PD-1 blockade in B-cell lymphomas. Blood 2018;131(1):68.

79. Chen R, Zinzani PL, Fanale MA, et al. Phase II study of the efficacy and safety of pembrolizumab for

relapsed/refractory classic Hodgkin lymphoma. J Clin Oncol 2017;35(19):2125–32.

80. Armand P, Shipp MA, Ribrag V, et al. Programmed death-1 blockade with pembrolizumab in patients with classical Hodgkin lymphoma after brentuximab vedotin failure. J Clin Oncol 2016;34(31):3733–9.

81. Niemeijer AN, Leung D, Huisman MC, et al. Whole body PD-1 and PD-L1 positron emission tomography in patients with non-small-cell lung cancer. Nature Com 2018;9(1):4664.

82. Nienhuis PH, Antunes IF, Glaudemans AWJM, et al. 18F-BMS986192 PET imaging of PD-L1 in metastatic melanoma patients with brain metastases treated with immune checkpoint inhibitors. A pilot study.

J Nucl Med 2022;63(6). https://doi.org/10.2967/jnumed.121.262368.

83. Niemeijer AL, Smit E, Bahce I, et al. Whole body PD-1 and PD-L1 PET in pts with NSCLC. Ann Oncol 2017; 28. https://doi.org/10.1093/annonc/mdx380.008.

84. Smit J, Borm FJ, Niemeijer ALN, et al. PD-L1 PET/CT imaging with radiolabeled durvalumab in patients with advanced-stage non-small cell lung cancer. J Nucl Med 2022;63(5). https://doi.org/10.2967/jnumed.121.262473.

85. Hatic H, Sampat D, Goyal G. Immune checkpoint inhibitors in lymphoma: challenges and opportunities. Ann Transl Med 2021;9(12). https://doi.org/10.21037/atm-20-6833.

Radioligand Therapy in Lymphoma
Past, Present, and Future

Ludmila Santiago Almeida, MD[a,b], Roberto C. Delgado Bolton, MD, PhD[b,c],
Victor Cabral Heringer, MD[a], Samuel de Souza Medina, MD[d],
Elba Etchebehere, MD, PhD[a,*]

KEYWORDS

• Radioligand • Therapy • Lymphoma • Immunotherapy • Theranostics

KEY POINTS

- Radiolabeled therapy in lymphoma has a great theranostics potential.
- Radioimmunotherapy with labeled monoclonal antibodies (MoAbs) anti-CD20 is underutilized despite its proven safety and efficacy as mono, consolidation, or combined therapy in NLH.
- MoAbs targeting CD22, CD37, and CD45 with radiation emitters like auger are expected to increase interest in the future.
- Radiolabeled peptides (such as targeting C-X-C chemokine receptor type 4) will probably be more easily adapted for theranostics due to easier labeling techniques.

INTRODUCTION

Lymphomas are a group of neoplastic diseases of the lymphoid tissue. They are divided into Hodgkin lymphoma (HL) and non-Hodgkin lymphoma (NHL). In 2023, an estimated 20,180 deaths would occur worldwide due to lymphomas.[1]

HL is an uncommon malignancy of B-cell origin with impressive cure rates for patients even with advanced disease. The death rate of HL reached levels as low as 1.3% in 1975 and in 2020 reached 0.2%.[1] The first treatments applied consisted of broad-field radiation therapy. Subsequently, the development of MOPP chemotherapy (vincristine, procarbazine, and prednisone) led to significant advances, with a 10 year survival rate of 66% in patients with advanced-stage disease. However,

because patients later evolved with toxic and fatal events, an alternate regimen was established: doxorubicin, bleomycin, vinblastine, and dacarbazine (ABVD). ABVD led to 5 year relative survival rates of nearly 89%. Therefore, although ongoing trials aim to improve treatment, especially in the relapse/refractory disease setting, the majority of the trials are aimed at NHL due to lower response rates.[1,2]

NHL, contrarily to HL, is a far more common and heterogeneous group of lymphoproliferative disorders.[1] Until the 1990s, the strategy for treating these lymphomas was quite challenging. Unlike the impressive cure rates of HL, chemotherapy only cures approximately one-half of patients with NHL. Thus, there is an ever-growing need to develop novel therapies to achieve better

[a] Division of Nuclear Medicine, University of Campinas (UNICAMP), Rua Vital Brasil 251, Campinas, 13083-888, Brazil; [b] Department of Diagnostic Imaging (Radiology) and Nuclear Medicine, University Hospital San Pedro and Centre for Biomedical Research of La Rioja, Outro Pl. San Pedro, 3, 26006 Logroño, La Rioja, España; [c] Servicio Cántabro de Salud, Av Herrera Oria, s/n, 39011 Santander, Cantabria, España; [d] Division of Hematology, Department of Internal Medicine, Faculty of Medical Sciences, Campinas University, R. Carlos Chagas, 480 - Cidade Universitária, Campinas, SP, 13083-878, Brazil
* Corresponding author. Division of Nuclear Medicine, UNICAMP, Rua Vital Brasil 251, Campinas, BRAZIL, 13083-888.
E-mail address: elba@unicamp.br

PET Clin 19 (2024) 475–494
https://doi.org/10.1016/j.cpet.2024.05.003

outcomes in patients with NHL, especially as the incidence of NHL has increased. Between 1970 and 1995, this increase was because of HIV infection; but more recently, it is in patients in the sixth and seventh decades of life, an aging population with multiple comorbidities.[3]

Brief History

Until the 1990s, treating lymphomas was quite challenging, and the role of nuclear medicine in lymphomas was restricted mainly to staging. Patients were staged with computed tomographic (CT) scans and gallium-67 scintigraphy, which, due to poor resolution, presented an estimated incorrect staging rate of 29% and 37%, respectively. Staging often had to be complemented with surgery, even in the pediatric population.[4] The staging strategy changed radically in later years with the advent of molecular imaging with PET/CT.[5]

Alavi and colleagues in 1984 demonstrated another essential application of nuclear medicine in oncohematological diseases. The authors used radiolabeled cells to investigate the normal cell kinetic patterns and analysis of migration changes induced by hematologic disorders.[6]

Until the early 2000s, mantle radiation was part of the treatment strategy, which involved irradiating a large body area, generally exceeding the target organs. In patients with more extensive disease, chemotherapy was combined.[7] Although relapse was reduced, there was no significant improvement in overall survival (OS), mainly due to side effects of radiation, such as a second neoplasm, sterility, and vascular degeneration.[8–10]

Monoclonal antibody (MoAb) development began in the 1980s and accelerated with the advent of hybridoma technology to produce purified MoAbs. This technology allowed MoAbs to target specific tumor-cell antigens. It opened new paths in therapy for hematological malignancies since MoAbs could now deliver antitumor agents such as chemotherapy, toxins, and radiation. The combination of an antibody labeled with a radionuclide to deliver cytotoxic radiation to a target cell is called radioimmunotherapy.[11]

RADIOIMMUNOTHERAPY

Since many lymphoma cells are radiosensitive, radiolabeling MoAbs to treat by targeting and irradiating at the cellular level (radioimmunotherapy) is an exciting option and a field in constant development.

Radioimmunotherapy has minimal side effects; outpatient treatment is possible with one single dose. Due to its safety profile and effectiveness, radioimmunotherapy has been applied as monotherapy or as a combination treatment with chemotherapy in both the myeloablative and non-myeloablative settings before transplant. Radioimmunotherapy is also used to treat the relapsed/refractory B-cell NHL as well as untreated patients with advanced follicular lymphomas or low-grade relapsed/refractory B-cell NHL.

Radioimmunotherapy also has the advantage of diagnostic imaging for planning and monitoring therapy (theragnostic approach).[12]

Although the cost of radioimmunotherapy is reported as a significant drawback, current treatments that demand patient visits, laboratory controls, and hospitalization due to substantial side effects have a lower cost–benefit than radioimmunotherapy.[13,14]

Despite the clear benefits of radioimmunotherapy over chemotherapy, after several decades since Food and Drug Administration (FDA) approval of MoAbs labeled with Iodine-131 (Bexxar - tositumomab and iodine I 131 tositumomab - GlaxoSmithKline Research Triangle Park, NC) or Yttrium-90 (Zevalin - ibritumomab tiuxetan Spectrum Pharmaceuticals, Henderson, NV) and indications incorporated in guidelines, its use is decreasing.[15] This fact may be caused by insufficient predictive and prognostic data and scarce phase III comparative trials. The reduction of radioimmunotherapy applications is also intimately related to the restricted availability and reimbursement of the radiotracer in many countries and to the difficulties in fulfilling requirements from the local Nuclear Regulatory Commissions since radioimmunotherapy dose delivery is only possible in facilities with permission to handle radioactive materials. **Table 1** describes the advantages and disadvantages of radioimmunotherapy.

In this review, we aim to introduce the types of MoAbs for radioimmunotherapy, discuss the radiation emitters' characteristics and the subsequent treatment strategies and discuss future directions of radioligand therapy (RLT) in lymphoma.

Monoclonal Antibodies

Antibodies are proteins produced by the immune system B cells binding to the cell surface markers known as antigens. A wide variety of antibodies or their fragments are developed in laboratories.[16]

Currently, the antibodies or their fragments can have any of 3 main structures: naked monoclonal antibodies (**Fig. 1**A), antibody–drug conjugates (**Fig. 1**B), and bispecific antibodies (**Fig. 1**C). These antibodies or their fragments can be obtained by any of 4 immunogenic origins: animal, chimeric,

Table 1
Advantages and disadvantages of radioimmunotherapy

Advantages	Disadvantages
Patient selection	Time-consuming in equipment
Dosimetry	Several visits
More personalized	Trained personnel
Treat what you see	Tracer availability
Outpatient regimen	Reimbursement
Single treatment dose	Cost
Effective	Reactions to cold, unlabeled MoAbs
Predicted reactions	Prior and post-HAMA laboratory controls
Predictive factors	Lack of prognostic factors
Tumor board	Oncologist prescription
Extensive literature on phase II trials	Lack of phase III trials
Safe	Lack of comparative trials
Suitable MoAb according to imaging	HAMA formation
PET/CT for monitoring	Degradation and unlabeled in vivo
Pretargeting radioimmunotherapy	Background activity
Development of MoAbs technology	Regulations and authorization
Few nonhematological effects	Few authorized centers

humanized, and fully human (**Fig. 2**). **Table 2** displays the characteristics of the MoAbs.[17,18]

Types of Radiation

When selecting the adequate radionuclide, key considerations are the energy of the emitted particles and the range of these particles in the tissues. A high linear energy transfer (LET) means a high amount of radiation energy is deposited per unit path length along the track of an ionizing particle. An alpha emitter has a higher LET than auger emitters, which in turn have a higher LET than beta emitters. A higher LET causes a progressively higher grade of direct cell death and sequentially a higher release of cell mediators measured by bystander effect.[19,20] The characteristics of different types of radiation and their biological effects are summarized in **Table 3** and in **Fig. 3**.

Targets for Radioligand Therapy in Lymphomas

Most clinically relevant targets until the present moment are radiolabeled anti-CD20 and, currently, labeled peptides to target C-X-C chemokine receptor type 4 (CXCR4) and other MoAbs (anti-CD22, anti-CD37, and anti-CD45).

Additional molecules have been radiolabeled in the past (CD90, ferritin, Lym-1, CD5, transferrin, CD19, CD22, anti-5-benzyl-1,3-thiazol-2-amine (LL2), CD30, anti-CD25, interleukin-2, CD37, CD79, and CD74) and can be found in the historical timeline provided in **Fig. 4**.

Targeting CD20

CD20 is a nonglycosylated phosphoprotein expressed on B cells that plays a role in B-cell activation and proliferation.[21] Preclinical studies on radioimmunotherapy with anti-CD20 MoAbs began in 1994 and several different antibodies have been labeled with a variety of isotopes such as I-131 (^{131}I), Y-90 (^{90}Y), Th-227, At-211, Re-188, Bi-213, and Lu-177 (^{177}Lu).[22–25] Pretargeting radioimmunotherapy systems were developed to reduce treatment toxicity, mainly by removing the free MoAbs from circulation, but they did not evolve in clinical practice[26] (**Fig. 5**).

The most prominent anti-CD20 is rituximab (FDA approval in 1997) for treating NHL.[15] Anti-CD20 labeled with ^{90}Y-ibritumomab (Zevalin) or ^{131}I-tositumomab (Bexxar) received FDA approval for the following applications: previously untreated patients with follicular NHL who achieved partial response or complete response (CR) to first-line chemotherapy (consolidation) and treatment of relapsed or refractory low-grade, follicular or transformed NHL.[15] The trials that applied radioimmunotherapy will be further discussed in later sections.

Targeting CD22 or anti-LL2

CD22 is a MoAb lectin and cell adhesion molecule found in B-lymphocytes, and LL2 is a B-cell (CD22)-specific immunoglobulin type G2a (IgG2a). The experience with radioimmunotherapy in B-cell lymphomas using the rapidly internalizing antibody, anti-CD22 (LL2), is limited and restricted to relapsed/refractory B-cell NHL. In the early 2000s, trials treating patients with epratuzumab (binds to the glycoprotein CD22 of B cells) labeled with Iodine-131 or Yttrium-90 demonstrated overall response rates (ORRs) that varied from 33% to 87%, with a more favorable profile when labeled with Yttrium-90.[27–29] Late adverse events include hypothyroidism in approximately 14% when applying Iodine-131 and human antimurine antibodies (HAMA) formation in 19%. From 2010 until 2017, the clinical trials that evaluated

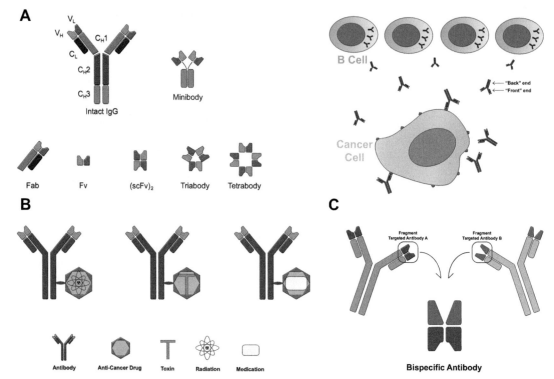

Fig. 1. Monoclonal antibodies according to structure. (*A*) Naked monoclonal antibodies. (*B*) Antibody–drug conjugates can carry drug, radiation, or toxin to increase action. (*C*) Bispecific antibodies can link different target cells together.

[90]Y-epratuzumab as either monotherapy or associated with chemo or other anti-CD20 MoAbs showed median progression-free survival (PFS) ranging from 9.5 to 19 months.[30,31] Although these results seem unimpressive, it is crucial to consider the highly priorly heavily treated subtype of the population.

Targeting CD37
CD37 is a protein expressed in B-cell lymphomas that mediates tumor survival signaling. In 1989, the therapeutic potential of ^{131}I-anti-CD37 was evaluated in 10 patients with refractory NHL, and although 4 patients attained CR (lasting 4–8 months), myelosuppression occurred 3 to 5 weeks after treatment in all 10 patients.[32] However, radioimmunotherapy with ^{177}Lu-lilotomab satetraxetan (anti-CD37) was conducted in 2018 and showed in 15 patients with relapsed CD37-positive indolent NHL that tumor dose is comparable to other radioimmunotherapy compounds.[33]

Targeting CD45
CD45 is a membrane glycoprotein expressed in most hematopoietic cells. The first phase I trial using radioimmunotherapy with ^{131}I-anti-CD45 studies for high-risk patients with refractory/resistant lymphoma began in 2019. A phase I trial of 16 patients

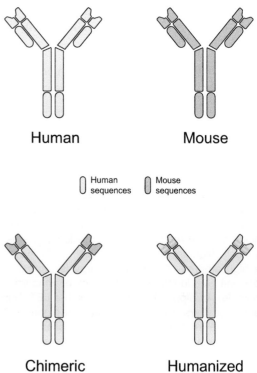

Fig. 2. Monoclonal antibodies according to immunogenic origin: animal, chimeric, humanized, or fully human.

Table 2
Characteristics of monoclonal antibodies according to structure and origin

Structure	Property
Naked monoclonal antibodies	It may have many structures according to the types and number of connecting chains. The most common is the Y shape
Antibody–drug conjugates	Can carry drugs, radiation, or toxins to increase action. Usually connected in a portion and applied in radioimmunotherapy
Bispecific antibodies	Structure with 2 regions and 2 different antibodies combined. It may link different target cells together

Immunogenic Origin	Nomenclature	Method of Obtainment
Animal	-omab	Extracted by hyperimmunized animals and purified or hybridomas (spleen cells with myeloma cells). They are problematic as therapeutic agents because of the immune reactions to the foreign mouse protein
Chimeric	-ximab	Engineering antibodies that replace mouse sequences for human sequences. Reduced immunogenicity
Humanized	-zumab	Only the complementarity determining regions of the variable (V) regions are of mouse-sequence origin
Fully human	-umab	Current state-of-the-art with fully human amino acid sequences carries a lower risk of inducing immune responses

followed by stem cell transplantation (SCT) demonstrated that nonhematologic toxicity was infrequent and CR occurred in 57% of patients.[34] In 2021, the combination of ^{90}Y-anti-CD45 with carmustine, etoposide, cytarabine, and melphalan (BEAM) and SCT in 21 patients demonstrated a median estimated 5 year OS of 68%, nonhematologic toxicities, and engraftment kinetics similar to the standard myeloablative therapies.[35]

Targeting C-X-C chemokine receptor type 4

CXCR4 are specific receptors for the CXCL12, a homeostatic chemokine that induces migration and activation of hematopoietic progenitor cells, thereby playing an essential role in regulating hematopoiesis.[21] The binding of CXCL12 to CXCR4 is involved in the process of tumor growth. CXCR4-targeted RLT with peptides using ^{177}Lu/^{90}Y-PentixaTher has recently evolved as a therapeutic option

Table 3
Characteristics of radionuclides for selection for treatment

	Beta	Alpha	Auger
	Few mm	40–100 μm	<100 ηm
Cross fire effect	+++++	+	—
Uniform radiation dose	+++++	++	—
Homogenous antigen expression	+	++	+++++
Affinity and specificity for the target	+	+++++	+++++
LET	0.2–2 keV/μm	50–230 keV/μm	1–23 keV/μm
RBE	+	+++++	++++
Stability in vivo	++	+++++	+++++
High specific activity	+	+++	+++++
Dependence of hypoxia, dose rate effects, and cell position	+++	—	—
Daughter products with extra emissions	—	+++++	—
Image	+++	+	+
Availability	+++++	++	—

Abbreviations: LET, linear energy transfer; mm, millimeters; RBE, relative biological effectiveness.

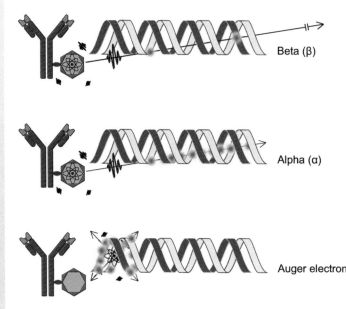

Fig. 3. Number of double strand breaks created due to radiation emission from radionuclides used for treatment increasing sequentially from beta, alpha, and auger emitters.

Beta (β)

Alpha (α)

Auger electrons

for patients with advanced hematological cancers.[36–38] A retrospective study in 690 patients with solid and hematological malignancies demonstrated that ^{68}Ga-pentixafor presented high lesion uptake (thus high CXCR4 expression), especially for marginal zone lymphoma.[39] The high tumor uptake of ^{68}Ga-pentixafor suggests the possibility of delivering high radiation doses with ^{177}Lu/^{90}Y-PentixaTher, a theranostic concept. Theranostic radioimmunotherapy is a promising field under investigation (**Fig. 6**A–C).

RADIOIMMUNOTHERAPY APPLICATIONS
Radioimmunotherapy in Relapsed/Refractory B-cell Non-Hodgkin Lymphoma in General

The benefit and rational use of radiolabeled MoAbs are summarized in **Table 4**.

Nonmyeloablative monotherapy

Knox and colleagues[40] pioneered applying ^{90}Y-ibritumomab in patients with relapsed/refractory B-cell NHL. Bone marrow reserve was the primary dependent factor of toxicity, and therefore, patients with baseline platelet counts less than 149,000/μL had a dose reduction from 0.4 to 0.3 mCi/kg.[41] Although OS was not determined, the ORR was 72%, and the complete response rate (CRR) was 33%.[40,41] Kaminski and colleagues[42] in 2000 demonstrated a similar CRR (34%) with OS of 42%, treating patients with relapsed/refractory B-cell NHL with ^{131}I-tositumumab (Bexxar). Turner and colleagues[43] treated patients with ^{131}I-rituximab and found CRR of 54%, ORR of 71%, and OS of 66% and reported toxicities with reversible hematologic myelosuppression in 4% of patients and hypothyroidism in 7% of patients.

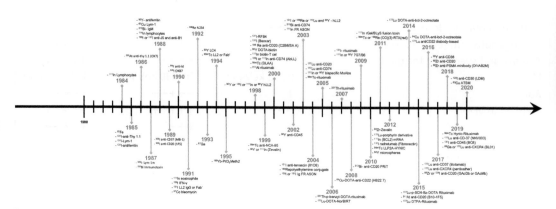

Fig. 4. Historical timeline of exploited targets for radioligand therapy for lymphoma represented by molecules that have been radiolabeled during years.

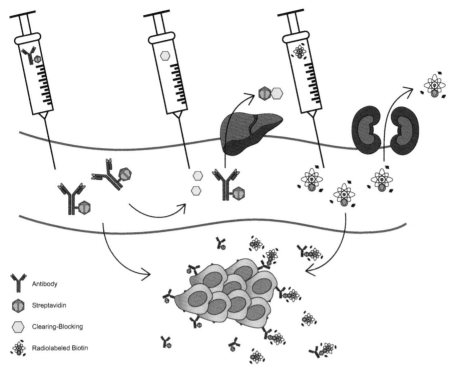

Fig. 5. Pretargeting radioimmunotherapy schematic representation of the "2 step" procedure. Antitumor immunoglobulin G (IgG)–streptavidin conjugate is given intravenously to localize to the tumor. One to 2 days after, a clearing agent is used to quickly remove the conjugate from the blood. Finally, a third injection with radiolabeled biotin is injected. The complex conjugates with high affinity to IgG–streptavidin in the tumor increasing the tumor-to-background ratio.

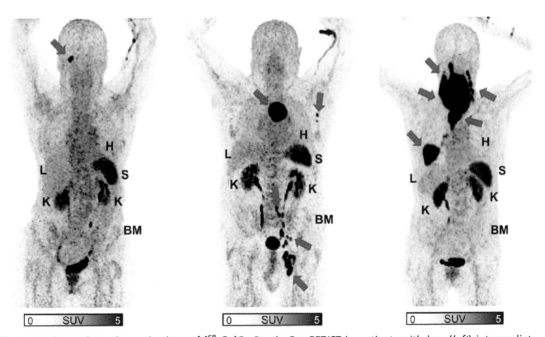

Fig. 6. Maximum intensity projections of [^{68}Ga]Ga-PentixaFor PET/CT in patients with low (*left*) intermediate (*middle*) and high (*right*) marginal lymphoma load. Red arrows indicate lymphoma manifestations.

Table 4
Radioimmunotherapy trials conducted with labeled B-cell-specific anti-CD20 monoclonal antibodies in relapse/refractory non-Hodgkin B-cell lymphoma subtypes

		Antibody	References	Design	N	Treatment	OS	PFS	ORR	CRR
Non-myeloablative	Monotherapy Relapse/refractory	90Y-ibritumomabomab	Knox et al,[40] 1996	Phase II	18	13.5–50 mCi	—	7 mo	72%	33%
		131I-tositumomab	Kaminski et al,[42] 2000	Phase I/II	59	75 cGy and 45 cGy (prior ASCT)	42%[a]	12 mo	71%	34%
		131I-rituximab	Turner et al,[43] 2003	Phase II	42	75 cGy (45–116 mCi)	66%[b]	14 mo	71%	54%
		90Y-ibritumomab	Gordon et al,[87] 2004	Phase I/II	51	0.2–0.4 mCi/kg	—	9.3 mo	73%	51%
	Combined Chemotherapy	131I-tositumomab	Press et al,[44] 2000	Phase I/II	52	20 Gy to 27 Gy + E + CTX	83%[b]	68%[b]	87%	77%
	Conditioning prior SCT relapse/refractory	90Y-ibritumomab	Shimoni et al,[45] 2007	Prospective	23	0.4 mCi/kg + HD-BEAM	67%[b]	52%[b]	95%	52%
		90Y-ibritumomab	Krishnan et al,[46] 2007	Phase II	41	0.4 mCi/kg + HD BEAM	89%[b]	69.8%[b]	65%	—
		90Y-ibritumomab	Winter et al,[47] 2009	Phase I	44	1–17 Gy + HD-BEAM	60%[a]	43%[c]	58%	37%
		131I-tositumomab	Chow et al,[48] 2020	Phase II	107	25 Gy + E + CTX	61%/71%/48% (Ag/In/MC)[e]	62%/64%/43% (Ag/In/MC)[e]	88%	82%
		90Y-ibritumomab	Mei et al,[49] 2023	Phase II	41	0.4 mCi/kg + F + M	63%[b]	61%[b]	51%	39%
	Other	90Y-ibritumomab	Othman et al,[88] 2023	Phase II	18	0.4 mCi/kg + ATG 1.5 mg/kg/d	66.7%[d]	—	100%	70.6%

		Study	Phase	n	Regimen				
Myeloablative	131I-tositumomab	Liu et al,[50] 1998	Phase II	29	280–785 mCi	68%[d]	42%[d]	86%	79%
Mono therapy	131I-tositumomab	Gopal et al,[51] 2007	Phase II	24	525 mCi	59%[c]	51%[c]	67%	54%
Combined Chemotherapy	131I-tositumomab	Gopal et al,[52] 2014	Phase I	36	471 mCi + F	54%[c]	53%[c]	85%	79%
Conditioning prior SCT relapse/refractory	131I-rituximab	Hohloch et al,[53] 2011	Phase II	9	243 mCi + Dexa-BEAM + HD-BEAM	67%[d]	64%[d]	88%	77%
	90Y-ibritumomab	Nademanee et al,[54] 2005	Phase I/II	31	71.6 mCi + HD-E + CTX	92%[b]	78%[b]	54%	—
	90Y-ibritumomab	Devizzi et al,[55] 2008	Phase II	30	0.8–1.2 mCi/kg + anthracycline or platinum + CTX + A	87%[c]	69%[c]	90%	83%
	90Y-ibritumomab	Bethge et al,[56] 2012	Phase II	20	0.6–0.8 mCi/kg + F + M + alemtuzumab	20%[c]	—	95%	20%

Abbreviations: A, cytarabine; AG, aggressive; ATG/TLI, antithymocyte globulin plus total lymphoid irradiation; BEAM, carmustine + etoposide + cytarabine + melphalan; CRR, complete response rate; CTX, cyclophosphamide; Dexa, dexamethasone; E, etoposide; F, fludarabine; HD, high-dose; In, indolent/low grade; MC, Mantle cell lymphoma; ORR, overall response rate; OS, overall survival; PFS, progression-free survival; R, rituximab; SCT, stem cell transplantation.

[a] 60 mo follow-up.
[b] 24 mo follow-up.
[c] 30 to 37.5 mo follow-up.
[d] 42 to 48 mo follow-up.
[e] 121 mo follow-up.

Table 5
Radioimmunotherapy monotherapy trials with labeled B-cell-specific anti-CD20 monoclonal antibodies in low-grade B-cell non-Hodgkin lymphoma subtypes

			Antibody	References	Design	N	ORR	CR	OS	PFS or TTP
Nonmyeloablative	Monotherapy	Untreated	^{131}I-tositumomab	Kaminski et al,[57] 2005	Phase II	76 (FL)	95%	75%	89% (5 y)	PFS: 59% (5 y)
			^{131}I-rituximab	Kesavan et al,[89] 2022	Phase II	68	98.5%	82.3%	NR (9.5 y)	—
			^{90}Y-ibritumomab	Illidge et al,[58] 2014	Phase II	74 (FL)	94.4%	58.3%	95% (3 y)	PFS: 58% (3 y) 40.2 mo
			^{90}Y-ibritumomab	Ibatici et al,[59] 2014	Prospective	50 (FL)	94%	86%	90% (3 y)	PFS: 63.4% (3 y)
			^{90}Y-ibritumomab	Rieger et al,[90] 2022	Phase II	59 (FL)	46.4%	40.4%	NR (9.6 y)	PFS:38.3% (8y)
			^{90}Y-ibritumomab	Samaniego et al,[60] 2014	Prospective	31	100%	97%	97% (4.6 y)	PFS: NR (4.6 y)
			^{90}Y-ibritumomab	Alhaj et al,[91] 2022	Retrospective	51	100%	94%	NR (5.3 y)	PFS: NR (5.3 y)
		Relapse or resistant	^{131}I-tositumomab	Vose et al,[61] 2000	Phase I/II	45	57%	32%	36 mo	9.9 mo
			^{131}I-tositumomab vs cold rituximab	Davis et al,[67] 2004	Phase II randomized	78	55% vs 19% (P = .002)	33% vs 8% (P = .012)	—	TTP: 6.3 vs 5.5 mo (P = .035)
			^{131}I-tositumomab	Buchegger et al,[62] 2006	Phase II	16	81%	50%	NR	PFS: 22.5 mo
			^{131}I-rituximab	Leahy et al,[63] 2006	Phase II	91	76%	53%	59% (4 y)	PFS: 13 mo
			^{131}I-rituximab	Illidge et al.[64] 2009	Phase I/II	16	94%	50%	—	TTP: 20 mo
			^{90}Y-ibritumomab	Witzig et al,[65] 1999	Phase I/II	51	67%	26%	—	TTP: 12.9 mo
			^{90}Y-ibritumomab	Schilder et al,[66] 2004	Phase I/II	30	83%	47%	NR	TTP: 9.4 mo
			^{90}Y-ibritumomab vs Cold rituximab	Gordon et al,[68] 2004	Phase III randomized	143	80% vs 56% (P = .002)	34% vs 20% (P = .04)	—	TTP: 15 vs 10.2 mo (P = .07)
			^{90}Y-ibritumomab	Choi et al,[92] 2023	Retrospective	347	88.6%	66%	NR (4.1 y)	PFS: 36 mo (4.1 y)

Abbreviations: CRR, complete response rate; FL, follicular; mo, months; N/A, not applicable/available; NR, not reached; ORR, overall response rate; OS, overall survival; PFS, progression-free survival; TTP, time-to-progression; y, years.

Table 6
Radioimmunotherapy combined therapy trials with labeled B-cell-specific anti-CD20 monoclonal antibodies in low-grade B-cell non-Hodgkin lymphoma subtypes

	Antibody	References	Design	N	Treatment	ORR	CRR	OS	PFS
Nonmyeloablative combined									
Untreated consolidation	131I-tositumomab	Press et al,[74] 2003	Phase II	77 FL	CHOP	90%	67%	97% (2 y)	81% (2 y)
	90Y-ibritumomab	Zinzani et al,[69] 2008	Phase II	20	F + mitoxantrone	100%	100%	100% (3 y)	89.5% (3 y)
	90Y-ibritumomab	Karmali et al,[70] 2011	Phase II	19	F + mitoxantrone + R	100%	70%	NR	47.2 mo
	90Y-ibritumomab	Zinzani et al,[71] 2008	Phase II	57 FL	F + mitoxantrone	98%	96.5%	100% (3 y)	76% (3 y)
	90Y-ibritumomab	Hainsworth et al,[72]	Phase II	39 FL	R-CHOP	98%	72%	6%	64%
	90Y-ibritumomab	López et al,[73] 2022	Phase II randomized	146 FL	Zevalin + R-CHOP vs R-CHOP + R maintenance	75% vs 90% (P = N/A)	66% vs 81% (P = .06)	58% vs 84.5% (10y) (P > .1)	50% vs 56% (10 y) (P > .1)
	90Y-ibritumomab	Morschhauser et al,[76] 2008	Phase III randomized	411 FL	Zevalin vs no treatment	100% vs 100%	77% vs 17.5% (P < .001)	—	36.5 vs 13.3 (P < .001)
Relapse or resistant	90Y-ibritumomab	Beaven et al,[93] 2012	Phase I	12	Bortezomib	50%	42%	NR	6.4 mo
	131I-tositumomab	Elstrom et al,[94] 2015	Phase I	25	Bortezomib	64%	44%	—	7 mo

Abbreviations: CHOP, cyclophosphamide + doxorubicin + vincristine + prednisolone; CRR, complete response rate; F, fludarabine; FL, follicular; mo, months; N/A, not applicable/available; ORR, overall response rate; OS, overall survival; PFS, progression-free survival; R, rituximab; y, years.

Nonmyeloablative combined therapy

The first phase I/II trial[44] that safely combined etoposide (E), cyclophosphamide (C), and ^{131}I-tositumumab (Bexxar) in 52 patients demonstrated similar ORR to a phase II trial[45] that treated 107 patients (88% vs 87%, respectively). In both trials, after a follow-up of 2 and 10.1 years, the median OS was 83% and 61%, respectively, with similar toxicities. Trials treating patients with ^{90}Y-ibritumomab (Zevalin) followed by high-dose BEAM plus SCT demonstrated an estimated 2 year OS ranging from 67% to 89%. All studies demonstrated toxicity and tolerability profiles similar to high-dose BEAM alone.[45–48] A recent phase II trial also confirmed that ^{90}Y-ibritumomab (Zevalin) associated with chemotherapy (fludarabine and melphalan) is safe.[49]

Myeloablative monotherapy

The monotherapy strategy in this group was designed as a precondition to perform SCT in patients with relapsed/resistant B-cell NHL. In 1998, Liu and colleagues[50] applied myeloablative doses of ^{131}I-tositumumab (Bexxar) (280–785 mCi) before SCT. Myeloablation with engraftment occurred between 9 and 15 days for all patients; no treatment-related deaths were found, and treatment was well tolerated.[50,51] Gopal and colleagues[51] treated 24 patients with the same protocol established by Liu and colleagues and found similar OS and PFS (59% vs 68% and 51% vs 42%, respectively).

Myeloablative combined therapy

The combined therapy strategy in this group was also designed as a precondition to perform SCT in patients with relapsed/resistant B-cell NHL. Trials combining myeloablative doses of ^{131}I-tositumumab (Bexxar), ^{131}I-rituximab, and ^{90}Y-ibritumomab (Zevalin) to several chemotherapy schemes found ORR ranging from 54% to 95% and CRR from 20% to 83%.[52–56] The OS ranged from 22 to 50.4 months, and the population that benefitted most were patients with low-grade NHL. The most

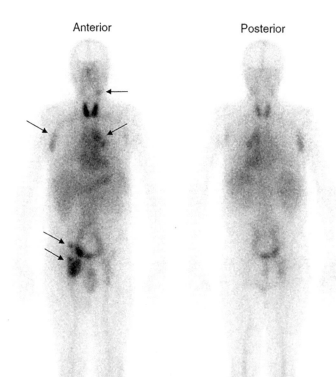

Anterior　　　　　　Posterior

R　　　　　　　L　　　　　　　R

Fig. 7. Anterior and posterior whole-body scans of patient with relapsed or refractory indolent NHL 6 days after injection of therapeutic ^{131}I-tositumomab. Antibody uptake is clearly visualized (*arrows*) in the left jugular, right axillar, left (*L*) mediastinal, right (*R*) iliac, and right inguinal adenopathies. Thyroid uptake was significant despite thyroid blockade. (*From* Buchegger F, Antonescu C, Delaloye AB, Helg C, Kovacsovics T, Kosinski M, Mach JP, Ketterer N. Long-term complete responses after 131I-tositumomab therapy for relapsed or refractory indolent non-Hodgkin's lymphoma. Br J Cancer. 2006 Jun 19;94(12):1770-6. https://doi.org/10.1038/sj.bjc.6603166. Epub 2006 May 9. PMID: 16685263; PMCID: PMC2361356.)

toxic regime with high mortality rates (11%) was associated with BEAM.[52,53]

Radioimmunotherapy in Low-Grade/Indolent B-Cell Non-Hodgkin Lymphoma

The initial trials described earlier paved the way for radioimmunotherapy in patients with low-grade/indolent B-cell NHL because the response rates in the subgroup of patients in those trials were higher. All subsequent trials described in later discussion evaluated nonmyeloablative doses of radioimmunotherapy. These studies are summarized in **Tables 5** and **6**.

Monotherapy in patients with untreated follicular lymphoma

In 2005, Kaminski and colleagues[57] treated advanced follicular lymphomas with ^{131}I-tositumumab (Bexxar) and achieved OS of 89%, CRR of 75%, and ORR of 85%. Trials using ^{90}Y-ibritumomab (Zevalin) found impressive response rates (OS = 90%–95%; ORR = 94%–95%).[58–60] Long-term remissions were found in all studies,

with reports of 70% of patients with CR remaining in remission from 4.3 to 7.7 years.[57] Hematologic toxicity was the most frequent adverse event, but with less than 3% grade III/IV nonhematological adverse.[57–60]

Monotherapy in patients with low-grade relapsed/resistant B-cell non-Hodgkin lymphoma

The scenario described in later discussion is the most explored field of radioimmunotherapy application due to the higher OS benefit compared to other therapeutic regimens. Within this field, some radioimmunotherapy regimens are more effective than others. For example, patients treated with ^{131}I-tositumumab (Bexxar) present ORRs ranging from 55% to 81%,[61,62] while ORR is slightly higher when treated with ^{131}I-rituximab (range:76%–94%),[63,64] and ^{90}Y-ibritumomab (Zevalin; range: 80%–83%).[65,66] The randomized trials in this scenario have also demonstrated radioimmunotherapy significant OS benefits compared to unlabeled rituximab[67,68] (**Fig. 7**, see **Table 5**).

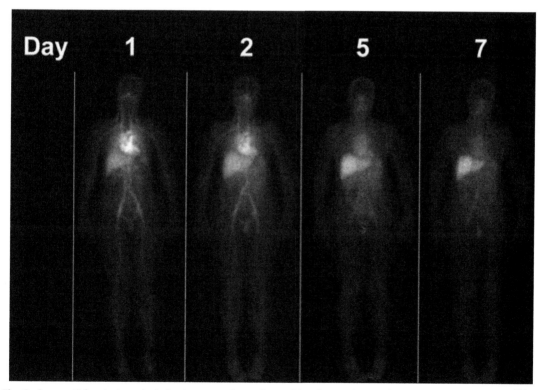

Fig. 8. Sequential anterior whole-body scans of a patient with advanced-stage follicular lymphoma using ^{111}In-ibritumomab tiuxetan for dosimetric purposes demonstrating normal, and no evidence of residual tumor after first-line remission. Patient was then submitted to treatment consolidation with ^{90}Y-ibritumomab tiuxetan. (This research was originally published in JNM. ADelaloye AB, Antonescu C, Louton T, Kuhlmann J, Hagenbeek A. Dosimetry of 90Y-ibritumomab tiuxetan as consolidation of first remission in advanced-stage follicular lymphoma: results from the international phase 3 first-line indolent trial. J Nucl Med. 2009 Nov;50(11):1837-43. https://doi.org/10.2967/jnumed.109.067587. © SNMMI.)

Table 7
Radioimmunotherapy trials with labeled B-cell-specific anti-CD20 monoclonal antibodies in high-grade DLB-Cell non-Hodgkin lymphoma

		Antibody	References	Design	N	Treatment	ORR	CR	OS	PFS or EFS
Nonmyeloablative combined therapy	Untreated/consolidation	90Y-ibritumomab	Zinzani et al,[77] 2008	Phase II	20 DLBCL	CHOP	100%	95%	95% (2 y)	PFS = 75% (2 y)
		90Y-ibritumomab	Stefoni et al,[78] 2016	Phase II	55	R-CHOP	80%	73%	38.9% (7.9 y)	PFS = 43.3% (7.9 y)
		90Y-ibritumomab	Yang et al,[79] 2012	Prospective	21 DLBCL	R-CHOP	80.9%	76%	85% (2.5 y)	PFS = 75% (2.5 y)
	Relapse	90Y-ibritumomab	Morschhauser et al,[80] 2007	Phase II	102 DLBCL	Group Ai = QT refractory Group Aii = QT relapse Group B = QT + R maintenance	Ai = 52% Aii = 53% B = 19%	AI = 24% AII = 39.5% B = 12%	AI = 21.4 mo AII = 22.4 mo B = 4.6 mo	AI = 5.9 mo (PFS) AII = 3.5 mo (PFS) B = 1.6 mo (PFS)
		90Y-ibritumomab	Arnason et al,[81] 2015	Phase II	25 DLBCL	R maintenance	36%	32%	8.1 mo	EFS = 2.5 mo
	Condition for SCT	90Y-ibritumomab	Chahoud et al,[95] 2018	Phase II 3 trials	113 DLBCL	Zevalin+ R-BEAM vs R-BEAM	100% vs 100% (P = 1)	85% vs 76.5% (P = .35)	73% vs 77% (P = .65)	(PFS) 65% vs 62% (P = .82)
	Relapse/refractory	90Y-ibritumomab	Hertzberg et al,[96] 2017	Phase II	143 DLBCL	R-CHOP ± R-ICE + Zevalin+ BEAM (nonresponders) vs R-CHOP + R maintenance (responders)	88% vs 95%	63% vs 95%	73% vs 77% (P = .65)	(PFS) 67% vs 74% (2 y) (P = .32)
		90Y-ibritumomab	Cabrero et al,[97] 2017	Phase II	20 Agg	F + M + thiotepa	72%	39%	44% (4 y)	PFS = 44% (4 y)

Abbreviations: Agg, aggressive; BEAM, carmustine + etoposide + cytarabine + melphalan; CHOP, cyclophosphamide + doxorubicin + vincristine + prednisolone; CRR, complete response rate; Dexa, dexamethasone; DLBCL, diffuse large B-cell lymphoma; EFS, event-free survival; F, fludarabine; mo, months; ORR, overall response rate; OS, overall survival; PFS, progression-free survival; QT, chemotherapy; R, rituximab; R-ICE, rituximab + ifosfamide + carboplatin + etoposide; Z, Zevalin (90Y-ibritumomab).

Combined therapy in patients with untreated low-grade B-cell non-Hodgkin lymphoma

Most studies in this population applied ^{90}Y-ibritumomab (Zevalin) combined with fludarabine and mitoxantrone ± unlabeled rituximab.[69–71] The second schema was the association of cyclophosphamide, vincristine, and prednisone ± doxorubicin and unlabeled rituximab (cyclophosfamide, doxorrubicine, vincristin e and prednisone plus Rituximab [R-CHOP]) in follicular lymphomas.[72–74] The ORRs and OS rates were extremely high for all the above-mentioned regimens (>90% and 96%, respectively).[69–75] A phase III randomized trial in 414 patients with follicular lymphoma treated with consolidation therapy with ^{90}Y-ibritumomab (Zevalin) versus placebo concluded that radioimmunotherapy is highly effective with no unexpected toxicities, prolongs PFS (36.5 vs. 13.3 months, respectively), and results in a higher rate of conversion of partial response to CR[76] (**Fig. 8**, see **Table 6**).

Radioimmunotherapy in High-Grade B-Cell Non-Hodgkin Lymphoma

The application of radioimmunotherapy in this population is restricted to combined treatment since chemotherapy alone has high response rates. The current evidence is related to the application of radioimmunotherapy in a nonmyeloablative scenario in both untreated and relapsed/refractory patients with diffuse large B-cell lymphoma (DLBCL; **Table 7**).

Combined with R-CHOP for untreated diffuse large B-cell lymphoma

Two trials applying ^{90}Y-ibritumomab (Zevalin) in untreated patients with DLBCL established this regimen's feasibility, tolerability, and efficacy with ORRs of 80% and 100% and OS of 95% and 85%. Transient neutropenia was the most frequent (60%) grade III/IV toxicity.[77–79]

Combined with chemotherapy for relapsed/refractory diffuse large B-cell lymphoma

A multicentric study demonstrated that ^{90}Y-ibritumomab (Zevalin) in patients with relapsed/refractory DLBCL after a nonspecified chemotherapy regimen has low ORRs (19%) in patients exposed to prior rituximab and better ORRs (53%) in patients not exposed to prior rituximab.[80,81]

FUTURE DIRECTIONS

Over the past decade, there has been a notable surge in the approval of groundbreaking therapies, specifically bispecific antibodies and chimeric antigen receptor (CAR) T-cell therapy. The latter stimulates the immune system's T cells, empowering

them to recognize and eliminate lymphoma cells, marking a significant advancement in clinical applications.[82] Although these novel treatment approaches present exciting and promising results, there are still challenges to overcome before becoming widely available, such as toxicities related to overactivation of T cells, antigen escape, and optimal positioning and combination with other treatments.[83]

In this continuously evolving scenario, RLT could still play an important role, especially in the challenging situations of heavily pretreated relapsed B-cell and T-cell lymphomas.

CXCR4-directed RLT, in combination with conditioning chemotherapy and allogeneic SCT, has been demonstrated to be a feasible approach in patients with relapsed DLBCL and peripheral T-cell lymphomas.[37,38,84] Radiolabeled bispecific MoAbs and CAR T cells help track antibodies and cell behavior in vivo and present the possibility of also being labeled with isotopes for treatment applications expanding RLT therapy strategies.[85,86]

In the coming years, there is a critical need for intensified efforts in advancing the development of clinical trials to investigate the safety and efficacy of CXCR4 RLT thoroughly. This exploration should encompass both standalone treatments and tandem therapy approaches. For instance, combining CXCR4 RLT with a tailored mixture of selective MoAbs and CAR T cells, specifically designed for individual patients, holds promising potential.

SUMMARY

Since the 1980s, radiolabeled cells have been instrumental in understanding the pathologic dynamics of hemato-oncological diseases. The evolution of this approach traversed the hybridoma technique in the 1990s, leading to numerous preclinical trials involving MoAbs. Subsequent clinical trials, predominantly in the 2000s, extensively explored MoAbs, focusing on anti-CD20 agents labeled with either ^{131}I (Bexxar) or ^{90}Y (Zevalin).

The FDA approved these therapies in 2002 and 2003, marking significant milestones recognizing their safety and enduring therapeutic responses. Despite this journey, there has been a consistent decline in prescriptions. Various factors contribute to this trend, encompassing availability issues, reimbursement challenges, regulatory complexities, the need for trained personnel, and intricate logistics.

Recent preclinical and clinical trials have shifted the spotlight onto novel antibodies, peptides, and further applications of known tracers. This renewed exploration may incentivize new suppliers to redirect their attention, potentially heralding the next wave of theragnostic trends soon.

DISCLOSURE

L.S. Almeida: This study was supported, in part, by the CapesPRInt (Institutional Program for Internationalization) scholarship given to Ludmila Santiago Almeida (reference number: PRINT – 88887.716546/2022-00) by the CAPES (Coordination for the Improvement of Higher Education Personnel) Foundation, within the Brazilian Ministry of Education, Government of Brazil (ludsantiagoalmeida@gmail.com). R.C. Delgado Bolton: rbiolton@gmail.com—Nothing to declare. V.C. Heringer: drv.cabralheringer@gmail.com—Nothing to declare. S. de Souza Medina: souzamedina@gmail.com—Nothing to declare. EE: elba@unicamp.br—CEPID – Cancer-Thera project (FAPESP # 2021/10,265–8) partly supports this study.

REFERENCES

1. Available at: https://seer.cancer.gov/statfacts/html. [Accessed 29 December 2023].
2. Roswarski JL, Longo DL. Hodgkin lymphoma: focus on evolving treatment paradigms. Best Pract Res Clin Haematol 2023;36(4):101510.
3. Available at: https://www.nccn.org/guidelines/guidelines-detail?category=1&id=1480. [Accessed 29 December 2023].
4. Lally KP, Arnstein M, Siegel S, et al. A comparison of staging methods for Hodgkin's disease in children. Arch Surg 1986;121(10):1125–7.
5. Gómez León N, Delgado-Bolton RC, Del Campo Del Val L, et al. Multicenter comparison of contrast-enhanced FDG PET/CT and 64-slice multi-detector-row CT for initial staging and response evaluation at the end of treatment in patients with lymphoma. Clin Nucl Med 2017;42(8):595–602.
6. Alavi JB, Hansell J. Labeled cells in the investigation of hematologic disorders. Semin Nucl Med 1984;14(3):208–25.
7. de Vos S. Historical overview and current state of art in diagnosis and treatment of Hodgkin's and Non-Hodgkin's Lymphoma. Pet Clin 2006;1(3):203–17.
8. King DJ, Ratcliffe MA, Dawson AA, et al. Fertility in young men and women after treatment for lymphoma: a study of a population. J Clin Pathol 1985;38(11):1247–51.
9. Cunningham J, Mauch P, Rosenthal DS, et al. Long-term complications of MOPP chemotherapy in patients with Hodgkin's disease. Cancer Treat Rep 1982;66(4):1015–22.
10. Nelson DF, Cooper S, Weston MG, et al. Second malignant neoplasms in patients treated for Hodgkin's disease with radiotherapy or radiotherapy and chemotherapy. Cancer 1981;48(11):2386–93.
11. Liu JK. The history of monoclonal antibody development - progress, remaining challenges and future innovations. Ann Med Surg (Lond) 2014;3(4):113–6.
12. Houghton A, Scheinberg D. Monoclonal antibodies in the treatment of hematopoietic malignancies. Semin Hematol 1988;25(3 Suppl 3):23–9.
13. Carson KR, Cook DF, Weidner SM. Impact of treatment sequencing on outcomes and costs in relapsed low-grade or follicular B-cell non-Hodgkin lymphoma. 2015 AVAHO Meeting; 2015. Abstract 33.
14. Alhaj Moustafa M, Borah BJ, Moriarty JP, et al. Yttrium-90 ibritumomab is cost-effective compared to bendamustine + rituximab in low-grade lymphomas. Clin Lymphoma, Myeloma & Leukemia 2023;23(4):259–65.
15. Available at: https://www.accessdata.fda.gov/. [Accessed 29 December 2023].
16. Available at: https://www.cancerresearch.org/treatment-types/targeted-antibodies. [Accessed 29 December 2023].
17. Ozaki S. Diabody. In: Schwab M, editor. Encyclopedia of cancer. Berlin, Heidelberg: Springer; 2011.
18. Harding FA, Stickler MM, Razo J, et al. The immunogenicity of humanized and fully human antibodies: residual immunogenicity resides in the CDR regions. mAbs 2010-Jun;2(3):256–65.
19. Bolcaen J, Kleynhans J, Nair S, et al. A perspective on the radiopharmaceutical requirements for imaging and therapy of glioblastoma. Theranostics 2021;11(16):7911–47.
20. Salih S, Alkatheeri A, Alomaim W, et al. Radiopharmaceutical treatments for cancer therapy, radionuclides characteristics, applications, and challenges. Molecules 2022;27(16):5231.
21. Available at: https://www.ncbi.nlm.nih.gov/mesh/. [Accessed 29 December 2023].
22. Dahle J, Bruland OS, Larsen RH. Relative biologic effects of low-dose-rate alpha-emitting 227Th-rituximab and beta-emitting 90Y-tiuexetan-ibritumomab versus external beam X-radiation. Int J Radiat Oncol Biol Phys 2008;72(1):186–92.
23. Aurlien E, Larsen RH, Kvalheim G, et al. Demonstration of highly specific toxicity of the alpha-emitting radioimmunoconjugate(211)At-rituximab against non-Hodgkin's lymphoma cells. Br J Cancer 2000;83(10):1375–9.
24. Park SI, Shenoi J, Pagel JM, et al. Conventional and pretargeted radioimmunotherapy using bismuth-213 to target and treat non-Hodgkin lymphomas expressing CD20: a preclinical model toward optimal consolidation therapy to eradicate minimal residual disease. Blood 2010;116(20):4231–9.
25. Thakral P, Singla S, Yadav MP, et al. An approach for conjugation of (177) Lu- DOTA-SCN- Rituximab (BioSim) & its evaluation for radioimmunotherapy of

relapsed & refractory B-cell non Hodgkins lymphoma patients. Indian J Med Res 2014;139(4):544–54.

26. Sharkey RM, Karacay H, Cardillo TM, et al. Improving the delivery of radionuclides for imaging and therapy of cancer using pretargeting methods. Clin Cancer Res 2005;11(19 Pt 2):7109s–21s.

27. Juweid ME, Stadtmauer E, Hajjar G, et al. Pharmacokinetics, dosimetry, and initial therapeutic results with 131I- and (111)In-/90Y-labeled humanized LL2 anti-CD22 monoclonal antibody in patients with relapsed, refractory non-Hodgkin's lymphoma. Clin Cancer Res 1999;5(10 Suppl):3292s–303s.

28. Behr TM, Wörmann B, Gramatzki M, et al. Low- versus high-dose radioimmunotherapy with humanized anti-CD22 or chimeric anti-CD20 antibodies in a broad spectrum of B cell-associated malignancies. Clin Cancer Res 1999;5(10 Suppl):3304s–14s.

29. Lindén O, Hindorf C, Cavallin-Ståhl E, et al. Dose-fractionated radioimmunotherapy in non-Hodgkin's lymphoma using DOTA-conjugated, 90Y-radiolabeled, humanized anti-CD22 monoclonal antibody, epratuzumab. Clin Cancer Res 2005;11(14):5215–22.

30. Morschhauser F, Kraeber-Bodéré F, Wegener WA, et al. High rates of durable responses with anti-CD22 fractionated radioimmunotherapy: results of a multicenter, phase I/II study in non-Hodgkin's lymphoma. J Clin Oncol 2010;28(23):3709–16.

31. Kraeber-Bodere F, Pallardy A, Maisonneuve H, et al. Consolidation anti-CD22 fractionated radioimmunotherapy with 90Y-epratuzumab tetraxetan following R-CHOP in elderly patients with diffuse large B-cell lymphoma: a prospective, single group, phase 2 trial. Lancet Haematol 2017;4(1):e35–45.

32. Press OW, Eary JF, Badger CC, et al. Treatment of refractory non-Hodgkin's lymphoma with radiolabeled MB-1 (anti-CD37) antibody. J Clin Oncol 1989;7(8):1027–38.

33. Blakkisrud J, Holtedahl JE, Løndalen A, et al. Biodistribution and dosimetry results from a phase 1 trial of therapy with the antibody-radionuclide conjugate 177Lu-lilotomab satetraxetan. J Nucl Med 2018;59(4):704–10.

34. Cassaday RD, Press OW, Pagel JM, et al. Phase I study of a CD45-targeted antibody-radionuclide conjugate for high-risk lymphoma. Clin Cancer Res 2019;25(23):6932–8.

35. Tuazon SA, Cassaday RD, Gooley TA, et al. Yttrium-90 anti-CD45 immunotherapy followed by autologous hematopoietic cell transplantation for relapsed or refractory lymphoma. Transplant Cell Ther 2021;27(1):57.e1–8.

36. Schottelius M, Osl T, Poschenrieder A, et al. [177Lu] pentixather: comprehensive preclinical characterization of a first CXCR4-directed endoradiotherapeutic agent. Theranostics 2017;7(9):2350–62.

37. Lapa C, Hänscheid H, Kircher M, et al. Feasibility of CXCR4-directed radioligand therapy in advanced diffuse large B-cell lymphoma. J Nucl Med 2019; 60(1):60–4.

38. Buck AK, Grigoleit GU, Kraus S, et al. C-X-C motif chemokine receptor 4-targeted radioligand therapy in patients with advanced T-cell lymphoma. J Nucl Med 2023;64(1):34–9. Epub 2022 Jun 23. PMID: 35738903; PMCID: PMC9841250.

39. Buck AK, Haug A, Dreher N, et al. Imaging of C-X-C motif chemokine receptor 4 expression in 690 patients with solid or hematologic neoplasms using 68Ga-pentixafor PET. J Nucl Med 2022;63(11): 1687–92. Epub 2022 Mar 3. PMID: 35241482.

40. Knox SJ, Goris ML, Trisler K, et al. Yttrium-90-labeled anti-CD20 monoclonal antibody therapy of recurrent B-cell lymphoma. Clin Cancer Res 1996; 2(3):457–70. PMID: 9816191.

41. Wiseman GA, White CA, Stabin M, et al. Phase I/II 90Y-Zevalin (yttrium-90 Ibritumomab , IDEC-Y2B8) radioimmunotherapy dosimetry results in relapsed or refractory non-Hodgkin's lymphoma. Eur J Nucl Med 2000;27(7):766–77. PMID: 10952488.

42. Kaminski MS, Estes J, Zasadny KR, et al. Radioimmunotherapy with iodine (131)I tositumomab for relapsed or refractory B-cell non-Hodgkin lymphoma: updated results and long-term follow-up of the University of Michigan experience. Blood 2000; 96(4):1259–66. PMID: 10942366.

43. Turner JH, Martindale AA, Boucek J, et al. 131I-Anti CD20 radioimmunotherapy of relapsed or refractory non-Hodgkins lymphoma: a phase II clinical trial of a nonmyeloablative dose regimen of chimeric rituximab radiolabeled in a hospital. Cancer Biother Radiopharm 2003;18(4):513–24. PMID: 14503945.

44. Press OW, Eary JF, Gooley T, et al. A phase I/II trial of iodine-131-tositumomab (anti-CD20), etoposide, cyclophosphamide, and autologous stem cell transplantation for relapsed B-cell lymphomas. Blood 2000;96(9):2934–42. PMID: 11049969.

45. Shimoni A, Zwas ST, Oksman Y, et al. Yttrium-90-ibritumomab tiuxetan (Zevalin) combined with high-dose BEAM chemotherapy and autologous stem cell transplantation for chemo-refractory aggressive non-Hodgkin's lymphoma. Exp Hematol 2007;35(4): 534–40. PMID: 17379063.

46. Krishnan A, Nademanee A, Fung HC, et al. Phase II trial of a transplantation regimen of yttrium-90 ibritumomab tiuxetan and high-dose chemotherapy in patients with non-Hodgkin's lymphoma. J Clin Oncol 2008;26(1):90–5. Epub 2007 Nov 19. PMID: 18025438.

47. Winter JN, Inwards DJ, Spies S, et al. Yttrium-90 ibritumomab tiuxetan doses calculated to deliver up to 15 Gy to critical organs may be safely combined with high-dose BEAM and autologous transplantation in relapsed or refractory B-cell non-Hodgkin's lymphoma. J Clin Oncol 2009;27(10):1653–9. Epub 2009 Mar 2. PMID: 19255322; PMCID: PMC2668971.

48. Chow VA, Rajendran JG, Fisher DR, et al. A phase II trial evaluating the efficacy of high-dose Radioiodinated Tositumomab (Anti-CD20) antibody, etoposide and cyclophosphamide followed by autologous transplantation, for high-risk relapsed or refractory non-hodgkin lymphoma. Am J Hematol 2020;95(7): 775–83. Epub 2020 Apr 22. PMID: 32243637.

49. Mei M, Palmer J, Tsai NN, et al. Results of a phase II trial of allogeneic hematopoietic stem cell transplantation using 90Y-ibritumomab (Zevalin) in combination with fludarabine and melphalan in patients with high-risk B-cell non-Hodgkin's lymphoma. Clin Lymphoma, Myeloma & Leukemia 2023;23(9): e268–76. Epub 2023 May 23. PMID: 37301631; PMCID: PMC10524945.

50. Liu SY, Eary JF, Petersdorf SH, et al. Follow-up of relapsed B-cell lymphoma patients treated with iodine-131-labeled anti-CD20 antibody and autologous stem-cell rescue. J Clin Oncol 1998;16(10): 3270–8. PMID: 9779701.

51. Gopal AK, Rajendran JG, Gooley TA, et al. High-dose [131I]tositumomab (anti-CD20) radioimmunotherapy and autologous hematopoietic stem-cell transplantation for adults > or = 60 years old with relapsed or refractory B-cell lymphoma. J Clin Oncol 2007;25(11):1396–402. Epub 2007 Feb 20. PMID: 17312330.

52. Gopal AK, Gooley TA, Rajendran JG, et al. Myeloablative I-131-tositumomab with escalating doses of fludarabine and autologous hematopoietic transplantation for adults age ≥ 60 years with B cell lymphoma. Biol Blood Marrow Transplant 2014;20(6): 770–5. Epub 2014 Feb 12. PMID: 24530971; PMCID: PMC4019701.

53. Hohloch K, Sahlmann CO, Lakhani VJ, et al. Tandem high-dose therapy in relapsed and refractory B-cell lymphoma: results of a prospective phase II trial of myeloablative chemotherapy, followed by escalated radioimmunotherapy with (131)I-anti-CD20 antibody and stem cell rescue. Ann Hematol 2011;90(11): 1307–15. Epub 2011 Mar 1. PMID: 21360108.

54. Nademanee A, Forman S, Molina A, et al. A phase 1/2 trial of high-dose yttrium-90-ibritumomab tiuxetan in combination with high-dose etoposide and cyclophosphamide followed by autologous stem cell transplantation in patients with poor-risk or relapsed non-Hodgkin lymphoma. Blood 2005;106(8): 2896–902. Epub 2005 Jul 7. PMID: 16002426; PMCID: PMC1895300.

55. Devizzi L, Guidetti A, Tarella C, et al. High-dose yttrium-90-ibritumomab tiuxetan with tandem stem-cell reinfusion: an outpatient preparative regimen for autologous hematopoietic cell transplantation. J Clin Oncol 2008;26(32):5175–82. Epub 2008 Oct 14. PMID: 18854569.

56. Bethge WA, von Harsdorf S, Bornhauser M, et al. Dose-escalated radioimmunotherapy as part of reduced intensity conditioning for allogeneic transplantation in patients with advanced high-grade non-Hodgkin lymphoma. Bone Marrow Transplant 2012;47(11):1397–402. Epub 2012 Apr 16. PMID: 22504934.

57. Kaminski MS, Tuck M, Estes J, et al. 131I-tositumomab therapy as initial treatment for follicular lymphoma. N Engl J Med 2005;352(5):441–9. PMID: 15689582.

58. Illidge TM, Mayes S, Pettengell R, et al. Fractionated 90Y-ibritumomab tiuxetan radioimmunotherapy as an initial therapy of follicular lymphoma: an international phase II study in patients requiring treatment according to GELF/BNLI criteria. J Clin Oncol 2014; 32(3):212–8. Epub 2013 Dec 2. PMID: 24297953.

59. Ibatici A, Pica GM, Nati S, et al. Safety and efficacy of (90) yttrium-ibritumomab-tiuxetan for untreated follicular lymphoma patients. An Italian cooperative study. Br J Haematol 2014;164(5):710–6. Epub 2013 Dec 17. PMID: 24344981.

60. Samaniego F, Berkova Z, Romaguera JE, et al. 90Y-ibritumomab tiuxetan radiotherapy as first-line therapy for early stage low-grade B-cell lymphomas, including bulky disease. Br J Haematol 2014; 167(2):207–13. Epub 2014 Jul 8. PMID: 25040450.

61. Vose JM, Wahl RL, Saleh M, et al. Multicenter phase II study of iodine-131 tositumomab for chemotherapy-relapsed/refractory low-grade and transformed low-grade B-cell non-Hodgkin's lymphomas. J Clin Oncol 2000;18(6):1316–23. PMID: 10715303.

62. Buchegger F, Antonescu C, Delaloye AB, et al. Long-term complete responses after 131I-tositumomab therapy for relapsed or refractory indolent non-Hodgkin's lymphoma. Br J Cancer 2006;94(12):1770–6. Epub 2006 May 9. PMID: 16685263; PMCID: PMC2361356.

63. Leahy MF, Seymour JF, Hicks RJ, et al. Multicenter phase II clinical study of iodine-131-rituximab radioimmunotherapy in relapsed or refractory indolent non-Hodgkin's lymphoma. J Clin Oncol 2006;24(27): 4418–25. Epub 2006 Aug 28. PMID: 16940276.

64. Illidge TM, Bayne M, Brown NS, et al. Phase 1/2 study of fractionated (131)I-rituximab in low-grade B-cell lymphoma: the effect of prior rituximab dosing and tumor burden on subsequent radioimmunotherapy. Blood 2009;113(7):1412–21. Epub 2008 Dec 12. PMID: 19074729.

65. Witzig TE, White CA, Wiseman GA, et al. Phase I/II trial of IDEC-Y2B8 radioimmunotherapy for treatment of relapsed or refractory CD20(+) B-cell non-Hodgkin's lymphoma. J Clin Oncol 1999;17(12): 3793–803. PMID: 10577851.

66. Schilder R, Molina A, Bartlett N, et al. Follow-up results of a phase II study of ibritumomab tiuxetan radioimmunotherapy in patients with relapsed or refractory low-grade, follicular, or transformed B-cell non-Hodgkin's lymphoma and mild thrombocytopenia. Cancer

Biother Radiopharm 2004;19(4):478–81. PMID: 15453962.

67. Davis TA, Kaminski MS, Leonard JP, et al. The radio-isotope contributes significantly to the activity of radioimmunotherapy. Clin Cancer Res 2004;10(23): 7792–8. PMID: 15585610.

68. Gordon LI, Witzig T, Molina A, et al. Yttrium 90-labeled ibritumomab tiuxetan radioimmunotherapy produces high response rates and durable remissions in patients with previously treated B-cell lymphoma. Clin Lymphoma 2004;5(2):98–101. PMID: 15453924.

69. Zinzani PL, Tani M, Fanti S, et al. A phase 2 trial of fludarabine and mitoxantrone chemotherapy followed by yttrium-90 Ibritumomab for patients with previously untreated, indolent, nonfollicular, non-Hodgkin lymphoma. Cancer 2008;112(4):856–62. PMID: 18189293.

70. Karmali R, Kassar M, Venugopal P, et al. Safety and efficacy of combination therapy with fludarabine, mitoxantrone, and rituximab followed by yttrium-90 Ibritumomab and maintenance rituximab as frontline therapy for patients with follicular or marginal zone lymphoma. Clin Lymphoma, Myeloma & Leukemia 2011;11(6):467–74. Epub 2011 Jun 22. PMID: 21700527.

71. Zinzani PL, Tani M, Pulsoni A, et al. Fludarabine and mitoxantrone followed by yttrium-90 Ibritumomab in previously untreated patients with follicular non-Hodgkin lymphoma trial: a phase II non-randomised trial (FLUMIZ). Lancet Oncol 2008;9(4):352–8. Epub 2008 Mar 14. PMID: 18342572.

72. Hainsworth JD, Spigel DR, Markus TM, et al. Rituximab plus short-duration chemotherapy followed by Yttrium-90 Ibritumomab tiuxetan as first-line treatment for patients with follicular non-Hodgkin lymphoma: a phase II trial of the Sarah Cannon Oncology Research Consortium. Clin Lymphoma Myeloma 2009;9(3): 223–8. PMID: 19525191.

73. López-Guillermo A, Canales MÁ, Dlouhy I, et al, PETHEMA/GELTAMO/GELCAB Spanish Intergroup. A randomized phase II study comparing consolidation with a single dose of ^{90}Y ibritumomab tiuxetan vs. maintenance with rituximab for two years in patients with newly diagnosed follicular lymphoma responding to R-CHOP. Long-term follow-up results. Leuk Lymphoma 2022;63(1):93–100. Epub 2021 Aug 30. PMID: 34459702.

74. Press OW, Unger JM, Braziel RM, et al. A phase 2 trial of CHOP chemotherapy followed by tositumomab/iodine I 131 tositumomab for previously untreated follicular non-Hodgkin lymphoma: Southwest Oncology Group Protocol S9911. Blood 2003;102(5):1606–12. Epub 2003 May 8. PMID: 12738671.

75. Delaloye AB, Antonescu C, Louton T, et al. Dosimetry of 90Y-ibritumomab tiuxetan as consolidation of first remission in advanced-stage follicular lymphoma: results from the international phase 3 first-line indolent trial. J Nucl Med 2009;50(11):1837–43. Epub 2009 Oct 16. PMID: 19837764.

76. Morschhauser F, Radford J, Van Hoof A, et al. Phase III trial of consolidation therapy with yttrium-90-ibritumomab tiuxetan compared with no additional therapy after first remission in advanced follicular lymphoma. J Clin Oncol 2008;26(32):5156–64. Epub 2008 Oct 14. PMID: 18854568.

77. Zinzani PL, Tani M, Fanti S, et al. A phase II trial of CHOP chemotherapy followed by yttrium 90 ibritumomab tiuxetan (Zevalin) for previously untreated elderly diffuse large B-cell lymphoma patients. Ann Oncol 2008;19(4):769–73. Epub 2008 Feb 25. PMID: 18303033.

78. Stefoni V, Casadei B, Bottelli C, et al. Short-course R-CHOP followed by (90)Y-Ibritumomab tiuxetan in previously untreated high-risk elderly diffuse large B-cell lymphoma patients: 7-year long-term results. Blood Cancer J 2016;6(5):e425. PMID: 27176801; PMCID: PMC4916298.

79. Yang DH, Kim WS, Kim SJ, et al. Pilot trial of yttrium-90 ibritumomab tiuxetan consolidation following rituximab, cyclophosphamide, doxorubicin, vincristine and prednisolone chemotherapy in patients with limited-stage, bulky diffuse large B-cell lymphoma. Leuk Lymphoma 2012;53(5):807–11. Epub 2011 Dec 7. PMID: 22035417.

80. Morschhauser F, Illidge T, Huglo D, et al. Efficacy and safety of yttrium-90 ibritumomab tiuxetan in patients with relapsed or refractory diffuse large B-cell lymphoma not appropriate for autologous stem-cell transplantation. Blood 2007;110(1):54–8. Epub 2007 Mar 26. PMID: 17387223.

81. Arnason JE, Luptakova K, Rosenblatt J, et al. Yttrium-90 ibritumomab tiuxetan followed by rituximab maintenance as treatment for patients with diffuse large B-cell lymphoma are not candidates for autologous stem cell transplant. Acta Haematol 2015;133(4):347–53. Epub 2015 Feb 7. PMID: 25677780.

82. Sterner RC, Sterner RM. CAR-T cell therapy: current limitations and potential strategies. Blood Cancer J 2021; 11(4):69. PMID: 33824268; PMCID: PMC8024391.

83. Falchi L, Vardhana SA, Salles GA. Bispecific antibodies for the treatment of B-cell lymphoma: promises, unknowns, and opportunities. Blood 2023;141(5): 467–80. PMID: 36322929; PMCID: PMC9936308.

84. Buck AK, Serfling SE, Kraus S, et al. Theranostics in hematooncology. J Nucl Med 2023;64(7):1009–16. Epub 2023 Jun 8. PMID: 37290799; PMCID: PMC10315699.

85. Wang XY, Wang Y, Wu Q, et al. Feasibility study of 68Ga-labeled CAR T cells for in vivo tracking using micro-positron emission tomography imaging. Acta Pharmacol Sin 2021;42(5):824–31. Epub 2020 Sep 8. PMID: 32901086; PMCID: PMC8115074.

86. Sharkey RM, Rossi EA, McBride WJ, et al. Recombinant bispecific monoclonal antibodies prepared by the dock-and-lock strategy for pretargeted radioimmunotherapy. Semin Nucl Med 2010;40(3):190–203. PMID: 20350628; PMCID: PMC2855818.

87. Gordon LI, Molina A, Witzig T, et al. Durable responses after Ibritumomab radioimmunotherapy for CD20+ B-cell lymphoma: long-term follow-up of a phase 1/2 study. Blood 2004;103(12):4429–31. Epub 2004 Mar 11. PMID: 15016644.

88. Othman T, Lowsky R, Richman C, et al. Yttrium-90 ibritumomab tiuxetan plus ATG/TLI for allogeneic hematopoietic cell transplantation in non-Hodgkin lymphoma. Bone Marrow Transplant 2023;58(10):1143–5. Epub 2023 Jun 30. PMID: 37391654.

89. Kesavan M, Zammar G, McQuillan JT, et al. Long-term efficacy and safety of chemotherapy-free first-line iodine-131-rituximab radioimmunotherapy of follicular lymphoma. Br J Haematol 2022;196(1):237–41. Epub 2021 Aug 8. PMID: 34368952.

90. Rieger K, De Filippi R, Lindén O, et al. 90-yttrium-ibritumomab tiuxetan as first-line treatment for follicular lymphoma: updated efficacy and safety results at an extended median follow-up of 9.6 years. Ann Hematol 2022;101(4):781–8. Epub 2022 Feb 12. PMID: 35150296; PMCID: PMC8913448.

91. Alhaj Moustafa M, Peterson J, Hoppe BS, et al. Real world long-term follow-up experience with yttrium-90 ibritumomab tiuxetan in previously untreated patients with low-grade follicular lymphoma and marginal zone lymphoma. Clin Lymphoma, Myeloma & Leukemia 2022;22(8):618–25. Epub 2022 Mar 17. PMID: 35400611.

92. Choi I, Okada M, Ito T. Real-world data from yttrium-90 ibritumomab tiuxetan treatment of relapsed or refractory indolent B-cell non-Hodgkin's lymphoma: J3Zi Study. Ann Hematol 2023;102(5):1149–58. Epub 2023 Mar 30. PMID: 36995403.

93. Beaven AW, Shea TC, Moore DT, et al. A phase I study evaluating ibritumomab tiuxetan (Zevalin®) in combination with bortezomib (Velcade®) in relapsed/refractory mantle cell and low grade B-cell non-Hodgkin lymphoma. Leuk Lymphoma 2012;53(2):254–8. Epub 2011 Sep 19. PMID: 21812533.

94. Elstrom RL, Ruan J, Christos PJ, et al. Phase 1 study of radiosensitization using bortezomib in patients with relapsed non-Hodgkin lymphoma receiving radioimmunotherapy with 131I-tositumomab. Leuk Lymphoma 2015;56(2):342–6. Epub 2014 Jun 17. PMID: 24730538; PMCID: PMC5176012.

95. Chahoud J, Sui D, Erwin WD, et al. Updated results of rituximab pre- and post-BEAM with or without 90Yttrium ibritumomab tiuxetan during autologous transplant for diffuse large B-cell lymphoma. Clin Cancer Res 2018;24(10):2304–11. Epub 2018 Feb 23. PMID: 29476021; PMCID: PMC5955837.

96. Hertzberg M, Gandhi MK, Trotman J, et al, Australasian Leukaemia Lymphoma Group (ALLG). Early treatment intensification with R-ICE and 90Y-ibritumomab tiuxetan (Zevalin)-BEAM stem cell transplantation in patients with high-risk diffuse large B-cell lymphoma patients and positive interim PET after 4 cycles of R-CHOP-14. Haematologica 2017;102(2):356–63. Epub 2016 Nov 10. PMID: 28143954; PMCID: PMC5286943.

97. Cabrero M, Martin A, Briones J, et al. Phase II study of yttrium-90-ibritumomab tiuxetan as part of reduced-intensity conditioning (with melphalan, fludarabine ± thiotepa) for allogeneic transplantation in relapsed or refractory aggressive B cell lymphoma: a GEL-TAMO trial. Biol Blood Marrow Transplant 2017;23(1):53–9. Epub 2016 Oct 19. PMID: 27771496.

Long-Axial Field-of-View PET Imaging in Patients with Lymphoma
Challenges and Opportunities

Clemens Mingels, MD[a,b,*], Hande Nalbant, MD[a], Hasan Sari, PhD[b,c], Felipe Godinez, PhD[a,d], Fatma Sen, MD, MSc[a], Benjamin Spencer, PhD[a], Naseem S. Esteghamat, MD, MS[e], Joseph M. Tuscano, MD[e], Lorenzo Nardo, MD, PhD[a]

KEYWORDS

- Total-body PET/CT • LAFOV PET • Lymphoma • [18F]FDG

KEY POINTS

- Long-axial field-of-view (LAFOV) systems have the potential to improve staging, prognostication, response to therapy assessment and early recurrence detection in the evaluation in patients with lymphoma.
- The current initial literature supports the use of LAFOV to perform (1) high image quality scans with reduced noise level, (2) low-dose imaging reducing patient radiation exposure; and (3) shorter scan durations mitigating or avoiding the need for anesthesia.
- In addition, the literature supports the feasibility of delayed imaging protocols. LAFOV scanners may also provide improved semiquantitative measurements compared to the analogous measurements obtained on short-axial field-of-view (SAFOV) scanners; however, the magnitude of difference and the clinical implication of this difference in measurements are not fully investigated and further studies are warranted.
- The potential to obtain new metrics for lymphoma assessment using LAFOV dynamic PET may be revealed in future research as well as the specific role of LAFOV in the assessment of new lymphoma-specific radio pharmaceutics.

INTRODUCTION

PET/computed tomography (CT) has been established for staging and restaging patients with lymphoma over nearly 2 decades.[1–3] [18F]Fluoro-2-deoxy-D-glucose ([18F]FDG) PET/CT is considered an essential imaging test during the initial workup of lymphoma, especially Hodgkin lymphoma (HL).[4]

Moreover, midtreatment imaging has prognostic value that has implications that optimize subsequent treatment that has now been incorporated in standard of treatment protocols for both early and advanced stage classic HL.[5,6] Of note, National Comprehensive Cancer Network (NCCN) guidelines state that radiation therapy planning is more precise by PET and MR imaging.[6,7] However, [18F]FDG PET/

[a] Department of Radiology, University of California Davis, Sacramento, CA, USA; [b] Department of Nuclear Medicine, Inselspital, Bern University Hospital, University of Bern, Bern, Switzerland; [c] Siemens Healthineers International AG, Zurich, Switzerland; [d] UC Cavis Comprehensive Cancer Center, University of California Davis, Sacramento, CA, USA; [e] Division of Malignant Hematology, Cellular Therapy & Transplantation, Department of Internal Medicine, University of California Davis, Sacramento, CA, USA
* Corresponding author. Department of Radiology, University of California Davis, 3195 Folsom Boulevard, Sacramento, CA 95816.
E-mail address: cmingels@ucdavis.edu

PET Clin 19 (2024) 495–504
https://doi.org/10.1016/j.cpet.2024.05.005
1556-8598/24/Published by Elsevier Inc.

CT's role in surveillance of patients with lymphoma is, according to the current NCCN guidelines, still unclear, and clinical or pathologic correlation is necessary for clinical decision management.[7]

PET technology is in continuous development. From the initial acquisition of PET only images, to the implementation of CT for attenuation correction, to the use of time of flight, and more recently, to the development of long-axial field-of-view (LAFOV) systems.[8,9] These systems are now installed worldwide.[10–17] These next-generation scanners enable (1) the possibility of improving image quality by providing low-noise, high-quality images and increasing lesion conspicuity; (2) imaging with lower injected activities, particularly important in the pediatric population and patients undergoing multiple follow-up studies; (3) imaging with shorter acquisition times, particularly important when trying to reduce anesthesia/sedation time or facilitating scanning patients suffering from claustrophobia or in pain when lying flat; (4) delayed imaging, which may exploit different kinetics between anatomic and pathologic tissue, in addition to allow following physiologic processes within several radiotracers half-lives (5–6 half-lives); and, moreover, (5) simultaneous assessment of lesions in part of the body far apart.

Improvements in image quality and sensitivity have enormous potential to change treatment strategies for lymphoma; however, there are limited data available investigating the effect of LAFOV systems on lymphoma imaging or on clinical implications.[18] This comprehensive literature review aims to evaluate challenges and opportunities of LAFOV PET/CT in assessing patients with lymphoma (**Fig. 1**). Specifically, this review will provide an overview of newly enabled protocols including (1) improved image quality, (2) low injected radiotracer dose PET images, (3) short acquisition times, (4) delayed imaging, and (5) LAFOV dynamic imaging protocols.[15,19] In addition, PET/CT quantitative measurements relevant to lymphoproliferative disease will be reported together with a possible perspective of new radiotracer imaging in patients with lymphoma.

IMPROVED IMAGE QUALITY

The increase in signal collection efficiency coupled together with high spatial resolution results in images of improved quality compared to conventional SAFOV scanners.[10,20] Moreover, the higher yield of coincident events has proven to reduce the image noise level significantly.[19,21,22] Due to the high coincident yield together with high spatial resolution, reconstructions employing very small voxels (>1 mm^3) can be accomplished without inheriting excessive noise given that the count density per voxel remains sufficiently high in LAFOV PET. Small voxel reconstructions of the total body (TB; or at least 1 m in length) may also result in additional challenges of reconstruction time, image data size, and image viewing without latency; however, it equips physicians with an improved capability to identify small lesions.[23] New pitfalls like an increased observance of physiologic gallbladder uptake need to be addressed properly when training physicians to interpret PET-images from these next-generation LAFOV scanners.[24]

LOWER INJECTED ACTIVITIES

LAFOV scanners have changed possibilities and workflows since their first introduction.[11,16,19] Higher sensitivity, yield of coincident events together with larger coverage of the body enabled clinicians to scan with less injected activity compared to SAFOV PET/CT.[10,25] Substantial dose reduction has become possible with these next-generation imaging devices.[19,20] Low-dose

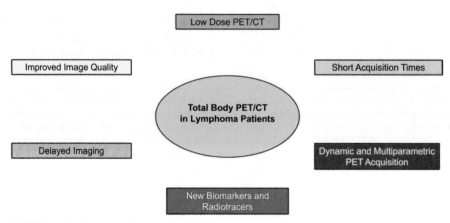

Fig. 1. TB PET/CT imaging features in patients with lymphoma.

scans are extremely valuable for patient populations at risk for high radiation burden like children.[26] Lymphoproliferative disease is one of the most common cancers affecting the pediatric population; therefore, it is critical to develop optimal clinical protocols for lymphoma imaging.[27] Low-dose LAFOV PET/CT imaging has proven to be feasible in children with only one-tenth of the clinical reference standard in a group of 33 children, 8 suffering from lymphoma.[28] **Fig. 2** shows an example from Mingels and colleagues of simulated low-dose images in a 9 year old male patient with HL.[26] This study found that a dose reduction of at least one-eighth (0.5 MBq/kg) of the clinical reference standard is possible without loss of diagnostic image quality. Further dose reductions up to 1/32nd of the reference standard were possible, but image quality was significantly impaired due to higher noise levels and lower signal-to-noise ratio (SNR).[26] Another population of patients that may benefit from reduction in radiation dose includes pregnant women. Van Sluis and colleagues presented a case of follicular lymphoma during pregnancy, which was successfully staged and restaged with a low dose [18F]FDG LAFOV PET/CT. In this case only one-tenth of the institutional injected activity was applied without loss of image quality.[29,30]

SHORTER ACQUISITION TIMES

Shortening acquisition times is possible with LAFOV scanners.[19,31] Shortening scan times is not only beneficial for PET centers as it may significantly increase throughput[14] but also can reduce motion artifacts and increase patients comfort.[32] In pediatric patients, the use of sedation or anesthesia is often necessary to obtain diagnostic images with SAFOV PET/CT. Short acquisition times may reduce or even avoid anesthesia in this patient population.[19] In a cohort of 270 pediatric patients, of whom the majority was referred for staging or restaging of lymphoma, the concept of short acquisition has shown to be feasible and a lower limit of 60 seconds acquisition was defined.[33] In the clinical routine, short acquisition durations may be useful to acquire diagnostic PET/CT images in patients with claustrophobia, patients affected by pain, or other patients who are not able to lie comfortably for the long periods typically required with multibed SAFOV PET.

Moreover, the multiple potential of LAFOV scanners can also be combined to optimize specific protocols. An example is the combination of a low-dose injection and short acquisition that was used to successfully scan a 10 week old newborn. Only 12 MBq [18F]FDG was injected with a scan time of 180 seconds, which allowed the avoidance of sedation.[34]

DELAYED IMAGING AND DUAL TIME IMAGING

Since the introduction of PET/CT in 2000, dual-time point (DTI) and delayed imaging protocols have been investigated to enhance the diagnostic accuracy of [18F]FDG PET/CT and to better differentiate between malignancy and benign processes.[35]

[18F]FDG uptake measurements depend on the time interval between the tracer administration and imaging. Tissues with high glucose turnover trap continuously increasing amounts of [18F]FDG. Increased cell proliferation rate and enhanced expression of some hexokinase enzymes and glucose transporters may also contribute to increased [18F]FDG uptake in tumor cells on delayed time-point imaging.[35]

In the past, a few reports described the increased [18F]FDG uptake in lymphoma lesions on delayed

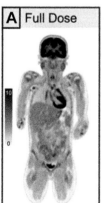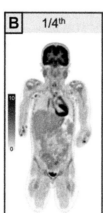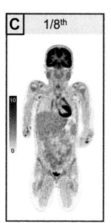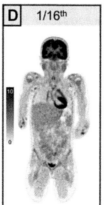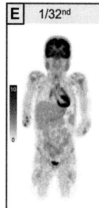

| A Full Dose | B 1/4th | C 1/8th | D 1/16th | E 1/32nd |

Fig. 2. Example of low-dose delayed TB PET/CT in a 9 year old patient with HL. Displayed are coronal PET-only example images of simulated dose reduction (up to 1/32nd of the reference standard) (*A–E*).

PET scans, and the usefulness of DTI in patients with malignant lymphoma.[36–38] More recently, Shinya and colleagues evaluated 524 lymphoma lesions in 43 patients comparing maximum standardized uptake value (SUV_{max}) and the retention index (RI) of SUV_{max} (RI_{max}) between different grades of lymphoma. They found that SUV_{max} of 2 hour delayed scan was significantly higher than on the clinical routine 1 hour scan.[39] Moreover, Nakayama and colleagues and Nielsen and colleagues reported in 2 different studies that delayed SUV_{max} and the SUV_{max}'s increase between early and delayed imaging showed significant potential to discriminate benign lymph nodes and malignant lymphoma lesions.[40,41] This may have significant implications by improving the staging accuracy with the potential to optimize management and reduce chemotherapeutic and/or radiation exposure. Subsequently, Lim and colleagues evaluated the connection between quantitative parameters extracted from DTI, including volumetric measurement (metabolic tumor volumes [MTVs] and metabolic volume different index) and some specific prognostic markers such as International Prognostic Index (IPI), Ann Arbor stage, and revised IPI particular to high-grade lymphoma.[42] RI_{max} differed significantly according to prognostic markers of malignant lymphoma. Also, quantitative measurements showed a significant inverse relationship to RI and weak negative connection with revised IPI. According to this preliminary study, the metabolic parameters could be useful imaging markers to predict patient prognosis in high-grade lymphoma before chemotherapy.[42]

In the past 5 years, a milestone was reached with the introduction and worldwide clinical implementation of LAFOV PET/CTs.[10,13,15,19] Whole body imaging with single bed position can enable high-quality delayed imaging, improved lesion detection, and even deeper insights of the tumor biology by allowing dynamic image acquisition of the entire body simultaneously.[13] In 2021, a small cohort of (n = 22) patients with lymphoma were assessed on a TB PET/CT with DTI. Lesion-based Deauville Scores trended to be slightly higher in 2 hour delayed scans than in a standard clinical routine 60 minute scans.[43] An example of a case of upstaging on the delayed 120 minute p.i. images is shown in **Fig. 3**. Moreover, partial volume-corrected total lesion glycolysis compared between 60 minutes and 120 minutes among patients with non-Hodgkin lymphoma (NHL) and patients with HL showed a statistically significant increase on delayed images.[35]

There is good agreement on delayed imaging that, background activity generally decreases and SUV_{max} increases in most FDG-avid lymphoma lesions.[41] Thus, SUV_{max} decreases in the inactive or chronic inflammation and some other benign lesions.[35] Therefore, DTI protocols might have the potential to increase the diagnostic accuracy of lymphoma PET/CT.[35]

SIMULTANEOUS AND DYNAMIC IMAGING OF LARGE PORTIONS OF THE BODY

TB or LAFOV dynamic PET imaging allows the simultaneous visualization and investigation of the dynamic processes of the radiotracers within the human body.[15] The dynamic PET data can be then analyzed using nonlinear compartmental models and linearized Patlak models.[44,45] LAFOV PET systems also allow extraction of image-derived input functions (IDIFs) from large blood pools such as aorta or left ventricle, allowing the application of [^{18}F]FDG dynamic imaging protocols without invasive blood sampling.[44,46] An example of Patlak images derived using an IDIF in a patient with lymphoma is shown in **Fig. 4**. However, due to the complexity of dynamic imaging protocols such as lengthened acquisition durations (ie, 60 minutes for [^{18}F]FDG), only very few publications have evaluated the impact of dynamic imaging in patients with lymphoma yet.

Introduction of LAFOV systems also enabled easier facilitation of abbreviated dynamic imaging methods, which can enable more practical protocols in busy clinical routines. Recent study has shown that abbreviated protocols that utilize population-based input functions can provide accurate tracer influx (K_i) values in tumor lesions in 20 minutes.[47–49] Recent research has also shown that dual time-window or dual-injection protocols might be able to provide accurate tracer delivery (K_1) and K_i values in certain scenarios.[48,50]

There is some evidence suggesting that dynamic imaging might be able to differentiate between inflammation and malignancy due to higher irreversible [^{18}F]FDG uptake in tumors lesions (Ki_{max}) compared to SUV_{max} images. However, a large overlap in semiquantitative measurements was detected limiting Ki_{max} image evaluation.[51] Of note, the impact of other parameters like metabolic rate of glucose consumption, MR_{FDG}, and time activity curves has not yet been evaluated in patients with lymphoma systematically.

LESION QUANTIFICATION IN TOTAL-BODY AND LONG-AXIAL FIELD-OF-VIEW PET/ COMPUTED TOMOGRAPHY
Standardized Uptake Values

Lesion segmentation and subsequently lesion quantification was performed since the introduction

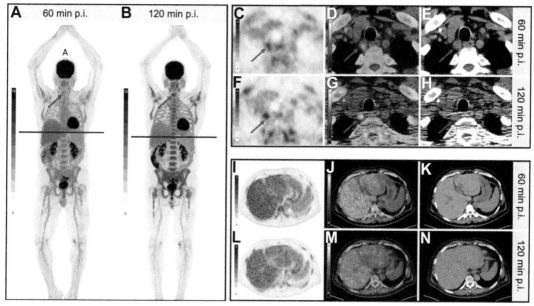

Fig. 3. Dual time point interim [^{18}F]FDG PET of a 57 year old male patient with Hodgkin lymphoma. (*A*) Image represents 60 minute and (*B*) 120 minute post injection (p.i.) maximum intensity projections (MIPs). PET-only (*C/F*), hybrid (*D/G*), and CT-only (*E/H*) images demonstrate an enlarged right lower cervical lymph node with SUV$_{max}$: 3.07 in 60 minutes (*C–E*) and a significant increase SUV$_{max}$: 3.55 120 minutes p.i. (*F–H*). The 60 minute (*I, J*) and 120 minute (*L–N*) p.i. PET-only (*I/L*), hybrid (*J/M*), and CT-only (*K/M*) images of the liver show a background activity decrease resulting in an upstaging of the cervical lymph node's (*red arrow*) Deauville score (3–4) as well as a scan-based upstaging of the treatment response group by Lugano criteria (complete metabolic response to partial metabolic response).

of hybrid PET/CT systems.[1] A common approach to quantify the [^{18}F]FDG uptake of a lymphoma lesion is to use SUV$_{max}$ and compare lesion uptake to reference organs. In lymphoma specifically, the visual Deauville scoring system is used, where lesion uptake is compared to liver and blood pool uptake and graded on a scale from 1 to 5.[2] Overall Deauville scoring can be grouped regarding treatment response in interim or end-of-treatment PET evaluation into different categories following the Lugano classification system.[3] Lesion quantification, Deauville scoring and grouping into response categories

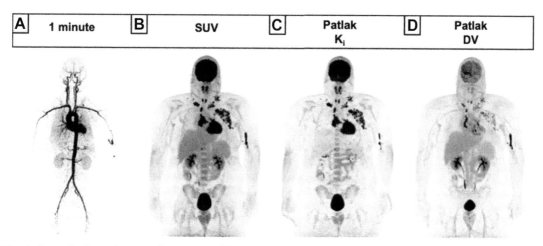

Fig. 4. Example dynamic MIPs of a 29 year old 130 kg male patient referred for lymphoma staging. (*A*) Image displays the 1 minute influx after injection of 398 MBq [^{18}F]FDG. (*B*) Image shows the SUV image. K$_i$ and the distribution volume (DV) are displayed in images C and D.

was shown to yield statistically higher prognostic value compared to stand-alone CT classifications.[52] Due to lower noise levels in LAFOV PET/CT, some publications emphasize that peak and mean SUV were more reliable throughout different scanner protocols.[21]

However, each of these classification systems has several limitations related to different uptake patterns of different lymphoma subtypes, different scan acquisition times (resulting in different noise level), different recontraction parameters as well as differences in lesion segmentation and different scanners.[10,11,16,21] Nevertheless, physicians have tried to identify cutoff values to associate with clinical outcomes. For example, in the LyMa-PET study for mantle cell lymphoma (MCL), SUV_{max} greater than 10.3 was associated with both poor progression-free survival (PFS) and decreased overall survival (OS).[53,54] Other semiquantitative measurements like ΔSUV_{max} were tested and have shown to be a possible alternative.[55] Other data suggest that combining SUV measurements with alternative parameters (eg, IPI) improves their value as an independent outcome predictor.[56] Nevertheless, all approaches showed some limitations, which led to a quest for other prognostic PET/CT biomarkers opening an opportunity for LAFOV PET/CT scanners.

Metabolic Tumor Volume and Total Metabolic Tumor Volume

Different approaches to quantify the tumor burden beyond the SUV measurements have resulted in the introduction of a new measure: MTV. MTV usually calculated by a 41% isocontour approach of the hottest vowel indicates the tumor activity and [^{18}F]FDG utilization of the lymphoma lesion.[57] Another described measure that takes into consideration all tumorous lesions is the total MTV (TMTV). LAFOV enables to simultaneously quantify lesions in different parts of the body, which is not possible when using SAFOV with either step-and-shoot or continuous bed motion techniques. Also, when assessing TMTV on the subcategory of LAFOV, TB PET/CT, the evaluation of the simultaneous TMTV, is different from the one obtained on a SAFOV scanner. The order of magnitude and the possible clinical implication associated with the difference in MTV and TMTV calculated on separately on a SAFOV and on a LAFOV scanner is still being studied.

As to prior assessment on SAFOV scanners, they have been reports indicating MTV cutoff values for the clinical outcome in patients with lymphoma. In HL, TMTV over 147 mL was prognostic for PFS and OS.[58] The PETAL trial revealed that a TMTV over 328 mL was an independent predictor of poor clinical outcome in patients with DLBCL.[59] However, the combination of TMTV with another prognostic factor (eg, ΔSUV_{max}, gene expression) was a more powerful predictor of clinical outcome. Nevertheless, MTV assessment is highly variable due to many different variables, including patient selection criteria, image processing algorithm, different segmentation methods, or different scanner types. Therefore, a challenge and opportunity in LAFOV PET/CT is to generate more homogeneous data that would optimize prediction of clinical outcomes. Since the entire body can be scanned in only one bed position, the TMTV might be less variable compared to conventional PET systems.

Moreover, new therapeutic approaches like chimeric antigen receptor (CAR) T-cell therapies have been recently implemented in the therapeutic regime of patients with lymphoma. There is already some evidence suggesting a beneficial role of [^{18}F]FDG PET/CT in the response prediction and evaluation. Murad and colleagues demonstrated that 2 PET/CT scans should be performed, one as baseline at the time of the decision and one after completion of bridging therapies.[60] Especially SUV measurements and TMTV assessed on the baseline PET/CT have shown to be predictive of OS and PFD. Moreover, baseline parameters at the time of decision have shown to be predictive for the development of treatment-related complication.[60–62] After CAR T-cell therapy, PET/CT is used to classify patients into treatment response groups to assess the long-term outcome.[63] Three month follow-up PET/CT can be used to identify possible therapy-related complications and determine early therapeutic efficacy.[60] Also in this case, there is now an opportunity for LAFOV scanners to challenge SAFOV scanners both as disease predictor and as predictor of therapy-related complications.

Radiomics

In radiology and especially tomography, lesion quantification plays a pivotal role. An approach of lesion quantification beyond routine analysis (ie, size or shape of a lymphoma lesion) has resulted in the concept of textural analysis. All those can be summarized under the term *Radiomics*. Radiomics epitomize the pursuit of precision medicine in combining image information with molecular and other biomarkers as a predictor for treatment response.[64] Few studies have evaluated yet the impact of radiomics analysis in lymphoma. In patients with diffuse large B cell lymphoma (DLBCL), some radiomic features have showed to be a promising outcome predictor when assessed on [18F]FDG PET/CT scans obtained before immunochemotherapy treatment.[65] In MCL, radiomic features combined with SUV measurements improved the prediction of 2 year PFS as well as the prediction of bone marrow involvement. Strongest results were found when combining radiomics imaging features with laboratory parameters.[66,67]

Another lesion characteristic in patients with lymphoma, which can be subsumed under the term radiomics is the distance between either different lymphoma lesions or between lymphoma lesions and a reference organ (eg, spleen).[68] In this publication, which included 290 DLBCL cases, the largest distance between lymphoma sites was a strong independent prognostic factor. There are different distance methods, which have been evaluated in patients with DLBCL: the Euclidean distance, Manhattan distance, and Chebychev distance.[69] However, the impact of each distance measure method for clinical evaluation is still unclear.

LONG-AXIAL FIELD-OF-VIEW PET/COMPUTED TOMOGRAPHY ENABLES IMAGING WITH NEW RADIOTRACERS

[18F]FDG is the main radiotracer for diagnosis and follow-up of patients with lymphoma. However, recent research has focused on targeting cancer cells on other receptors and molecules, leading to the development of new radiotracers beyond FDG.[56,70] Possible target mechanisms in patients with lymphoma, which have been identified for imaging, are accelerated cancer cell replication with, for example, amino acid tracers (eg, [18F]-fluoro-thymidine or [18F]-fludarabine), the fatty acid synthesis with choline or acetate tracers, and the protein synthesis, for example, with [11C]-methionine. Moreover, cell surface markers like chemokine receptors (eg, CXCR4), immune checkpoint inhibitors (like PD-L1), or cluster of differentiation (CD) are possible targets for imaging (eg, CD20, CD22, CD30, or CD37).[56] Furthermore, T-cell receptor targeting radiolabeled antibodies might be explored in clinical studies in patients with lymphoma.[71,72] Additionally, recent developments have led to a new imaging approach of targeting the tumor environment. This resulted in the development of a radiotracer, which shows increased fibroblast-activation-protein inhibitors (FAPI) that characterize upregulation of cancer-associated fibroblasts.[73] FAPI has shown to be a possible diagnostic agent to detect lymphoma lesions.[74] Moreover, FAPI might be also a promising "theranostic" radiopharmaceutical.[75] LAFOV PET/CT

can help to establish imaging protocols and dosimetry of these new radiotracers.[14]

SUMMARY

LAFOV systems have the potential to improve staging, prognostication, response to therapy assessment and early recurrence detection in the evaluation in patients with lymphoma. The current initial literature supports the use of LAFOV to perform (1) high image quality scans with reduced noise level; (2) low-dose imaging reducing patient radiation exposure; and (3) shorter scan durations mitigating or avoiding the need for anesthesia. In addition, the literature supports the feasibility of delayed imaging protocols. LAFOV scanners may also provide improved semiquantitative measurements compared to the analogous measurements obtained on SAFOV scanners; however, the magnitude of difference and the clinical implication of this difference in measurements are not fully investigated and further studies are warranted. The potential to obtain new metrics for lymphoma assessment using LAFOV dynamic PET may be revealed in future research as well as the specific role of LAFOV in the assessment of new lymphoma-specific radio pharmaceutics.

DISCLOURE

Research reported in this publication was supported by the National Institutes of Health, United States under award number R01CA249422. The study was also supported by the In Vivo Translational Imaging Shared Resources with funds from NCI P30CA093373 and by the Fred and Julia Rusch Foundation for Nuclear Medicine Research and Education. Dr H. Nalbant's funding is partially provided by United Imaging Healthcare's Fellowship Gift. L. Nardo is PI of service agreement with United Imaging Healthcare. L. Nardo is site PI of clinical trials supported by Novartis Pharmaceuticals Corporation, United States. L. Nardo is PI of a clinical trial supported by Telix Pharmaceuticals. L. Nardo is PI of a clinical trial supported by Lantheus Medical Imaging, United States. L. Nardo is PI of a clinical trial supported by GE Healthcare, United States. L. Nardo is Co-PI of a clinical trial supported by Lilly, United States. L. Nardo has a speaker engagement agreement with Lilly. UC Davis has a share revenue agreement with United Imaging Healthcare. H. Sari is a full-time employee of Siemens Healthcare AG, Switzerland. UC Davis has a revenue sharing agreement with United Imaging Healthcare. F. Sen is PI of clinical research sponsored by Biogen, United States. All other authors have no conflicts of interest to report.

REFERENCES

1. Beyer T, Townsend DW, Brun T, et al. A combined PET/CT scanner for clinical oncology. J Nucl Med 2000;41(8):1369–79.
2. Barrington SF, Mikhaeel NG, Kostakoglu L, et al. Role of imaging in the staging and response assessment of lymphoma: consensus of the international conference on malignant lymphomas imaging working group. J Clin Oncol 2014;32(27):3048–58.
3. Cheson BD, Fisher RI, Barrington SF, et al. Recommendations for initial evaluation, staging, and response assessment of Hodgkin and non-Hodgkin lymphoma: the Lugano classification. J Clin Oncol 2014;32(27):3059–68.
4. Eichenauer DA, Aleman BMP, André M, et al. Hodgkin lymphoma: ESMO Clinical Practice Guidelines for diagnosis, treatment and follow-up. Ann Oncol 2018;29:iv19–29.
5. Zanoni L, Bezzi D, Nanni C, et al. PET/CT in non-hodgkin lymphoma: an update. Semin Nucl Med 2023;53(3):320–51.
6. Zelenetz AD, Gordon LI, Abramson JS, et al. NCCN Guidelines® insights: B-cell lymphomas, version 6.2023: featured updates to the NCCN guidelines. J Natl Compr Cancer Netw 2023;21(11):1118–31.
7. Hoppe RT, Advani RH, Ai WZ, et al. Hodgkin lymphoma, version 2.2015. J Natl Compr Cancer Netw 2015;13(5):554–86.
8. Vandenberghe S, Moskal P, Karp JS. State of the art in total body PET. EJNMMI Phys 2020;7(1):35.
9. Alberts I, Prenosil G, Sachpekidis C, et al. Digital versus analogue PET in [68Ga]Ga-PSMA-11 PET/CT for recurrent prostate cancer: a matched-pair comparison. Eur J Nucl Med Mol Imaging 2020;47(3):614–23.
10. Alberts I, Hünermund JN, Prenosil G, et al. Clinical performance of long axial field of view PET/CT: a head-to-head intra-individual comparison of the Biograph Vision Quadra with the Biograph Vision PET/CT. Eur J Nucl Med Mol Imaging 2021;48(8):2395–404.
11. Prenosil GA, Sari H, Fürstner M, et al. Performance characteristics of the biograph vision quadra PET/CT system with a long axial field of view using the NEMA NU 2-2018 standard. J Nucl Med 2022;63(3):476–84.
12. Karp JS, Viswanath V, Geagan MJ, et al. PennPET explorer: design and preliminary performance of a whole-body imager. J Nucl Med 2020;61(1):136–43.
13. Pantel AR, Viswanath V, Daube-Witherspoon ME, et al. PennPET explorer: human imaging on a whole-body imager. J Nucl Med 2020;61(1):144–51.
14. Alberts I, Sari H, Mingels C, et al. Long-axial field-of-view PET/CT: perspectives and review of a revolutionary development in nuclear medicine based on clinical experience in over 7000 patients. Cancer Imag 2023;23(1):28.
15. Mingels C, Caobelli F, Alavi A, et al. Total-body PET/CT or LAFOV PET/CT? Axial field-of-view clinical classification. Eur J Nucl Med Mol Imaging 2023;51(4):951–3.
16. Spencer BA, Berg E, Schmall JP, et al. Performance evaluation of the uEXPLORER total-body PET/CT scanner based on NEMA NU 2-2018 with additional tests to characterize PET scanners with a long axial field of view. J Nucl Med 2021;62(6):861–70.
17. van Sluis J, van Snick JH, Brouwers AH, et al. EARL compliance and imaging optimisation on the Biograph Vision Quadra PET/CT using phantom and clinical data. Eur J Nucl Med Mol Imaging 2022;49(13):4652–60.
18. Alberts I, Seibel S, Xue S, et al. Investigating the influence of long-axial versus short-axial field of view PET/CT on stage migration in lymphoma and non-small cell lung cancer. Nucl Med Commun 2023;44(11):988–96.
19. Badawi RD, Shi H, Hu P, et al. First human imaging studies with the EXPLORER total-body PET scanner. J Nucl Med 2019;60(3):299–303.
20. Mingels C, Weissenrieder L, Zeimpekis K, et al. FDG imaging with long-axial field-of-view PET/CT in patients with high blood glucose-a matched pair analysis. Eur J Nucl Med Mol Imaging 2024;51(7):2036–46.
21. Mingels C, Weidner S, Sari H, et al. Impact of the new ultra-high sensitivity mode in a long axial field-of-view PET/CT. Ann Nucl Med 2023;37(5):310–5.
22. Calderón E, Schmidt FP, Lan W, et al. Image quality and quantitative PET parameters of low-dose [18F] FDG PET in a long axial field-of-view PET/CT scanner. Diagnostics 2023;13(20):3240.
23. Mingels C, Sari H, Gözlügöl N, et al. Long-axial field-of-view PET/CT for the assessment of inflammation in calcified coronary artery plaques with [68 Ga] Ga-DOTA-TOC. Eur J Nucl Med Mol Imaging 2023;51(2):422–33 [Internet].
24. Calabro' A, Abdelhafez YG, Triumbari EKA, et al. 18F-FDG gallbladder uptake: observation from a total-body PET/CT scanner. BMC Med Imaging 2023;23(1):9.
25. Slart RHJA, Tsoumpas C, Glaudemans AWJM, et al. Long axial field of view PET scanners: a road map to implementation and new possibilities. Eur J Nucl Med Mol Imaging 2021;48(13):4236–45.
26. Mingels C, Spencer BA, Nalbant H, et al. Accepted: dose reduction in pediatric oncology patients with delayed total-body FDG PET/CT. J Nucl Med 2024; jnumed(124):267521.
27. Agarwal S. Pediatric cancers: insights and novel therapeutic approaches. Cancer 2023;15(14):3537.
28. Zhao YM, Li YH, Chen T, et al. Image quality and lesion detectability in low-dose pediatric 18F-FDG scans using total-body PET/CT. Eur J Nucl Med Mol Imaging 2021;48(11):3378–85.

29. Calais J, Hapdey S, Tilly H, et al. Hodgkin's disease staging by FDG PET/CT in a pregnant woman. Nucl Med Mol Imaging 2014;48(3):244–6.

30. Van Sluis J, Bellido M, Glaudemans AWJM, et al. Long axial field-of-view PET for ultra-low-dose imaging of non-hodgkin lymphoma during pregnancy. Diagnostics 2022;13(1):28.

31. Alberts I, Sachpekidis C, Prenosil G, et al. Digital PET/CT allows for shorter acquisition protocols or reduced radiopharmaceutical dose in [18F]-FDG PET/CT. Ann Nucl Med 2021;35(4):485–92.

32. Katal S, Eibschutz LS, Saboury B, et al. Advantages and applications of total-body PET scanning. Diagnostics 2022;12(2):426.

33. Zhang Q, Hu Y, Zhou C, et al. Reducing pediatric total-body PET/CT imaging scan time with multimodal artificial intelligence technology. EJNMMI Phys 2024;11(1):1.

34. Van Rijsewijk ND, Van Leer B, Ivashchenko OV, et al. Ultra-low dose infection imaging of a newborn without sedation using long axial field-of-view PET/CT. Eur J Nucl Med Mol Imaging 2023;50(2):622–3.

35. Cheng G, Torigian DA, Zhuang H, et al. When should we recommend use of dual time-point and delayed time-point imaging techniques in FDG PET? Eur J Nucl Med Mol Imaging 2013;40(5):779–87.

36. Kubota K, Itoh M, Ozaki K, et al. Advantage of delayed whole-body FDG-PET imaging for tumour detection. Eur J Nucl Med 2001;28(6):696–703.

37. Ahmadzadehfar H, Sabet A, Näke K, et al. Dual-time F-18 FDG-PET/CT imaging for diagnosis of occult non-Hodgkin lymphoma in a patient with esophageal cancer. Clin Nucl Med 2009;34(3):168–70.

38. Jeanguillaume C, Metrard G, Rakotonirina H, et al. Delayed [(18)F]FDG PET imaging of central nervous system lymphoma: is PET better than MRI? Eur J Nucl Med Mol Imaging 2006;33(11):1370–1.

39. Shinya T, Fujii S, Asakura S, et al. Dual-time-point F-18 FDG PET/CT for evaluation in patients with malignant lymphoma. Ann Nucl Med 2012;26(8):616–21.

40. Nielsen A, Mylam K, Pedersen L, et al. Dual time point 18F-FDG PET/CT in patients on suspicion of malignant lymphoma. J Nucl Med 2014;55(supplement 1):1581.

41. Nakayama M, Okizaki A, Ishitoya S, et al. Dual-time-point F-18 FDG PET/CT imaging for differentiating the lymph nodes between malignant lymphoma and benign lesions. Ann Nucl Med 2013;27(2):163–9.

42. Lim DH, Lee JH. Relationship between dual time point FDG PET/CT and clinical prognostic indexes in patients with high grade lymphoma: a pilot study. Nucl Med Mol Imaging 2017;51(4):323–30.

43. Abdelhafez Y, Sen F, Tuscano J, et al. Differences in Deauville scores generated using 60- and 120-minute uptake times on Total-Body 18F-FDG PET/CT scans. J Nucl Med 2021;62(supplement 1):1680.

44. Sari H, Mingels C, Alberts I, et al. First results on kinetic modelling and parametric imaging of dynamic 18F-FDG datasets from a long axial FOV PET scanner in oncological patients. Eur J Nucl Med Mol Imaging 2022;49(6):1997–2009.

45. Wang G, Nardo L, Parikh M, et al. Total-body PET multiparametric imaging of cancer using a voxelwise strategy of compartmental modeling. J Nucl Med 2022;63(8):1274–81.

46. Zhang X, Xie Z, Berg E, et al. Total-body dynamic reconstruction and parametric imaging on the uEXPLORER. J Nucl Med 2020;61(2):285–91.

47. Sari H, Eriksson L, Mingels C, et al. Feasibility of using abbreviated scan protocols with population-based input functions for accurate kinetic modeling of [18F]-FDG datasets from a long axial FOV PET scanner. Eur J Nucl Med Mol Imaging 2023;50(2):257–65.

48. Wu Y, Feng T, Zhao Y, et al. Whole-body parametric imaging of 18 F-FDG PET using uEXPLORER with reduced scanning time. J Nucl Med 2022;63(4):622–8.

49. Van Sluis J, Van Snick JH, Brouwers AH, et al. Shortened duration whole body 18F-FDG PET Patlak imaging on the Biograph Vision Quadra PET/CT using a population-averaged input function. EJNMMI Phys 2022;9(1):74.

50. Viswanath V, Sari H, Pantel AR, et al. Abbreviated scan protocols to capture 18F-FDG kinetics for long axial FOV PET scanners. Eur J Nucl Med Mol Imaging 2022;49(9):3215–25.

51. Skawran S, Messerli M, Kotasidis F, et al. Can dynamic whole-body FDG PET imaging differentiate between malignant and inflammatory lesions? Life 2022;12(9):1350.

52. Trotman J, Barrington SF, Belada D, et al. Prognostic value of end-of-induction PET response after first-line immunochemotherapy for follicular lymphoma (GALLIUM): secondary analysis of a randomised, phase 3 trial. Lancet Oncol 2018;19(11):1530–42.

53. Bailly C, Carlier T, Berriolo-Riedinger A, et al. Prognostic value of FDG-PET in patients with mantle cell lymphoma: results from the LyMa-PET Project. Haematologica 2020;105(1):e33–6.

54. Bodet-Milin C, Bailly C, Meignan M, et al. Predictive power of FDG-PET parameters at diagnosis and after induction in patients with mantle cell lymphoma, interim results from the LyMa-PET project, conducted on behalf of the lysa group. Blood 2015;126(23):335.

55. Rekowski J, Hüttmann A, Schmitz C, et al. Interim PET evaluation in diffuse large B-cell lymphoma using published recommendations: comparison of the Deauville 5-point scale and the ΔSUVmax method. J Nucl Med 2021;62(1):37–42.

56. Al Tabaa Y, Bailly C, Kanoun S. FDG-PET/CT in lymphoma: where do we go now? Cancer 2021;13(20):5222.

57. Basu S, Zaidi H, Salavati A, et al. FDG PET/CT methodology for evaluation of treatment response in lymphoma: from "graded visual analysis" and "semi-quantitative SUVmax" to global disease burden assessment. Eur J Nucl Med Mol Imaging 2014; 41(11):2158–60.

58. Cottereau AS, Versari A, Loft A, et al. Prognostic value of baseline metabolic tumor volume in early-stage Hodgkin lymphoma in the standard arm of the H10 trial. Blood 2018;131(13):1456–63.

59. Schmitz C, Hüttmann A, Müller SP, et al. Dynamic risk assessment based on positron emission tomography scanning in diffuse large B-cell lymphoma: post-hoc analysis from the PETAL trial. Eur J Cancer 2020;124:25–36.

60. Murad V, Kohan A, Ortega C, et al. Role of FDG PET/CT in patients with lymphoma treated with CAR T-cell therapy: current concepts. AJR Am J Roentgenol 2023;222(3):e2330301.

61. Cohen D, Luttwak E, Beyar-Katz O, et al. [18F]FDG PET-CT in patients with DLBCL treated with CAR-T cell therapy: a practical approach of reporting pre- and post-treatment studies. Eur J Nucl Med Mol Imaging 2022;49(3):953–62.

62. Vercellino L, Di Blasi R, Kanoun S, et al. Predictive factors of early progression after CAR T-cell therapy in relapsed/refractory diffuse large B-cell lymphoma. Blood Adv 2020;4(22):5607–15.

63. Kuhnl A, Roddie C, Kirkwood AA, et al. Early FDG-PET response predicts CAR-T failure in large B-cell lymphoma. Blood Adv 2022;6(1):321–6.

64. Gillies RJ, Kinahan PE, Hricak H. Radiomics: images are more than pictures, they are data. Radiology 2016;278(2):563–77.

65. Aide N, Fruchart C, Nganoa C, et al. Baseline 18F-FDG PET radiomic features as predictors of 2-year event-free survival in diffuse large B cell lymphomas treated with immunochemotherapy. Eur Radiol 2020; 30(8):4623–32.

66. Mayerhoefer ME, Riedl CC, Kumar A, et al. Radiomic features of glucose metabolism enable prediction of outcome in mantle cell lymphoma. Eur J Nucl Med Mol Imaging 2019;46(13):2760–9.

67. Mayerhoefer ME, Riedl CC, Kumar A, et al. [18F]FDG-PET/CT radiomics for prediction of bone marrow involvement in mantle cell lymphoma: a retrospective study in 97 patients. Cancer 2020;12(5):1138.

68. Girum KB, Cottereau AS, Vercellino L, et al. Tumor location relative to the spleen is a prognostic factor in lymphoma patients: a demonstration from the re-marc trial. J Nucl Med 2024;65(2):313–9.

69. Cottereau AS, Meignan M, Nioche C, et al. New approaches in characterization of lesions dissemination in DLBCL patients on baseline PET/CT. Cancer 2021;13(16):3998.

70. Omidvari N, Jones T, Price PM, et al. First-in-human immunoPET imaging of COVID-19 convalescent patients using dynamic total-body PET and a CD8-targeted minibody. Sci Adv 2023;9(41):eadh7968.

71. Study to evaluate CD8 PET imaging as a marker of immune response to stereotactic body radiation therapy (ELIXR). Available at: https://clinicaltrials.gov/study/NCT05371132?cond=Solid%20Tumor&term=CD8%20PET&intr=radiation&rank=1.

72. 89Zr-Df-IAB22M2C PET/CT in patients with selected solid malignancies or Hodgkin's lymphoma. Available at: https://www.clinicaltrials.gov/study/NCT03107663.

73. Lindner T, Loktev A, Altmann A, et al. Development of quinoline-based theranostic ligands for the targeting of fibroblast activation protein. J Nucl Med 2018; 59(9):1415–22.

74. Jin X, Wei M, Wang S, et al. Detecting fibroblast activation proteins in lymphoma using 68Ga-FAPI PET/CT. J Nucl Med 2022;63(2):212–7.

75. Watabe T, Liu Y, Kaneda-Nakashima K, et al. Theranostics targeting fibroblast activation protein in the tumor stroma: 64Cu- and 225Ac-labeled FAPI-04 in pancreatic cancer xenograft mouse models. J Nucl Med 2020;61(4):563–9.

FDG-PET/CT Imaging in Chimeric Antigen Receptor–Engineered T-Cell Treatment in Patients with B-Cell Lymphoma: Current Evidence

Elisabetta Maria Abenavoli, MD[a], Flavia Linguanti, MD[b,c],
Laurent Dercle, MD, PhD[d], Valentina Berti, MD[c], Egesta Lopci, MD, PhD[e,*]

KEYWORDS

- B-cell lymphoma • Non-Hodgkin lymphoma • CAR-T • FDG • PET/CT • Response
- Adverse events

KEY POINTS

- [18F]-FDG PET/computed tomography stands as a cornerstone in the enhancement of patient care throughout all stages of chimeric antigen receptor-engineered (CAR) T-cell therapy.
- Prognostic and predictive markers obtained from baseline FDG PET offer insights into patient outcomes, enabling the identification of individuals who might derive long-term benefit most from CAR T-cell therapy.
- Early evaluations with FDG PET at 1 and 3 months posttreatment are paramount for gauging response to therapy.

INTRODUCTION

The Food and Drug Administration (FDA) has approved 4 different chimeric antigen receptor-engineered (CAR) T-cell therapies for patients diagnosed with B-cell lymphomas (**Fig. 1**) in the last 5 years[1–5]: BREYANZI (lisocabtagene maraleucel), KYMRIAHTM (tisagenlecleucel), YESCARTATM (axicabtagene ciloleucel), and TECARTUSTM (brexucabtagene autoleucel). The role of CAR T-cell therapy is constantly expanding in hematological malignancies as well as solid tumors.[6,7] This is demonstrated by the first CAR-T products used for multiple myeloma and called ABECMA (idecabtagene vicleucel) and CARVYKTITM (ciltacabtagene autoleucel) that have been recently FDA approved[8–11] (**Table 1**).

The implementation of CAR T cells has created the need to unravel biomarkers that can allow for optimal tailoring of therapeutic strategies to individual patients. Such biomarkers could enhance risk stratification, prognostication, prediction of response, response assessment, and prediction/diagnosis of immune-related adverse events.

Predictive biomarkers could forecast the likelihood of a patient to respond to CAR T-cell therapy before treatment initiation. By identifying biomarkers

[a] Nuclear Medicine Unit, Careggi University Hospital, Largo Brambilla 3, 50134 Florence, Italy; [b] Nuclear Medicine Department, Ospedale San Donato, Via Pietro Nenni 20, Arezzo 52100, Italy; [c] Nuclear Medicine Unit, Department of Experimental and Clinical Biomedical Sciences "Mario Serio", University of Florence, Largo Brambilla 3, Florence 50134, Italy; [d] Department of Radiology, New York-Presbyterian Hospital, Columbia University Vagelos College of Physicians and Surgeons, 622 West 168th Street, New York, NY 10032, USA; [e] Nuclear Medicine Unit, IRCCS-Humanitas Research Hospital, Via Manzoni 56, Rozzano, Milano CAP 20089, Italy
* Corresponding author.
E-mail address: egesta.lopci@cancercenter.humanitas.it

PET Clin 19 (2024) 505–513
https://doi.org/10.1016/j.cpet.2024.05.006
1556-8598/24/© 2024 Elsevier Inc. All rights are reserved, including those for text and data mining, AI training, and similar technologies.

pet.theclinics.com

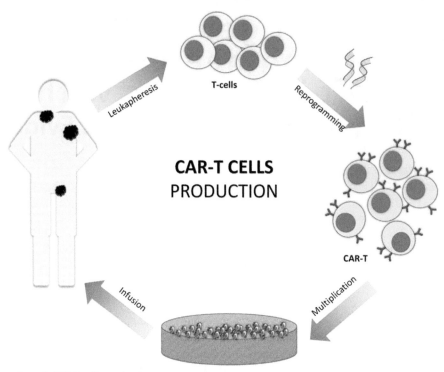

Fig. 1. Overview of CAR T-cell production.

associated with treatment response or resistance, clinicians could select the most appropriate candidates for CAR T-cell therapy. For example, biomarkers such as tumor mutational burden, expression levels of certain antigens (eg, CD19, BCMA, or B-cell maturation antigen), cytokine profiles, or genetic markers can help predict response to treatment.[13]

Table 1
Principal indications of the commercially available CAR T-cell therapy[6,12]

CAR-T Product	First Approval	Target	Indication	Pharmaceutical Company
Kymriah® (tisagenlecleucel)	2017	CD19	B-cell ALL LBCL DLBCL FL	Novartis Pharmaceuticals Corp.
Yescarta® (axicabtagene ciloleucel)	2017	CD19	LBCL DLBCL FL	Kite Pharma, Inc.
Tecartus® (brexucabtagene autoleucal)	2020	CD19	B-cell ALL MCL	Kite Pharma, Inc.
Breyanzi® (lisocabtagene maraleucel)	2021	CD19	LBCL	Juno Therapeutics, Inc.
Abecma® (idecabtagene vicleucel)	2021	BCMA	MM	Bristol Myers Squibb
Carvykti® (ciltacabtagene autoleucel)	2022	BCMA	MM	Janssen Biotech, Inc.

Abbreviations: ALL, acute lymphoblastic leukemia; BCMA, B-cell maturation antigen; CAR T cells, chimeric antigen receptor-engineered T cells; CD19, cluster of differentiation 19; DLBCL, diffuse large B-cell lymphoma; FL, follicular lymphoma; LBCL, large B-cell lymphoma; MCL, mantle cell lymphoma; MM, multiple myeloma.

Linguanti F, Abenavoli EM, Berti V, Lopci E. Metabolic Imaging in B-Cell Lymphomas during CAR-T Cell Therapy. Cancers (Basel). 2022 Sep 27;14(19):4700; and Chen YJ, Abila B, Mostafa Kamel Y. CAR-T: What Is Next? Cancers (Basel). 2023 Jan 21;15(3):663. https://doi.org/10.3390/cancers15030663.

Prognostic biomarkers provide information about the likelihood of disease progression or relapse independent of treatment. These biomarkers assist in stratifying patients into risk groups, enabling clinicians to develop personalized monitoring and treatment plans. Biomarkers like baseline disease burden, tumor microenvironment characteristics, T-cell fitness, and markers of immune exhaustion can help predict long-term outcomes and guide posttreatment surveillance strategies.[14–16]

The early prediction and identification of adverse events is a critical aspect of CAR T-cell therapy.[13] In particular, neurotoxicity, often associated with cytokine release syndrome (CRS), is a frequent and potentially severe adverse event following CAR T-cell therapy. Predicting and monitoring and neurotoxicity could enhance patient safety during treatment.

The current literature supports the pivotal role of [^{18}F]-FDG PET/computed tomography (CT) to assess CAR T-cell therapy response in lymphomas. This imaging modality, already proven effective in evaluating traditional treatments, offers valuable insights into treatment efficacy. The response evaluation on [^{18}F]-FDG PET/CT, usually performed following the Lugano 2014 criteria[17] in patients diagnosed with lymphoma, is assessed at approximately 4 time points: 1, 3 (**Fig. 2**), 6, and 12 months after CAR T cells infusion.[6,17]

This comprehensive review aims to demonstrate the pivotal role that [^{18}F]-FDG PET/CT imaging can play to enhance the care of patients treated with CAR T-cell therapy. To this end, this review deciphers evidence showing the diagnostic, prognostic, predictive, and theragnostic value of [^{18}F]-FDG PET/CT-derived parameters.

BASELINE BIOMARKERS FOR RESPONSE TO CHIMERIC ANTIGEN RECEPTOR-ENGINEERED T CELLS

Several groups have explored the predictive and prognostic value of metabolic parameters in patients treated with CAR T-cell therapy and, especially, the role of baseline [^{18}F]-FDG PET/CT scans in predicting the outcome and thus assisting in the selection of patients benefiting from the treatment.

Recently, Georgi and colleagues[18] have confirmed the prognostic value of total metabolic tumor volume (TMTV) in PET baseline (PET-0) reported by previous publications.[19–21] The authors have found that a value of 25 mL for TMTV in PET-0 could be an optimal discrimination between patients with complete metabolic response (CMR) and non-CMR in PET after 1 month of infusion

(PET-1). Furthermore, SUVmax in PET-0 seems to be also predictive for early response. The patients with CMR in PET-1 showed significantly lower values for SUVmax (median 5.1) in their PET-0 than patients with non-CMR (median 21.2). Also Ababneh and colleagues[22] confirmed that low metabolic tumor volume (MTV) and low total lesion glycolysis (TLG) pre-CAR T are predictive of CMR post-CAR T, and they also evaluated the predictive value of pre-CAR T and post-CAR T metabolic parameters on survival, demonstrating that high TLG pre-CAR T and high MTV pre-CAR T were significantly correlated with shorter overall survival (OS) and shorter progression-free survival (PFS), but only high TLG pre-CAR T was identified to be an independent risk factor for worse PFS in multivariate analysis.

Another interesting new parameter measured recently in PET is standardized maximum tumor dissemination (sDmax), defined by the distance separating the 2 most distant FDG-avid lesions standardized on the body surface. Marchal and colleagues[23] were the first to evaluate its prognostic value before treatment with CAR T cells. In their study, sDmax was found as the only feature independently associated with OS; the median OS was significantly longer in the group of patients with sDmax of 0.15 m^{-1} or lesser compared to that of patients with sDmax greater than 0.15 m^{-1}. Differently from previous studies, TMTV was only an independent prognostic factor for progression (TMTV > 36 mL), but not for OS.

Other quantitative predicting features are those derived from texture analysis of either PET-metabolic and CT-morphologic imaging data. In this setting, Reinert and colleagues[24] investigated the value of CT-textural features and volume-based PET parameters in comparison to serologic markers for response prediction in patients with diffuse large B-cell lymphoma (DLBCL) undergoing CD19-CAR T-cell therapy. At baseline, "entropy" on CT-texture analysis was lower in patients achieving CMR compared to patients achieving partial response (PR). In contrast, "uniformity" was higher in patients with CMR compared to patients with PR, suggesting that increasing tumor tissue homogeneity in the baseline imaging could extend the chances of achieving CMR.

PET/COMPUTED TOMOGRAPHY IN RESPONSE EVALUATION AT M1 AND M3

Assessing disease status at month 1 after infusion (M1) is crucial for predicting the long-term efficacy of CAR T-cell therapy. However, interpreting PET scans at this time point can be challenging due to inflammation triggered by the CAR T cells.

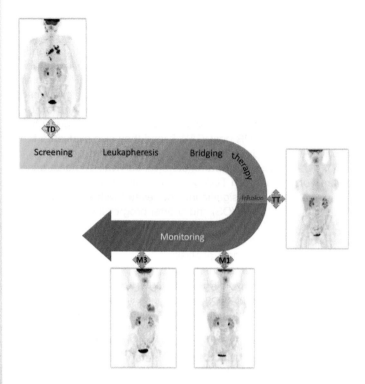

Fig. 2. Time line for CAR T-cell therapy and corresponding [^{18}F]-FDG PET/CT schedules at time of decision (TD) before leukapheresis and bridging therapy, followed by time of transfusion (TT), when CAR T cells are administered to the patient. Subsequent monitoring is performed at M1 (1 month after CAR T-cell infusion), and M3 (3 months evaluation after CAR T-cell infusion).

Patients showing disease progression at M1 are typically considered nonresponders and may require alternative options. Yet, the prognosis for patients with Deauville score 4 or 5 (DS4 or DS5) at M1 without clinical progression remains unclear. The significant interest in determining the prognostic value of early disease assessment at M1 is justified to facilitate prompt initiation of salvage therapy or other treatments. Various approaches have been undertaken to address this issue.[25–28]

Kuhln and colleagues[29] after initial PET evaluation according to the 5 point DS system, subclassified DS4 in order to distinguish between inflammatory changes after bridging radiotherapy as DS4RT. DS categories were significantly linked to the durability of response, revealing a 15% risk of early progression for DS 1/2, 32% for DS3, 37% for DS4, and 100% for DS5. While patients achieving early DS 1/2 remission demonstrated excellent long-term outcomes, those with DS3 to 4 responses faced a 31% risk of early relapse, rising to 46% for patients with DS4 when cases with radiation therapy (RT)-related activity (DS4RT) were excluded. The DS4RT group, characterized by focal uptake in RT filed, behaved similarly to DS1/2 cases regarding risk of progression, which was 10% at 6 months (M6) of 10% (vs 46% for the remaining DS4 cases). In contrast to DS4, all patients with DS5 at M1 progressed by month 3 (M3). Classifying these patients as "responders"

or "indeterminate" creates unrealistic expectations, and treatment decisions should not be delayed until formal confirmation of progressive disease (PD), especially if the disease is responsive to RT.

Alzaki and colleagues[30] evaluated patients with PR and stable disease (SD) at M1 from infusion and showed that 26% of them converted to a CMR. Among 95 patients with a D3 CR, 76% remained in CMR. The only factor at M1 associated with conversion from PR/SD to subsequent CMR was a lower SUVmax. All M1 patients with SUVmax greater than 10 ended in disease progression, with 100% sensitivity and 52% specificity.

Lutfi and colleagues[31] confirmed these findings and combined baseline and M1 parameters, showing that lower SUVmax values at M1, lower TMTV at both baseline and M1, and lower TLG at baseline are the most predictive imaging factors for CMR in patients in PR at 1 month. These results suggest that there might be inherent qualities of the tumor itself, such as FDG-avidity and metabolic volume, serving as surrogates for tumor virulence and microenvironment, which ultimately determine the outcome.

In the real-world multicenter study conducted by Galtier and colleagues,[32] the metabolic response evaluated by [^{18}F]-FDG PET/CT at M1 was found to be a significant predictor of outcome in 75% of patients. The PET/CT results, assessed using Deauville criteria with a positivity threshold set at DS5, were prognostic of both PFS and OS, with DS5 PET-positive patients having a 7 fold higher risk of PFS compared to DS 1-4 PET-negative patients. Among patients with DS4, only a minority experienced adverse outcomes, despite exhibiting high residual uptake. This suggests that residual uptake may not necessarily indicate residual tumoral activity, as observed in other lymphomas under different treatments. Most patients experiencing relapse or death were in the DS5 group, which were characterized by extremely high residual uptake, possibly reflecting the aggressiveness or microenvironmental activity of the lymphoma. Additionally, the difference in metabolic activity, calculated using ΔSUVmax with a cut-off of 70%, did not maintain its prognostic value in multivariate analysis, potentially leading to false-positive results in this population.

In the same study, PET/CT evaluation at M3 predicted PFS in 57% of the patients, but not OS, suggesting the pivotal role of early metabolic response in identifying patients with poor outcomes, which would need prompt consideration of alternative or combined treatment. Such findings align with previous trials' results, where partial responders at M3 had outcomes like complete responders.

De Boer and colleagues[33] thoroughly investigated the resemblance between CAR T-cell therapy and immunotherapy with checkpoint inhibitors, highlighting the possibility of unconventional imaging patterns like pseudo-progression and sarcoid-like reactions (SLRs) that can mimic residual/recurrent lymphoma. Through evaluation of the Dutch CAR-T tumor board and the clinical, radiological, and pathologic analyses of CD19-directed CAR-T-treated patients, 2 imaging reactions, an SLR and a histiocytic reaction (HR), were identified. They focused on patients showing [18F]-FDG PET/CT abnormalities suspected for SLR or HR during routine response evaluations post CAR T-cell therapy. Out of 236 patients, the estimated incidences of SLRs and HRs were 4.7% and 3.8%, respectively. Moreover, 49.2% of patients experienced PD following CAR T-cell therapy.

Another important aspect under evaluation is the role of lymphoid organ activity as assessed by molecular imaging. Derlin and colleagues[34] discovered that early metabolic changes in lymphoid organs between PET before transfusion CAR T cell and PET at M1 were predictive of treatment outcomes. Patients showing a significant decrease in lymphoid organ glucose metabolism, particularly in the spleen and lymph nodes, demonstrated poor responses to CAR T-cell therapy. Interestingly, the metabolic activity of Waldeyer's ring did not correlate with treatment outcomes, possibly due to its susceptibility to fluctuations driven by local immunologic responses to antigens. These findings may be associated with limited in vivo expansion of CAR T cell, or depletion of off-target CD19+ B cells, disrupting crucial immune networks for antitumor response.

BASELINE PREDICTIVE BIOMARKERS FOR IMMUNE EFFECTOR CELL-ASSOCIATED NEUROTOXICITY SYNDROME AND CYTOKINE RELEASE SYNDROME

The advancement of CAR T-cell therapy, while promising, encounters obstacles in the form of treatment-related toxicities, particularly CRS and immune effector cell-associated neurotoxicity syndrome (ICANS). CRS is often influenced by patient-related factors, such as high tumor burden, previous infections, elevated levels of C-reactive protein or ferritin, and thrombocytopenia. The other significant side effect is ICANS, affecting approximately 20% to 60% of patients, with risk factors including previous neurologic disease, organ dysfunction, older age, and severe CRS. A typical subacute progression of neurologic symptoms may manifest in patients experiencing severe ICANS, characterized by early signs, such as expressive aphasia, dysgraphia or paleography, frontal release signs, behavioral disinhibition, and apathy, which may progress to a dysexecutive syndrome, akinetic mutism, and ultimately a coma state.[35–38] However, studies have shown high rates of readmission within 30 days, predominantly due to fever. Incidences of CRS and ICANS in outpatient settings mirror those reported in pivotal trials.

The impact of tumor burden on patient outcomes has been extensively studied in patients with lymphoma, particularly in first-line treatment. The significance of the tumor growth rate (TGR) before treatment, especially TGR pre-baseline on survival outcomes after CAR T-cell therapy has recently been demonstrated. However, it is associated with occurrence of CRS, but it remains uncertain whether dynamic TGR can predict severity of CRS and ICANS.[39]

To date, significant correlation between [18F]-FDG PET/CT quantitative measurements before CAR T-cell therapy and adverse effects following infusion represents an important aspect to be evaluated. Specifically, tumor burden, as indicated by high TLG and high MTV, was correlated to the development of CRS events and associated with grade 3 or higher CRS.[20,22,23,40,41] Regarding neurologic toxicity, high MTV and SUV were correlated with any grade of ICANS and high grade of ICANS events, respectively.[22,40,42]

Another aspect that has been evaluated was how [18F]-FDG uptake of the healthy immune system structures could predict immune-related adverse events. Marchal and colleagues[23] found that hepatic SUVmean greater than 2.5 was linked to CRS grade 2 to 4, and spleen SUVmean greater than 1.9 correlated with grade 2 to 4 ICANS. Liver and spleen are known to play pivotal roles in immune function, with hepatic inflammation contributing to CRS severity.

NEUROTOXICITY IMAGING PATTERNS

The role of [18F]-FDG PET/CT imaging in diagnosing neurotoxicity is controversial. Evidence supporting frontal lobe involvement is bolstered by brain [18F]-FDG PET/CT scans, which consistently reveal prevalent frontal hypometabolism in most cases. Notably, in the first published case series, various patterns of hypometabolism were correlated with findings using different diagnostic tools. For instance, Rubin and colleagues[43] cohort demonstrated elevated flow velocities at transcranial Doppler ultrasound, which correlated with electroencephalogram (EEG) abnormalities and regional [18F]-FDG PET/CT hypometabolism, but absence of structural lesions. Within this cohort, among various PET hypometabolic patterns observed, the most prevalent finding was the presence of diffuse hypometabolism, consistently involving temporal and frontal lobes. This observation was further corroborated in the evaluation of a male patient with DLBCL experiencing ICANS, where global brain hypometabolism was evident, particularly marked in the left hemisphere and frontal regions, with significant reduction compared to a normal population. This hypometabolism was associated with diffuse slowing on EEG and unremarkable MR imaging findings.[44]

As Vernier and colleagues[45] suggested in their report, the presence of hypometabolism on PET coupled with the absence of abnormal MR imaging findings is pivotal in the evaluation of CAR T-cell neurotoxicity. Diffuse EEG abnormalities were noted in conjunction with no observable alterations on the brain MR imaging. On the 14th day post-infusion, a [18F]-FDG PET/CT brain scan was conducted, revealing bilateral and diffuse hypometabolism, predominantly in the parietal and temporal cortex, while excluding the limbic and cerebellar lobes. Four months following CAR T-cell infusion, a subsequent brain PET/CT scan showed only prefrontal and temporal hypometabolism.

Moreover, the Bologna group in the CARNON NEUTRAL protocol[46] confirmed a robust correlation between laboratory inflammatory biomarkers, clinical features of CRS, and neurotoxicity. Remarkably, all patients who experienced ICANS presented with CRS either preceding or concurrent with neurotoxicity, and severe CRS invariably led to neurotoxicity, aligning the evidence supporting cytokine-mediated neuroinflammation as the primary underlying mechanism of ICANS. EEG and brain [18F]-FDG PET/CT findings also indicated a predominant involvement of the frontal lobe through qualitative and quantitative analyses. Predominant frontal hypometabolism was defined as bilateral frontal lobe hypometabolism, either isolated or accompanied by less significant diffuse cerebral hypometabolism.

Finally, an added value of Morbelli and colleagues research[47] was the specific evaluation of brain metabolism in patients with CRS, who have not experienced ICANS. These patients showed sparser and smaller clusters of hypometabolism with a generally less prominent involvement of the frontal cortex. This less extended pattern of hypometabolism was also in keeping with the capability of [18F]-FDG PET/CT to mirror disease severity in neurocognitive disorders. In this regard, ICANS showed an extended and bilateral hypometabolic pattern mainly involving the orbitofrontal cortex, frontal dorsolateral cortex, and anterior cingulate. CRS without ICANS showed significant hypometabolism in less extended clusters mainly involving bilateral medial and lateral temporal lobes, posterior parietal lobes, anterior cingulate, and cerebellum. When compared, ICANS showed a more prominent hypometabolism in the orbitofrontal and frontal dorsolateral cortex in both hemispheres than CRS.

Another aspect to consider in this kind of studies is the suggestion by Beuchat and colleagues[48] that [18F]-FDG PET/CT functional images were primarily obtained from patients with focal neurologic symptoms or focal EEG abnormalities. This selection bias complicates interpreting whether reported hypoperfusion/hypometabolism directly relates to focal clinical findings or extends to broader neurotoxicity. It remains uncertain whether similar metabolic changes occur in patients undergoing CAR T-cell treatment without neurotoxicity.

Addressing this issue requires thorough data analysis, considering factors such as patient demographics, treatment protocols, and potential confounding variables. Comparative studies with control groups or longitudinal assessments could help clarify the relationship between metabolic changes observed on [18F]-FDG PET/CT scans and clinical outcomes following CAR T-cell therapy. Collaborative efforts and methodological rigor are essential for accurately understanding neurotoxicity and its mechanisms in this context.

SUMMARY

[18F]-FDG PET/CT stands as a cornerstone in the enhancement of patient care throughout all stages of CAR T-cell therapy. This review elucidates the substantial clinical utility of diverse biomarkers extracted from FDG PET such as glucose metabolism within tumor lesions and healthy tissues, including the liver and lymphoid structures. Prognostic and predictive markers obtained from baseline FDG PET offer insights into patient outcomes, enabling the identification of individuals who might derive long-term benefit most from CAR T-cell therapy. Early evaluations with FDG PET at 1 and 3 months posttreatment are paramount for gauging response to therapy. Furthermore, 2-Deoxy-2-[18F]fluoroglucose ([18F]-FDG) PET/CT shows potential in forecasting significant toxicities, with increasing interest in its application for brain scans to evaluate ICANS, underscoring its promise in advancing personalized treatment strategies in CAR T-cell therapy.

CLINICS CARE POINTS

- CAR T-cell therapy represents a innovative treatment approach for relapsed/refractory B-cell lymphomas.
- Imaging plays a crucial role in the assessment of CAR T-cell therapy benefit and for the identification of related adverse events.

REFERENCES

1. Viardot A, Wais V, Sala E, et al. Chimeric antigen receptor (CAR) T-cell therapy as a treatment option for patients with B-cell lymphomas: perspectives on the therapeutic potential of Axicabtagene ciloleucel. Cancer Manag Res 2019;11:2393–404.
2. Available at: https://www.fda.gov/vaccines-blood-biologics/cellular-gene-therapy-products/breyanzi-lisocabtagene-maraleucel.
3. Available at: https://www.fda.gov/vaccines-blood-biologics/cellular-gene-therapy-products/tecartus-brexucabtagene-autoleucel.
4. Available at: https://www.fda.gov/vaccines-blood-biologics/cellular-gene-therapy-products/yescarta.
5. Available at: https://www.fda.gov/vaccines-blood-biologics/cellular-gene-therapy-products/kymriah-tisagenlecleucel.
6. Linguanti F, Abenavoli EM, Berti V, et al. Metabolic imaging in B-cell lymphomas during CAR-T cell therapy. Cancers (Basel) 2022;14(19):4700.
7. Maalej KM, Merhi M, Inchakalody VP, et al. CAR-cell therapy in the era of solid tumor treatment: current challenges and emerging therapeutic advances. Mol Cancer 2023;22(1):20.
8. Fischer L, Grieb N, Platzbecker U, et al. CAR T cell therapy in multiple myeloma, where are we now and where are we heading for? Eur J Haematol 2024;112(1):19–27.
9. Rasche L, Hudecek M, Einsele H. CAR T-cell therapy in multiple myeloma: mission accomplished? Blood 2024;143(4):305–10.
10. Mullard A. FDA approves first BCMA-targeted CAR-T cell therapy. Nat Rev Drug Discov 2021; 20(5):332.
11. Xiang X, He Q, Ou Y, et al. Efficacy and safety of CAR-modified T cell therapy in patients with relapsed or refractory multiple myeloma: a meta-analysis of prospective clinical trials. Front Pharmacol 2020;11:544754.
12. Chen YJ, Abila B, Mostafa Kamel Y. CAR-T: what is Next? Cancers (Basel) 2023;15(3):663.
13. Yang J, Zhou W, Li D, et al. BCMA-targeting chimeric antigen receptor T-cell therapy for multiple myeloma. Cancer Lett 2023;553:215949.
14. Cai F, Zhang J, Gao H, et al. Tumor microenvironment and <scp>CAR-T</scp> cell immunotherapy in B-cell lymphoma. Eur J Haematol 2024;112(2):223–35.
15. Ventin M, Cattaneo G, Maggs L, et al. Implications of high tumor burden on chimeric antigen receptor T-cell immunotherapy. JAMA Oncol 2024;10(1):115.
16. Golubovskaya V, Wu L. Different subsets of T cells, memory, effector functions, and CAR-T immunotherapy. Cancers (Basel) 2016;8(3):36.
17. Cheson BD, Fisher RI, Barrington SF, et al. Recommendations for initial evaluation, staging, and response assessment of Hodgkin and non-Hodgkin lymphoma: the Lugano classification. J Clin Oncol 2014;32(27):3059–67.
18. Georgi TW, Kurch L, Franke GN, et al. Prognostic value of baseline and early response FDG-PET/CT in patients with refractory and relapsed aggressive B-cell lymphoma undergoing CAR-T cell therapy. J Cancer Res Clin Oncol 2023;149(9):6131–8.
19. Vercellino L, Di Blasi R, Kanoun S, et al. Predictive factors of early progression after CAR T-cell therapy in relapsed/refractory diffuse large B-cell lymphoma. Blood Adv 2020;4(22):5607–15.
20. Dean EA, Mhaskar RS, Lu H, et al. High metabolic tumor volume is associated with decreased efficacy of axicabtagene ciloleucel in large B-cell lymphoma. Blood Adv 2020;4(14):3268–76.
21. Iacoboni G, Simó M, Villacampa G, et al. Prognostic impact of total metabolic tumor volume in large

B-cell lymphoma patients receiving CAR T-cell therapy. Ann Hematol 2021;100(9):2303–10.

22. Ababneh HS, Ng AK, Abramson JS, et al. Metabolic parameters predict survival and toxicity in chimeric antigen receptor T-cell therapy-treated relapsed/refractory large B-cell lymphoma. Hematol Oncol 2024;42(1):e3231.

23. Marchal E, Palard-Novello X, Lhomme F, et al. Baseline [18F]FDG PET features are associated with survival and toxicity in patients treated with CAR T cells for large B cell lymphoma. Eur J Nucl Med Mol Imaging 2024;51(2):481–9.

24. Reinert CP, Perl RM, Faul C, et al. Value of CT-textural features and volume-based PET parameters in comparison to serologic markers for response prediction in patients with diffuse large B-cell lymphoma undergoing CD19-CAR-T cell therapy. J Clin Med 2022;11(6):1522.

25. Abramson JS, Palomba ML, Gordon LI, et al. Lisocabtagene maraleucel for patients with relapsed or refractory large B-cell lymphomas (TRANSCEND NHL 001): a multicentre seamless design study. Lancet 2020;396(10254):839–52.

26. Chong EA, Ruella M, Schuster SJ. Five-year outcomes for refractory B-cell lymphomas with CAR T-cell therapy. N Engl J Med 2021;384(7):673–4.

27. Schuster SJ, Svoboda J, Chong EA, et al. Chimeric antigen receptor T cells in refractory B-cell lymphomas. N Engl J Med 2017;377(26):2545–54.

28. Neelapu SS, Locke FL, Bartlett NL, et al. Axicabtagene ciloleucel CAR T-cell therapy in refractory large B-cell lymphoma. N Engl J Med 2017;377(26):2531–44.

29. Kuhnl A, Roddie C, Kirkwood AA, et al. Early FDG-PET response predicts CAR-T failure in large B-cell lymphoma. Blood Advances 2022;6:321–6.

30. Al Zaki A, Feng L, Watson G, et al. Day 30 SUVmax predicts progression in patients with lymphoma achieving PR/SD after CAR T-cell therapy. Blood Adv 2022;6(9):2867–71.

31. Lutfi F, Goloubeva O, Kowatli A, et al. Imaging biomarkers to predict outcomes in patients with large B-cell lymphoma with a day 28 partial response by 18F-FDG PET/CT imaging following CAR-T therapy. Clin Lymphoma Myeloma Leuk 2023;23(10):757–63.

32. Galtier J, Vercellino L, Chartier L, et al. Positron emission tomography-imaging assessment for guiding strategy in patients with relapsed/refractory large B-cell lymphoma receiving CAR T cells. Haematologica 2023;108(1):171–80.

33. de Boer JW, Pennings ERA, Kleinjan A, et al. Inflammatory reactions mimic residual or recurrent lymphoma on [18F]FDG-PET/CT after CD19-directed CAR T-cell therapy. Blood Adv 2023; 7(21):6710–6.

34. Derlin T, Schultze-Florey C, Werner RA, et al. 18F-FDG PET/CT of off-target lymphoid organs in CD19-targeting chimeric antigen receptor T-cell therapy for relapsed or refractory diffuse large B-cell lymphoma. Ann Nucl Med 2021;35(1):132–8.

35. Nie EH, Ahmadian SS, Bharadwaj SN, et al. Multifocal demyelinating leukoencephalopathy and oligodendroglial lineage cell loss with immune effector cell-associated neurotoxicity syndrome (ICANS) following CD19 CAR T-cell therapy for mantle cell lymphoma. J Neuropathol Exp Neurol 2023;82(2):160–8.

36. Cook MR, Dorris CS, Makambi KH, et al. Toxicity and efficacy of CAR T-cell therapy in primary and secondary CNS lymphoma: a meta-analysis of 128 patients. Blood Adv 2023;7(1):32–9.

37. Bachy E, Le Gouill S, Di Blasi R, et al. A real-world comparison of tisagenlecleucel and axicabtagene ciloleucel CAR T cells in relapsed or refractory diffuse large B cell lymphoma. Nat Med 2022; 28(10):2145–54.

38. Hayden PJ, Roddie C, Bader P, et al. Management of adults and children receiving CAR T-cell therapy: 2021 best practice recommendations of the European society for blood and marrow transplantation (EBMT) and the joint accreditation committee of ISCT and EBMT (JACIE) and the European haematology association (EHA). Ann Oncol 2022;33(3):259–75.

39. Winkelmann M, Blumenberg V, Rejeski K, et al. Predictive value of pre-infusion tumor growth rate for the occurrence and severity of CRS and ICANS in lymphoma under CAR T-cell therapy. Ann Hematol 2024;103(1):259–68.

40. Wang J, Hu Y, Yang S, et al. Role of fluorodeoxyglucose positron emission tomography/computed tomography in predicting the adverse effects of chimeric antigen receptor T cell therapy in patients with non-Hodgkin lymphoma. Biol Blood Marrow Transplant 2019;25(6):1092–8.

41. Wright CM, LaRiviere MJ, Baron JA, et al. Bridging radiation therapy before commercial chimeric antigen receptor T-cell therapy for relapsed or refractory aggressive B-cell lymphoma. Int J Radiat Oncol Biol Phys 2020;108(1):178–88.

42. Wu X, Pertovaara H, Korkola P, et al. Glucose metabolism correlated with cellular proliferation in diffuse large B-cell lymphoma. Leuk Lymphoma 2012;53(3):400–5.

43. Rubin DB, Danish HH, Ali AB, et al. Neurological toxicities associated with chimeric antigen receptor T-cell therapy. Brain 2019;142(5):1334–48.

44. Paccagnella A, Farolfi A, Casadei B, et al. 2-[18F]FDG-PET/CT for early response and brain metabolic pattern assessment after CAR-T cell therapy in a diffuse large B cell lymphoma patient with ICANS. Eur J Nucl Med Mol Imaging 2022;49(3):1090–1.

45. Vernier V, Ursu R, Belin C, et al. Hypometabolism on brain FDG-PET as a marker for neurotoxicity after

CAR T-cell therapy: a case report. Rev Neurol (Paris) 2022;178(3):282–4.

46. Pensato U, Amore G, Muccioli L, et al. CAR t-cell therapy in BOlogNa–NEUrotoxicity TReatment and Assessment in Lymphoma (CARBON–NEUTRAL): proposed protocol and results from an Italian study. J Neurol 2023;270(5):2659–73.

47. Morbelli S, Gambella M, Raiola AM, et al. Brain FDG-PET findings in chimeric antigen receptor T-cell therapy neurotoxicity for diffuse large B-cell lymphoma. J Neuroimaging 2023;33(5):825–36.

48. Beuchat I, Danish HH, Rubin DB, et al. EEG findings in CAR T-cell-associated neurotoxicity: clinical and radiological correlations. Neuro Oncol 2022;24(2):313–25.

New PET Tracers for Symptomatic Myeloma

Sambit Sagar, MD, Dikhra Khan, MD, Kanankulam Velliangiri Sivasankar, MD, Rakesh Kumar, MD, PhD*

KEYWORDS

- PET/CT • New PET tracer • Multiple myeloma

KEY POINTS

- Pentixafor, a peptide with high affinity for chemokine receptor 4, labeled with gallium-68 for PET imaging, holds promise in prognostic stratification and aiding in patient selection for radiotargeted therapy in multiple myeloma (MM).
- Daratumumab, targeting CD38, has been radiolabeled with positron emitters like zirconium-89 or copper-64, offering a potent PET tracer for MM imaging, allowing visualization of known and unknown osseous myeloma sites.
- Amino acid tracers like 11C-methionine and 18F-fluciclovine show potential in MM imaging due to their uptake mechanisms in plasma cells involved in immunoglobulin production, although 11C-methionine's short half-life poses logistical challenges.
- Choline PET, particularly with 11C-choline, demonstrates sensitivity in detecting myeloma lesions, potentially surpassing ^{18}F-fluorodeoxyglucose (^{18}F-FDG) PET. However, availability remains limited.
- Tracers like 11C-methionine and 11C-thiothymidine show enhanced sensitivity over 18F-FDG, indicating their potential for evaluating tumor growth in MM. However, studies with 18F-FLT (fluorothymidine) PET/CT have shown variable results due to high background activity within the bone marrow compartment.

INTRODUCTION

Multiple myeloma (MM) is a complex and heterogeneous disease that poses diagnostic challenges due to its varied clinical manifestations. It is characterized by the monoclonal proliferation of plasma cells leading to the production of monoclonal antibodies and end-organ damage.[1] The hallmark clinical presentation has been described as CRAB, which includes hypercalcemia, renal involvement, anemia, and bone lesions.[2] According to the latest GLOBOCON 2020 (Global Cancer Observatory) data, MM is the 23rd most common malignancy in India and the 15th most common malignancy in the United States causing 0.85% of malignancy-related deaths in the Asian subcontinent and 2.2% in the Northern American Continent.[3] The median age at diagnosis of MM is approximately 70 years.[4] There are no known associated risk factors like obesity, smoking, or alcohol consumption associated with MM,[5] and male individuals are known to be affected 1.5 times more than women globally. The revised diagnostic criteria by the International Myeloma Working Group Diagnostic Criteria for MM and related plasma cell disorders are used for diagnosis,[6] and imaging modalities including skeletal surveys are used to detect skeletal lesions.

Diagnostic Nuclear Medicine Division, Nuclear Medicine, All India Institute of Medical Sciences, New Delhi, Delhi, India
* Corresponding author.
E-mail address: rkphulia@hotmail.com

PET Clin 19 (2024) 515–524
https://doi.org/10.1016/j.cpet.2024.06.001

Conventional imaging techniques, such as radiograph, MR imaging, and computed tomography (CT), have limitations in detecting early bone lesions and assessing disease activity. PET imaging, utilizing radiotracers like 18F-fluorodeoxyglucose (^{18}F-FDG) and other novel agents (**Table 1**), has shown promise in addressing some of the limitations.[7] The 2 main staging systems applied for MM are the international staging system (ISS) and the Durie–Salmon system (DSS), and both ISS and DSS systems are known to assess the tumor burden, but neither ISS nor DSS takes into consideration the biology of the disease, which determines the overall survival (OS),[8] and to tackle that, The revised ISS was introduced, which combines elements of tumor burden (ISS) and disease biology.[9] This review explores the applications, advancements, and significance of PET in MM diagnosis and monitoring.

^{18}F-FLUORODEOXYGLUCOSE PET/ COMPUTED TOMOGRAPHY IMAGING

18F-FDG PET/CT provides valuable information about the extent of bone involvement, extramedullary disease (EMD), and metabolic activity, aiding in accurate staging and risk stratification. The integration of PET findings with other clinical and laboratory parameters enhances the precision of disease characterization.[10] 18F-FDG PET/CT has shown good sensitivity and specificity for the detection of both medullary disease and EMD.[11] 18F-FDG PET/CT helps assess the metabolic burden and activity of MM in different stages of the disease due to its ability to differentiate between metabolically active and inactive lesions, thereby guiding treatment response assessment.[12]

FLUORODEOXYGLUCOSE PET/COMPUTED TOMOGRAPHY FOR STAGING

18F-FDG PET/CT is being increasingly used as imaging modality for the whole-body assessment of MM. The reported sensitivity and specificity for the assessment of medullary and EMD extent ranges from 80% to 100%.[13–15] 18F-FDG PET/CT (**Fig. 1**) when compared to other imaging modalities has superior detection to skeletal survey or whole-body x-ray (WBXR). 18F-FDG PET/CT is comparable to MR imaging in disease staging although the sensitivity of PET/CT in the spine was inferior to MR imaging, underestimating the disease in one-third of the patients; on the contrary, 18F-FDG PET/CT had an advantage of detecting sites of active disease in areas outside the field of view of MR imaging.[16] Currently, there is a dearth of large prospective study comparing 18F-FDG PET/CT with whole-body CT. The French IMAJEM prospective study revealed no difference in the detection of bone lesions at diagnosis between PET/CT and MR imaging with the former being positive in 95% and the latter in 91% of the patients.[17] Use of whole-body CT is less favored compared to MR imaging due to higher radiation exposure. Therefore, the use of

---

Table 1
Novel targeted radiotracers explored for multiple myeloma

Type of Radiotracer	Target/Metabolism	Radiopharmaceuticals
Chemokine receptor imaging	CXCR4	[^{68}Ga]Ga-pentixafor
Integrin receptor imaging	Integrins $\alpha 4\beta 1$ (also called VL4)	^{64}Cu-CB-TE1A1P-LLP2A
Immuno PET/CT	Transmembrane glycoprotein CD38	[^{64}Cu]-daratumumab [^{89}Zr]-daratumumab
Amino-acid tracer	Amino acid metabolism	[^{11}C]methionine [^{18}F]-fluoro-ethyl-tyrosine ([^{18}F]FET) [^{18}F]-fluciclovine
Lipid tracer	Cell membrane synthesis Fatty acid metabolism Cell membrane synthesis	[^{11}C]-choline [^{11}C]-acetate [^{18}F]-fluorocholine
Nucleoside tracer	Thymidine kinase activity	[^{11}C]-thiothymidine [^{18}F-Fluorothymidine]
Miscellaneous	Bone matrix Tumor vasculature Hypoxia Anti-CD-38 antibody VEGF	[^{18}F]fluoride [^{68}Ga]Ga-PSMA [^{18}F]-FAZA [^{89}Zr]-DFO-daratumumab [^{89}Zr]-bevacizumab

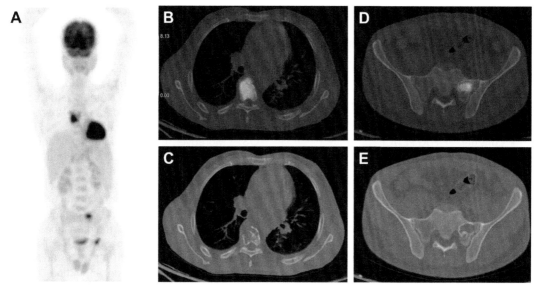

Fig. 1. A 48 year old male patient presented with bilateral lower limb neuropathy with significant weight loss. After clinical examination, patients was referred for 18F-FDG PET/CT for further evaluation. MIP (maximum intensity projection) image (*A*) shows focal FDG uptake in dorsal vertebrae, left pelvic bone. Axial images reveal lytic lesions in the D5 and D6 vertebrae (*B, C*), sacrum (*D, E*) and left acetabulum. HPE from D5 vertebrae revealed plasmacytoma. Final diagnosis of MM with the involvement of medullary component of bone was made.

low-dose CT combined whole-body FDG PET allows for the whole-body assessment along with the delineation of CT characteristics and detection of lytic lesions, their extent, and the extent of FDG avidity. In the consensus statement by the IMWG (**Table 2**), it was noted that although whole-body low-dose CT is the preferred method for the detection of lytic bone lesions in MM, FDG PET should be considered as an option, because of its ability to identify lytic lesions and extramedullary masses, and in cases with WBXR-negativity and unavailability of whole-body MR imaging, 18F-FDG PET/CT was recommended for the differentiation between active and smoldering MM.[11] In one study, 18F-FDG PET/CT was compared with PET/MR imaging, which showed comparable results for most of the parameters in terms of tracer uptake quantitation and lesion detection; however, there was a significant difference between maximum standardized uptake value (SUVmax) of lesions with 18F-FDG PET/CT being on the higher side.[18]

RESPONSE ASSESSMENT AND PROGNOSTICATION

18F-FDG PET/CT is considered the gold standard for treatment monitoring and response assessment in MM.[11] In the IMAJEM trial, the French group assessed the utility of PET/CT following induction treatment (consisting of lenalidomide, bortezomib, and dexamethasone) and before

lenalidomide maintenance in a cohort of 134 patients with MM. The study demonstrated that achieving normalization of 18F-FDG PET/CT scans after 3 cycles of induction therapy correlated with enhanced progression-free survival (PFS). Furthermore, patients who achieved normalization of PET findings before initiating lenalidomide maintenance exhibited prolonged PFS and OS compared to those who did not experience normalization of their PET results.[17] The significance of 18F-FDG PET/CT in evaluating therapeutic response at various stages of MM treatment has been underscored by the Bologna group. Specifically, their findings emphasize that the persistence of intense FDG uptake, indicated by factors such as the number of focal lesions, SUVmax, and the presence of EMD (**Fig. 2**), following thalidomide/dexamethasone induction therapy serves as an early indicator of unfavorable long-term clinical outcomes. Additionally, achieving a complete response on 18F-FDG PET/CT (**Fig. 3**) post-autologous stem-cell transplantation (ASCT) is associated with superior PFS and OS compared to cases where 18-FDG uptake persists. Notably, the prognostic value of 18F-FDG PET/CT persists even at the time of relapse, as patients with positive 18F-FDG PET/CT scans exhibit significantly shorter survival durations compared to those with negative 18F-FDG PET/CT results.[19] The same group later in a group of 282 patients showed that attainment of 18F-FDG PET/CT negativity by 3 months after the last cycle of first-line treatment (chemotherapy, novel agents with or without ASCT) significantly influenced both PFS and OS.[20] In their study, Bartel and colleagues demonstrated, for the first time, in a cohort of 239 patients with MM undergoing initial treatment with novel agents and double ASCT, that the existence of more than 3 FDG-avid focal lesions was intricately linked to biological behavior and genomics of myeloma. Notably, this factor emerged as the primary independent parameter, correlating significantly with inferior PFS and OS.[13] Moreover, the IMAJEM study underscored the independent and adverse prognostic significance of EMD for both PFS and OS in a cohort of 134 patients who underwent treatment with a combination of lenalidomide, bortezomib, and dexamethasone, either with or without ASCT, followed by lenalidomide maintenance.[17] In a study conducted by Zamagni and colleagues, involving 192 patients with MM who underwent thalidomide-dexamethasone induction therapy followed by double ASCT, the research revealed that the baseline presence of a minimum of 3 focal lesions, a SUVmax exceeding 4.2 in the hottest lesion, and the existence of EMD had detrimental effects on 4 year PFS estimates. Moreover, SUVmax exceeding 4.2 and the presence of EMD were also associated with significantly shorter OS.[19] The prognostic significance of the 3 well-established PET risk factors has been recently reaffirmed in a prospective study involving 48 patients with MM undergoing induction treatment and ASCT. Additionally, this study demonstrated that adverse PFS in the disease is not only linked to quantitative PET parameters derived from focal lesions but also extends to those obtained from reference bone marrow samples.[21] Currently, minimal residual disease (MRD) within the bone marrow is identified using either multicolor flow cytometry (MFC) or next-generation sequencing technologies.[7] In a recent retrospective study involving 103 newly diagnosed patients with MM, outcome prediction was analyzed using a combination of 18F-FDG PET/CT and MRD assessment by MFC. The study not only reaffirmed the individual benefits—specifically in terms of PFS—associated with achieving negativity by MFC and 18F-FDG PET/CT but also demonstrated that the combined negativity by both techniques significantly improved PFS compared to each method alone. This underscores the potential complementary role between PET/CT and MFC in the context of MRD detection.[22] FDG imaging has known limitations in oncological imaging due to potential false positives (arising from inflammation, postsurgical areas, recent chemotherapy use, fractures, and so forth) and false negatives (associated with hyperglycemia, recent administration of high-dose

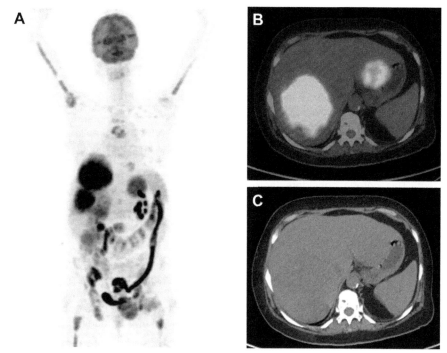

Fig. 2. FDG PET/CT of a known case of MM showing (*A, B,C*) extramedullary involvement in liver with (*A*) MIP image showing diffuse patchy marrow involvement.

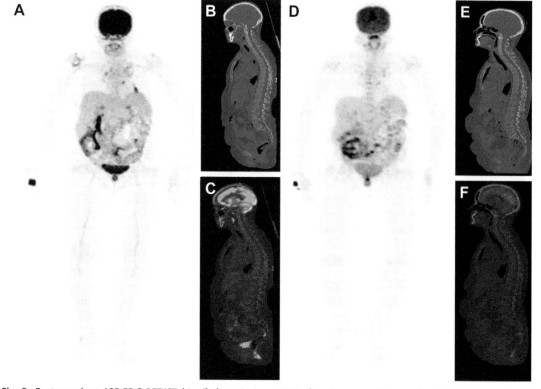

Fig. 3. Pretransplant 18F-FDG PET/CT (*A−C*) done in June 2021 showing no evidence of metabolically active disease. Posttransplant 18F-FDG PET/CT (*D–F*) done in September 2023 revealed no evidence of metabolically active disease signifying the prognostic role of 18F-FDG PET/CT in pretransplant evaluation.

steroids, and so forth). Most importantly, false-negative results for detecting skull lesions occurs, due to intense physiologic uptake in the brain that makes delineation of uptake in small lesions and low-grade lesions difficult. Challenges also arise from the absence of established criteria for interpreting 18F-FDG PET/CT scans in MM, leading to low interobserver reproducibility in result interpretation. To standardize the interpretation of 18F-FDG PET/CT, the Bologna group recently introduced the Italian Myeloma criteria for PET Use (IMPeTUs), which adopts the Deauville 5 point system. This criteria considers factors such as the number and location of focal lesions, the presence of EMD, and the extent of diffuse bone marrow involvement. Initial findings from the application of IMPeTUs indicate potential improvements in interobserver reproducibility in scan interpretation; however, further studies are required to validate these results.[23] In a retrospective series comprising 40 confirmed relapsed patients, the Nantes' group observed that the independent presence of a minimum of 6 focal lesions in the peripheral skeleton emerged as an adverse prognostic factor, influencing both PFS and OS according to multivariate analysis.[24]

OTHER PET TRACERS
Chemokine Receptor 4 (Pentixafor PET/Computed Tomography)

Expressed on hematopoietic stem and progenitor cells within the bone marrow, the chemokine receptor 4 (CXCR4) is a G-protein-coupled receptor. CXCR4 plays a crucial role in cell migration, the homing of hematopoietic stem cells back to the bone marrow, angiogenesis, and cell proliferation. Pentixafor, a peptide exhibiting high affinity for CXCR4, stands out as a highly promising tracer. It can undergo labeling with gallium-68 [^{68}Ga] for PET imaging, and alternatively, it can be labeled with a beta-emitting isotope, such as lutetium-177, for therapeutic applications. Its expression is linked to disease progression and is indicative of a poor prognosis in MM.[25] One study showed that a positive [^{68}Ga]Ga-pentixafor scan was also associated with poorer OS ($P = .009$).[26] Given the constraints posed by the limited scope of available small-scale studies, [^{68}Ga]Ga-pentixafor PET/CT may offer utility in prognostic stratification and aiding in patient selection for radiotargeted therapy as a theragnostic imaging agent. However, its value for diagnostic purposes is more uncertain, particularly considering the absence of data for assessing MRD. Eight patients with advanced-stage MM and EMD were subjected to molecular radiotherapy utilizing CXCR4 ([177Lu]pentixather). [177Lu]pentixather was administered concurrently with chemotherapy and ASCT and initial results showed that the treatment was well tolerated and demonstrated antimyeloma activity.[27]

Immuno-PET/Computed Tomography

The transmembrane integrin receptor, very late antigen 4 (VLA-4), is implicated in angiogenesis, metastasis, and resistance to chemotherapy.[28] The integrins $\alpha 4\beta 1$ (VLA-4) and $\alpha 4\beta 7$ are currently of special interest due to their crucial roles in MM cells. Recent findings indicate that integrin $\alpha 4\beta 7$ consistently adopts an active conformation in MM cells. Chimeric antigen receptor T-cell therapy targeting the activated state of integrin $\beta 7$ is emerging as a promising novel treatment approach for relapsed or refractory MM.[29]

The transmembrane glycoprotein CD38 is universally expressed on all MM cells and serves as the direct target for immunotherapy with daratumumab. For MM imaging, daratumumab has been labeled with a positron emitter like zirconium-89 or copper-64, enabling PET imaging to assess receptor status and potential to assess target and therapy monitoring.[30]

Amino Acid Tracers

Amino acid tracers hold significant appeal as biomarkers, partly because of their potential uptake mechanism in MM cells involved in immunoglobulin production. Among these tracers, [11C]methionine has been extensively investigated, revealing notable uptake in plasma cells.[31] Data indicate that [11C]methionine PET/CT exhibits greater sensitivity compared to 18F-FDG PET/CT in detecting MM lesions.[32] However, the use of [11C]methionine is constrained by its short half-life (20 minutes), necessitating on-site cyclotron production of the radiopharmaceutical.

[18F]fluoro-ethyl-tyrosine ([18F]FET) serves as an amino acid tracer employed in the diagnosis of brain tumors . Similar to [11C]methionine, [18F]FET is taken up and integrated into newly synthesized proteins. Nevertheless, data derived from cell lines indicate a comparatively low relative uptake of [18F]FET in comparison to [^{11}C]methionine and [18F]fluorodeoxyglucose ([18F]FDG). Both [11C]methionine and [18F]FDG surpass [18F]FET by 7 to 20 fold and 3.5 to 5 fold, respectively.[33]

Another amino acid tracer for PET imaging of myeloma that has recently gained attraction is [18F]fluciclovine. [18F]fluciclovine is analogous to leucine, which is Food and Drug Administration (FDA)-approved for imaging of prostate cancer and has demonstrated similar uptake patterns to [11C]methionine.[34]

Furthermore, in a recently published article by Lapa and colleagues, [11C]methionine PET was shown to outperform [11C]choline PET. In this study involving 18 patients with a history of MM and one patient with solitary bone plasmacytoma, [11C]methionine detected more intramedullary MM lesions with higher lesion-to-muscle ratios compared to [11C]choline PET.[35]

Lipid Tracers

Choline, a constituent of phosphatidylcholine, serves as an indicator of plasma membrane synthesis. It can be labeled with both ^{11}C and ^{18}F isotopes, and choline PET finds clinical utility primarily in the diagnosis of prostate cancer. Nanni and colleagues reported higher sensitivity of ^{11}C-choline PET imaging than [18F]FDG in detecting myeloma lesions.[36]

[11C]acetate PET has demonstrated superiority over [18F]FDG in detecting focal and diffuse symptomatic MM. In a study involving 35 patients with confirmed and untreated MM who underwent imaging with both [11C]acetate and [18F]FDG PET, [11C]acetate PET identified significantly more patients with diffuse and focal symptomatic MM.[37] [11C]choline/[18F]fluorocholine and [11C]acetate may play a niche role in imaging MM; however, their overall utility is not fully established and availability remain limited.

Nucleoside Tracers

Nucleoside analog tracers have been investigated as markers for evaluating tumor growth. The uptake of these tracers is indirectly associated with the rate of DNA synthesis and can reflect the high cell cycling activity within tumors.[38] Both [11C]methionine and [11C]thiothymidine demonstrate a higher number of positive lesions compared to [18F]FDG, with no significant disparities observed between the findings of [11C]methionine and [11C]thiothymidine. Some study highlights the enhanced sensitivity of nucleoside analogs in comparison to [18F]FDG.[39] Studies with ^{18}F-FLT PET/CT have shown variable results with a high background activity within the bone marrow compartment, thereby complicating the assessment of bone marrow lesions.[40]

Other Tracers

[18F]fluoride is recognized as a highly sensitive and specific radiotracer biomarker of bone remodeling. Its substantial uptake and distribution in newly diagnosed patients with MM have been proposed to hold prognostic significance.[41] Studies utilizing [18F]fluoride PET/CT for this patient population vary in methodology for assessing uptake and extent. For instance, Zedeh and colleagues employed an adaptive thresholding algorithm to automatically compute the total metabolic active volume in 37 patients with suspected treatment-demanding MM. They observed that a high metabolic active volume was linked to inferior OS.[42]

Prostate-specific membrane antigen (PSMA) can be labeled with either gallium-68 or fluorine-18 and can be imaged using PET. The ability of [^{68}Ga]Ga-PSMA to image MM has been reported, which is intriguing due to its potential use as a theragnostic pair with agents like [^{177}Lu]PSMA. However, as more specific and promising targets emerge in the imaging of MM, the value of PSMA PET may be limited and requires further evaluation. Other angiogenesis tracer like [89]Zr-bevacizumab has also been tried for MM (Clinicaltrials.gov NCT01859234).

Microvessel density has been established to correlate with disease progression in MM.[43] Leveraging this approach, de Waal and colleagues utilized the PET tracer 1-α-D: -(5-deoxy-5-[^{18}F]-fluoroarabinofuranosyl)-2-nitroimidazole (^{18}F-FAZA), which accumulates in tumor hypoxia. The authors investigated 5 patients with relapsed MM using both ^{18}F-FDG PET and ^{18}F-FAZA PET. Despite all patients showing positive ^{18}F-FDG PET scans, ^{18}F-FAZA PET did not reveal any lesions, indicative of the limited performance of this tracer in the assessment of patients with MM.[44]

The membrane glycoprotein cluster of differentiation 38 (CD38) is highly expressed by almost all myeloma cells, while its expression on normal hematopoietic cells remains relatively low. CD38 serves as a well-established therapeutic target in MM. Daratumumab, an FDA-approved therapeutic monoclonal antibody, binds directly to CD38, providing clinical benefits to patients with MM.

Daratumumab was radiolabeled with [89]Zr using deferoxamine (DFO), resulting in the PET agent [89]Zr-DFO-daratumumab. The outcomes of a phase I first-in-human study involving [89]Zr-DFO-daratumumab PET/CT imaging in 6 patients with MM demonstrated successful whole-body PET visualization of MM. Focal tracer uptake was observed in both previously known and unknown sites of osseous myeloma, consistent with effective CD38-targeted immunoPET imaging of myeloma in human patients.[45]

FUTURE PERSPECTIVE
PET/MR Imaging

PET/MR imaging technology has emerged over the years that either replaces the conventional

CT scan with MR imaging for attenuation correction or combines dedicated imaging with PET. In the context of MM, the theoretic and practical advantages of conducting single-shot simultaneous ^{18}F-FDG PET/MR imaging are considerable. However, there is a scarcity of published data on this approach to date. A preliminary retrospective study demonstrated that whole-body PET/MR imaging offered optimal diagnostic performance. Nonetheless, the study did not provide a comparison between PET/MR imaging and PET/CT. Further trials are required to assess the diagnostic and prognostic performance of PET/MR imaging in patients with MM.[46]

Radiomics and Artificial Intelligence

The potential prognostic significance of 18F-FDG PET–derived radiomics at baseline in newly diagnosed MM was recently investigated for the first time. This exploration occurred through a combined analysis of 2 independent prospective European phase III trials, utilizing a random survival forest approach.[47] Despite the inclusion of numerous image features, clinical parameters, and histopathologic data, radiomics did not feature in the final prognosis model. However, they were among the most predictive variables. Further investigations into the potential prognostic value of textural features in MM using the random-survival-forest approach are set to commence soon. This will involve a larger cohort of patients participating in the multicenter international CASSIOPET study.[48] Regarding machine learning, artificial intelligence, and radiomics, many studies are retrospective, and dealing with a small pool of patients poses challenges regarding data reliability. Data mutability becomes a significant concern in such scenarios. Furthermore, the operational performance of these systems with interlaboratory and intralaboratory variability remains largely unknown. Additionally, current artificial intelligence techniques lack transparency in their elaboration processes. Stakeholders may be unaware of how artificial intelligence techniques reached specific conclusions, leading to potential trust issues, especially when critical decisions are based on these conclusions. Consequently, the application of artificial intelligence in clinical settings of MM is still in a preliminary phase.

SUMMARY

PET has evolved as a valuable imaging modality in MM, offering improved sensitivity and specificity in initial staging, treatment response assessment, and prognostication. As technology advances and new radiotracers are developed, PET imaging is poised to play an increasingly integral role in the multidisciplinary management of MM.

DISCLOSURE

No disclosure/conflict of interest.

CLINICS CARE POINTS

- Pentixafor for Prognostic Stratification: Pentixafor, a peptide with high affinity for CXCR4 labeled with gallium-68, is promising for prognostic stratification in multiple myeloma (MM). It aids in patient selection for radiotargeted therapy, providing a potential theragnostic imaging agent for MM management.

- Daratumumab as a Potent PET Tracer: Daratumumab, targeting CD38 and radiolabeled with positron emitters like Zirconium-89 or Copper-64, offers a potent PET tracer for MM imaging. This allows for the visualization of known and unknown osseous myeloma sites, enhancing the accuracy of MM detection and monitoring.Amino Acid Tracers for MM Imaging.

- Amino acid tracers like 11C-methionine and 18F-fluciclovine show potential in MM imaging due to their uptake mechanisms in plasma cells involved in immunoglobulin production. Despite logistical challenges with 11C-methionine's short half-life, these tracers can enhance the sensitivity of MM lesion detection.

- Choline PET for Detecting Myeloma Lesions: Choline PET, particularly with 11C-choline, demonstrates higher sensitivity in detecting myeloma lesions compared to traditional 18F-FDG PET. However, the availability of this tracer remains limited, posing challenges for widespread clinical application.

- Response Assessment with FDG PET/CT: FDG PET/CT is considered the gold standard for treatment monitoring and response assessment in MM. Achieving normalization of FDG PET/CT scans after induction therapy correlates with enhanced progression-free survival (PFS) and overall survival (OS), highlighting its significance in therapeutic response evaluation.

REFERENCES

1. Jurczyszyn A, Suska A. Multiple myeloma. Encycl. Biomed. Gerontol 2019;2:461–78.

2. Michels TC, Petersen KE. Multiple myeloma: diagnosis and treatment. Am Fam Physician 2017;95: 373–83.

3. Ferlay J, Ervik M, Lam F, et al. Global cancer observatory: cancer today. Lyon, France: International Agency for Research on Cancer; 2020.

4. Palumbo A, Anderson K. Multiple myeloma. N Engl J Med 2011;364(11):1046–60.

5. Cowan AJ, Allen C, Barac A, et al. Global burden of multiple myeloma: a systematic analysis for the global burden of disease study 2016. JAMA Oncol 2018;4:1221–7.

6. Rajkumar SV. Updated diagnostic criteria and staging system for multiple myeloma. Am. Soc. Clin. Oncol. Educ. Book 2016;35:e418–23.

7. Kumar S, Paiva B, Anderson KC, et al. International Myeloma Working Group consensus criteria for response and minimal residual disease assessment in multiple myeloma. Lancet Oncol 2016;17(8): e328–46.

8. Greipp PR, Miguel JS, Durie BG, et al. International staging system for multiple myeloma. J Clin Oncol 2005;23:3412–20.

9. Palumbo A, Avet-Loiseau H, Oliva S, et al. Revised international staging system for multiple myeloma: a report from international myeloma working group. J Clin Oncol 2015;33:2863–9.

10. Zamagni E, Nanni C, Gay F, et al. 18F-FDG PET/CT focal, but not osteolytic, lesions predict the progression of smoldering myeloma to active disease. Leukemia 2016;30(2):417–22.

11. Cavo M, Terpos E, Nanni C, et al. Role of 18F-FDG PET/CT in the diagnosis and management of multiple myeloma and other plasma cell disorders: a consensus statement by the International Myeloma Working Group. Lancet Oncol 2017;18:e206–17.

12. Zamagni E, Cavo M. The role of imaging techniques in the management of multiple myeloma. Br J Haematol 2012;159:499–513.

13. Bartel TB, Haessler J, Brown TL, et al. F18-fluorodeoxyglucose positron emission tomography in the context of other imaging techniques and prognostic factors in multiple myeloma. Blood 2009;114: 2068–76.

14. Van Lammeren-Venema D, Regelink JC, Riphagen II, et al. 18F-fluoro-deoxyglucose positron emission tomography in assessment of myeloma-related bone disease: a systematic review. Cancer 2012;118: 1971–81.

15. Lu YY, Chen JH, Lin WY, et al. FDG PET or PET/CT for detecting intramedullary and extramedullary lesions in Multiple Myeloma: a systematic review and meta-analysis. Clin Nucl Med 2012;37:833–7.

16. Zamagni E, Nanni C, Patriarca F, et al. A prospective comparison of 18F-fluorodeoxyglucose positron emission tomography-computed tomography, magnetic resonance imaging and whole-body planar radiographs in the assessment of bone disease in newly diagnosed multiple myeloma. Haematologica 2007;92:50–5.

17. Moreau P, Attal M, Caillot D, et al. Prospective evaluation of magnetic resonance imaging and [18F] fluorodeoxyglucose positron emission tomography-computed tomography at diagnosis and before maintenance therapy in symptomatic patients with multiple myeloma included in the IFM/DFCI 2009 trial: results of the IMAJEM study. J Clin Oncol 2017;35(25):2911.

18. Sachpekidis C, Hillengass J, Goldschmidt H, et al. Comparison of (18)F-FDG PET/CT and PET/MRI in patients with multiple myeloma. Am J Nucl Med Mol Imaging 2015;5(5):469–78. PMID: 26550538; PMCID: PMC4620174.

19. Zamagni E, Patriarca F, Nanni C, et al. Prognostic relevance of 18-F FDG PET/CT in newly diagnosed multiple myeloma patients treated with up-front autologous transplantation. Blood 2011;118: 5989–95.

20. Zamagni E, Nanni C, Mancuso K, et al. PET/CT improves the definition of complete response and allows to detect otherwise unidentifiable skeletal progression in multiple myeloma. Clin Cancer Res 2015;21(19):4384–90.

21. Sachpekidis C, Merz M, Kopp-Schneider A, et al. Quantitative dynamic 18F-fluorodeoxyglucose positron emission tomography/computed tomography before autologous stem cell transplantation predicts survival in multiple myeloma. Haematologica 2019; 104(9):e420.

22. Alonso R, Cedena MT, Gómez-Grande A, et al. Imaging and bone marrow assessments improve minimal residual disease prediction in multiple myeloma. Am J Hematol 2019;94(8):853–61.

23. Nanni C, Versari A, Chauvie S, et al. Interpretation criteria for FDG PET/CT in multiple myeloma (IMPeTUs): final results. IMPeTUs (Italian myeloma criteria for PET USe). Eur J Nucl Med Mol Imag 2018;45:712–9.

24. Jamet B, Bailly C, Carlier T, et al. Added prognostic value of FDG-PET/CT in relapsing multiple myeloma patients. Leuk Lymphoma 2018;60:222–5. https://doi.org/10.1080/10428194.2018.1459602.

25. Vande Broek I, Leleu X, Schots R, et al. Clinical significance of chemokine receptor (CCR1, CCR2, and CXCR4) expression in human myeloma cells: the association with disease activity and survival (vol 91, pg 200, 2006). Haematologica 2007;92(1):136.

26. Kuyumcu S, Isik EG, Tiryaki TO, et al. Prognostic significance of 68Ga-Pentixafor PET/CT in multiple myeloma recurrence: a comparison to 18F-FDG PET/CT and laboratory results. Ann Nucl Med 2021;35(10):1147–56.

27. Lapa C, Herrmann K, Schirbel A, et al. CXCR4-directed endoradiotherapy induces high response

rates in extramedullary relapsed Multiple Myeloma. Theranostics 2017;7(6):1589.

28. Hatano K, Kikuchi J, Takatoku M, et al. Bortezomib overcomes cell adhesion-mediated drug resistance through downregulation of VLA-4 expression in multiple myeloma. Oncogene 2009;28(2):231–42.

29. Hosen N, Yoshihara S, Takamatsu H, et al. Expression of activated integrin β7 in multiple myeloma patients. Int J Hematol 2021;114(1):3–7.

30. Caserta E, Chea J, Minnix M, et al. Copper 64–labeled daratumumab as a PET/CT imaging tracer for multiple myeloma. Blood 2018;131(7):741–5.

31. Dankerl A, Liebisch P, Glatting G, et al. Multiple myeloma: molecular imaging with 11 C-methionine PET/CT—initial experience. Radiology 2007;242(2):498–508.

32. Morales-Lozano MI, Viering O, Samnick S, et al. 18F-FDG and 11C-Methionine PET/CT in newly diagnosed multiple myeloma patients: comparison of volume-based PET biomarkers. Cancers 2020;12(4):1042.

33. Lückerath K, Lapa C, Spahmann A, et al. Targeting paraprotein biosynthesis for non-invasive characterization of myeloma biology. PLoS One 2013;8(12):e84840.

34. Ono M, Oka S, Okudaira H, et al. Comparative evaluation of transport mechanisms of trans-1-amino-3-[18F] fluorocyclobutanecarboxylic acid and L-[methyl-11C] methionine in human glioma cell lines. Brain Res 2013;1535:24–37.

35. Lapa C, Kircher M, Da Via M, et al. Comparison of 11C-choline and 11C-methionine PET/CT in multiple myeloma. Clin Nucl Med 2019;44(8):620–4.

36. Nanni C, Zamagni E, Cavo M, et al. 11C-choline vs. 18F-FDG PET/CT in assessing bone involvement in patients with multiple myeloma. World J Surg Oncol 2007;5:68.

37. Ho CL, Chen S, Leung YL, et al. 11C-acetate PET/CT for metabolic characterization of multiple myeloma: a comparative study with 18F-FDG PET/CT. J Nucl Med 2014;55(5):749–52.

38. Agool A, Schot BW, Jager PL, et al. 18F-FLT PET in hematologic disorders: a novel technique to analyze the bone marrow compartment. J Nucl Med 2006;47(10):1592–8.

39. Okasaki M, Kubota K, Minamimoto R, et al. Comparison of 11 C-4′-thiothymidine, 11 C-methionine, and 18 F-FDG PET/CT for the detection of active lesions of multiple myeloma. Ann Nucl Med 2015;29:224–32.

40. Sachpekidis C, Goldschmidt H, Kopka K, et al. Assessment of glucose metabolism and cellular proliferation in multiple myeloma: a first report on combined 18 F-FDG and 18 F-FLT PET/CT imaging. EJNMMI Res 2018;8:1–9.

41. Czernin J, Satyamurthy N, Schiepers C. Molecular mechanisms of bone 18F-NaF deposition. J Nucl Med 2010;51(12):1826–9.

42. Zadeh MZ, Seraj SM, Østergaard B, et al. Prognostic significance of 18F-sodium fluoride in newly diagnosed multiple myeloma patients. American Journal of Nuclear Medicine and Molecular Imaging 2020;10(4):151.

43. Rajkumar SV, Mesa RA, Fonseca R, et al. Bone marrow angiogenesis in 400 patients with monoclonal gammopathy of undetermined significance, multiple myeloma, and primary amyloidosis. Clin Cancer Res 2002;8(7):2210–6.

44. de Waal EG, Slart RH, Leene MJ, et al. 18F-FDG PET increases visibility of bone lesions in relapsed multiple myeloma: is this hypoxia-driven? Clin Nucl Med 2015;40(4):291–6.

45. Ulaner G, Sobol N, O'Donoghue J, et al. Preclinical development and First-in-human imaging of 89Zr-Daratumumab for CD38 targeted imaging of myeloma.

46. Burns R, Mulé S, Blanc-Durand P, et al. Optimization of whole-body 2-[18 F] FDG-PET/MRI imaging protocol for the initial staging of patients with myeloma. Eur Radiol 2022;1:1–2.

47. Jamet B, Morvan L, Nanni C, et al. Random survival forest to predict transplant-eligible newly diagnosed multiple myeloma outcome including FDG-PET radiomics: a combined analysis of two independent prospective European trials. Eur J Nucl Med Mol Imag 2021;48:1005–15.

48. Kraeber-Bodéré F, Zweegman S, Perrot A, et al. Prognostic value of positron emission tomography/computed tomography in transplant-eligible newly diagnosed multiple myeloma patients from CASSIOPEIA: the CASSIOPET study. Haematologica 2023;108(2):621.

Symptomatic Myeloma
PET, Whole-Body MR Imaging with Diffusion-Weighted Imaging or Both

Alice Rossi, MD[a], Arrigo Cattabriga, MD[b,c], Davide Bezzi, MD[d,*]

KEYWORDS

- WB-MR imaging • Diffusion imaging • FDG PET-CT • Myeloma • Functional imaging

KEY POINTS

- At baseline, whole-body MR (WB-MR) imaging had a high rate of detection of focal and diffuse pattern of bone marrow infiltration in myeloma.
- PET/computed tomography (CT) remains the imaging modality of choice for monitoring treatment response.
- Imaging technique standardization is fundamental through Italian criteria for myeloma for PET–CT use (IMPeTUS Criteria) and WB-MRI Myeloma Response Assessment and Diagnosis System guidelines.

INTRODUCTION

The diagnosis of multiple myeloma (MM) is based on a wide range of features ("CRAB criteria") and includes hypercalcemia (C), renal failure (R), anemia (A), and the presence of one or more osteolytic bone lesions (B) on whole-body radiograph (WBXR), low-dose whole-body computed tomography (WBCT) or 18F-fluorodeoxyglucose (FDG) PET/computed tomography (CT), and pathologic evidence of bone marrow infiltration by monoclonal plasma cells or extramedullary plasmacytoma.[1] In 2014, the International Myeloma Working Group (IMWG) updated the criteria for the diagnosis of MM by adding 3 biomarkers of malignancy (SLiM criteria). SLiM criteria include 60% or greater plasma cell infiltration of the bone marrow (S), involved/uninvolved serum-free light chain ratio of 100(Li) or greater, and greater than 1 clear focal lesion (FL) on MR imaging 5 mm or greater (M).[2] Bone destruction of approximately 50% to 75% is required for bone lesions to be detected by

WBXR. For this reason, international guidelines now recommend WBCT, axial MR (Ax-MR) imaging or whole-body MR (WB-MR) imaging, and PET/CT as imaging modalities for diagnostic suspicion of MM.[3] WBCT is the first option for baseline imaging in MM according to the IMWG guidelines. However, functional imaging modalities are sensitive methods for assessing disease in bone and extramedullary disease (EMD), and they can quantify bone disease before bone damage.[4] They have therefore acquired a major role with respect to WBCT.

FLs identified by WB-MR imaging and PET/CT are focal accumulations of plasma cells and are distinct from the lytic lesions detected by low-dose CT, where bone destruction has already occurred.[3] PET/CT can be considered as an alternative to WBCT if available, and WB-MR imaging should be used if the PET/CT scan is negative or inconclusive.[3] However, recent improvements, such as diffusion-weighted imaging (DWI) with the derived quantitative apparent diffusion

[a] Radiology Unit, IRCCS Istituto Romagnolo per lo Studio dei Tumori (IRST) "Dino Amadori", Meldola, Italy;
[b] Department of Radiology, IRCCS Azienda Ospedaliero-Universitaria di Bologna; [c] Dipartimento di Scienze Mediche e Chirurgiche, Via Massarenti 9, 40138 Bologna, Italy; [d] Nuclear Medicine Unit, AUSL Romagna, Italy
* Corresponding author. Medicina nucleare di Forlì, via Carlo Forlanini, 34 - Forlì (FC)47100 - Italy
E-mail address: davide.bezzi@auslromagna.it

PET Clin 19 (2024) 525–534
https://doi.org/10.1016/j.cpet.2024.05.004
1556-8598/24/© 2024 Elsevier Inc. All rights are reserved, including those for text and data mining, AI training, and similar technologies.

coefficient (ADC) maps and bone marrow fat fraction (FF) percentage quantification using the Dixon technique, elevated WB-MR imaging to a multiparametric technique that allows both better baseline staging and response assessment in myeloma patients.[5] In the next studies, we will try to make a brief comparison between PET/CT and MR imaging, with a focus on the new potentialities of the WB-MR imaging technique, in order to analyze the available scientific data and to hypothesize their future role, probably complementary, in the MM.

18F-FLUORODEOXYGLUCOSE-PET/computed TOMOGRAPHY AND WHOLE-BODY-MR IMAGING FOR BASELINE EVALUATION AND AS PROGNOSTIC FACTORS

PET/CT and WB-MR imaging provide different and complementary functional information about the tissue under investigation. WB-MR imaging is based on the examination of the water and fat composition of tissues, whereas PET/CT is based on information from the metabolic activity of cells. The strengths of PET/CT lie in its faster acquisition times and relative simplicity of interpretation and quantification. Advantages of WB-MR imaging include its lack of pre-scan dietary requirements and of exposure to radioactive tracers. Indeed WB-MR imaging is also well accepted by patients (68.7% prefer WB-MR imaging while 7.4% PET/CT in a case history including 41.8% of myeloma patients).[6] On the other hand, the complexity of multiparametric (mp) WB-MR imaging that combines morphologic images with "functional" information leaves room for variability in its interpretation and quantification, requiring longer training and strict adherence to guidelines to ensure imaging quality (repeatability and reproducibility).[7] PET/CT allows a whole-body evaluation to be performed in one session, while ensuring a sensitivity and specificity in detecting bone damage and EMD in the range of 80% to 100%. However, the most important advantage of PET/CT is its ability to distinguish between metabolically active and inactive lesions, providing important prognostic information both at initial diagnosis and after completion of therapy.[8] Ax-MR imaging has been the reference method for the assessment of "skeletal-related events" and complications in MM. Previous studies have compared the detection rates of PET/CT and Ax-MR imaging in patients with newly diagnosed MM (NDMM),[9–11] with most of the additional lesions detected by PET/CT being outside the field of view of MR imaging. These studies have also shown that Ax-MR imaging is superior to PET/CT in the diagnosis of diffuse disease.[10,11] However, a larger prospective study of 134 patients did not find any statistically significant difference in the diagnosis of bone involvement.[12] WB-MR imaging is superior to Ax-MR imaging, inclusion of the skull, humerus, thorax, and femur in the scan helps to identify more than 50% of lesions.[13]

WB-MR imaging performed along Myeloma Response Assessment and Diagnosis System (MY-RADS) guidelines for acquisition, interpretation, and reporting in myeloma can further increase the diagnostic confidence.[14] FLs and diffuse disease (BM) present high signal intensity on high b-value DWI, pathologic ADC values due to increased cellularity and decreased fat content,[15] thus WB-MR imaging presents a sensitivity of 68% to 100% and specificity of 83% to 100% in non-treated patients.[14] Indeed, whole-body functional imaging with PET/CT or WB-MR imaging plays a key role in the identification of patients with NDMM in need of treatment. Comparison of the detectability of FLs in a recently published prospective study has shown that WB-MR imaging overall detects more FLs than FDG PET/CT and powerfully detects the BM and correlates with tumor burden and molecular markers of risk.[16] Reports agree that PET/CT appears to be superior in detecting FLs in the upper extremities, ribs, and scapulae, while WB-MR imaging appears to be better at analyzing the skull, spine, and pelvis.[16–18] Indeed, the high physiologic uptake of FDG in the brain complicates the analysis of the cranial region; within the spine, the sensitivity of PET-CT may be compromised by its lower spatial resolution; in addition, multiple millimeter lesions on WB-MR imaging may translate as diffuse uptake on PET-CT. When comparing the 2 techniques, there are 3 points that we believe need to be confirmed and validated in future studies.

First, the impact on a per-patient basis and on the clinical management of patients. It should be acknowledged that approximately 10% of patients with NDMM have "false"-negative findings on PET/CT.[19] In such patients, PET/CT is not appropriate to assess metabolic activity, and WB-MR imaging may have a complementary role. A previous large study of 227 NDMM found that around 10% of patients had positive WB-MR imaging but no apparent disease on PET/CT.[20] This phenomenon was related to the gene encoding hexokinase-2, which catalyzes the first step of glycolysis, which was significantly lower expressed in PET false-negative cases. However, the presence of disease was defined as diffuse and/or focal activity, it is unclear whether patients in this study had positive WB-MR imaging because of BM undetected by PET-CT or non-FDG-avid FLs. In addition, this subgroup of patients may have a more favorable progression-free survival (PFS) than those with positive PET/CT findings.[21] Alberge and colleagues demonstrated that normal or negative PET/CT scan results are associated with specific expression of glucose metabolism genes and with a subgroup of low-grade bone disease.[22] A recent study has shown that although WB-MR imaging had higher sensitivity than PET/CT in 40 NDMM, PET/CT had a higher impact on clinical decisions[23]; however, only a minority of patients had WB-MR imaging and DWI sequences.[24] Another prospective study on 30 patients with NDMM found that although WB-MR imaging detected more FLs compared to PET/CT, there was no difference in the diagnosis of bone disease on a per-patient basis.[17] This is in contrast to another retrospective study that reported a per-patient detection rate of bone disease of 69.6% for PET/CT versus 91.3% for WB-MR imaging.[18] However, the addition of PET/CT to the clinical data increased the number of patients treated to 40 out of 46 (87.0%) versus 43 out of 46 (93.5%) for WB-MR imaging, with no statistically significant difference in the clinical decision to treat. In a Messiou and colleagues' study, WB-MR imaging and PET/CT helped to identify at least one FL in 83% and 60% of participants, respectively.[16] However, the clinical impact was not assessed, and the inclusion criteria required that all participants had MM requiring treatment, thus limiting participants with a lower disease burden. In a recent prospective study by Jamet and colleagues (n = 52), evaluating the performance of FDG-PET/MR imaging, PET, and MR imaging was equally effective in detecting patients with FL (69% vs 75%) and BM (62% for both) in the symptomatic MM group.[25]

Second, the ability of the 2 techniques to detect paramedullary disease (PMD) and EMD, which are known to have a significant impact on patient prognosis. EMD is pathologic plasmacytomas involving only soft tissues (pleura, liver, mammary gland, lymph nodes); it differs from PMD, consisting of soft tissue plasmacytomas arising from bone lesions.[26]

In Rasche and colleagues, using WB-MR imaging, only 11 out of 23 patients with EMD according to PET-CT scans were identified. This discrepancy was mainly due to solitary PET-avid lymph nodes suspicious for EMD, which were either too small or considered nonspecific/nonreactive on WB-MR imaging.[27]

In contrast, in Chen and colleagues,[28] 23 of the 49 patients (12 with NDMM and 11 previously treated for MM) were confirmed to have PMD/EMD; 17 patients had the same number of PMD/EMD on both imaging modalities, whereas 3 patients had more lesions on WB-MR imaging and the other 3 patients had more lesions on PET/CT. WB-MR imaging appeared to have a sensitivity close to that of PET/CT and added value in detecting some non-FDG-avid EMD (spinal canal, nerve root, and abdominal lymph nodes), although it was less sensitive in detecting mediastinal lymph nodes. Furthermore, due to the small sample size, the study did not investigate WB-MR imaging detection in various organs typically reported in previous PET/CT studies, such as lung, perinephric region, spleen, breast, and adrenal gland.

In a Gomez and colleagues' study, 6 patients with MM presented with lymphatic involvement, all correctly detected by FDG-PET/CT, but only 1 by DW-MR imaging.[29] In a Messiou and colleagues' study, only 1 participant (1.7%) had EMD (pancreatic and subcutaneous) detected by both modalities.[16] However, it should be emphasized that the number of EMDs at diagnosis is estimated to be low (1.75%–4.75%), and it may be difficult to study these data in small groups.[19]

Third, the impact of WB-MR imaging results on the baseline prognostic outcome of MM compared to PET/CT is still not clear, due to the lack of direct imaging study comparing the 2 methods in this setting. Currently, PET/CT is considered first line in the baseline prognostic imaging assessment of patients. In 2 recent meta-analyses, analyzing 1690 and 2589 patients, respectively, the impact of PET/CT on prognosis was strongly confirmed. Among several PET/CT parameters, the presence of EMD, FLs more than 3, and high FDG uptake were associated with shorter overall survival (OS) and PFS. The first meta-analysis suggested that the prognostic values may not differ significantly between patients eligible for autologous steam cell transplantation (ASCT) and those not eligible for ASCT.[30,31] Recently, from a biological point of view, Rasche and colleagues suggested that in all patients with PET/CT FLs more than 3, relapse is driven by multiple surviving subclones, indicating that a higher number of PET-positive FLs at baseline are associated with a higher degree of spatial clonal heterogeneity.[32] In addition, several studies have investigated the prognostic impact of metabolic tumor volume and total lesion glycolysis, although there is no consensus on their applicability in clinical practice. The main limitation is the standardization of the criteria used to delineate the areas affected by the disease and, consequently, to quantify the tumor burden (several calculations based on fixed standardized uptake value (SUV), 40% of SUVmax, and background red marrow). On the other hand, the use of Artificial Intelligence in PET images of patients with MM could improve standardization of metabolic-volumes but is still in its early stages.[19] Regarding

Ax-MR imaging, a study in 611 patients showed that more than 7 FLs had a negative impact on OS. Furthermore, the combination of more than 7 FLs on MR imaging with cytogenetic abnormalities defined a group with a poor prognosis.[33]

These data have recently been confirmed in an independent study, although the same study found a higher threshold (>25 FLs) for patients undergoing WB-MR imaging with similar treatments.[34] Regarding WB-MR imaging, in 404 transplant-eligible patients undergoing baseline WB-MR imaging, Rasche and colleagues found that the presence of more than 3 large FLs (>5 cm^2) was a strong independent prognostic factor for PFS and OS.[27] This pattern, seen in 13.8% of patients, was independent of the Revised-International Staging System (R-ISS), gene expression profiling-based risk score, gain (1q), or EMD. One explanation is that the presence of multiple large FLs reflects an increased level of intra-patient genomic heterogeneity, which is more likely to be associated with the emergence of drug-resistant subclones. Furthermore, the ADC value is believed to reflect the cell density of MM lesions and can correlate WB-MR imaging with quantitative markers of tumor burden. A retrospective series of 380 patients with NDMM supports that ADC can stratify patients with MM and better predict their prognosis as an independent risk factor for PFS and OS (ADC <0.4886, 0.4886 ≤ ADC <0.6545, 0.6545 ≤ ADC <0.7750, and ADC ≥0.7750).[35] In addition, Kim and colleagues recently developed and proposed a semiquantitative WB-MR imaging scoring system to estimate tumor burden in patients with NDMM. In a prospective group (n = 39), the score increased with ISS stage and R-ISS stage.[36] Limitations are that it was not validated as an independent prognostic factor with prospective survival data due to the short, limited follow-up period. In our opinion, the abovementioned studies highlight the current complementary role of the 2 methods. The sensitivity of WB-MR imaging seems to play a greater role in the detection of FLs and diffuse bone marrow infiltration pattern, especially in low-risk and low-glucose expression profiles. On the contrary, PET/CT seems to play a more crucial role in the assessment of the baseline prognostic profile and should be considered as fundamental in the evaluation of EMD, given the more limited data on WB-MR imaging (Table 1).

FDG-PET/CT AND WHOLE-BODY-MR IMAGING FOR RESPONSE ASSESSMENT AND MINIMAL RESIDUAL DISEASE EVALUATION

Current guidelines suggest that PET/CT should be considered the preferred imaging modality for monitoring treatment response in MM, due to its ability to distinguish between metabolically active and inactive sites of MM.[3] But considering the MM spatial heterogeneity and the evolving patterns of relapse especially in the era of new therapeutic options, the role of WB-MR imaging should be considered.[37]

For NDMM with FLs, it is well known that normalization of PET/CT after induction and before maintenance is a positive prognostic factor for PFS and OS,[19,23,38] as the prognosis of these patients appears to be the same as that of patients without lesions at diagnosis.[39]

Homogenization and standardization of post-therapy PET/CT interpretation, in particular the refinement of the definition of complete metabolic response (CMR) and its integration into MM staging systems, are increasingly supported by the Italian criteria for myeloma for PET use (IMPeTUs). These criteria are a comprehensive evaluation including various semiquantitative parameters (SUVmax, PET-FLs, CT lytic lesions, fracture lesions, PMD/EMD disease) and are based on the 5 point Deauville scale (D5-PS), just as for lymphoma.[40]

Sachpekidis and colleagues demonstrated the reproducibility of IMPeTUs in 47 patients with NDMM[41]; a large analysis based on 2 prospective imaging substudies in 228 transplant-eligible patients with NDMM referred at baseline and at pre-maintenance, reported the results of all PET/CT scans according to the IMPeTUs criteria and used the D5-PS to describe BM (BM score [BMS]) and FLs uptake (FL score [FLS]).[42] Both FS and BMS less than 4, tested in univariate and multivariate analyses, were strong predictors of prolonged PFS and OS (FS < 4 vs >4: OS estimate at 60 months, 77.7% vs 64.1%; BMS < 4 vs >4: OS estimate at 60 months, 76.7% vs 52.1%). Recently, a sub-analysis of the multicenter, randomized phase II FORTE trial in transplant-eligible patients with NDMM (n = 109) demonstrated the applicability and validity of the D5-PS criteria to define PET CMR and its impact on post-treatment patient outcomes.[43] On the other hand, there are difficulties with conventional MR imaging in differentiating residual disease. The FLs uptake of PET/CT changes rapidly after the start of MM treatment, despite morphologic stability of MM bone lesions, the FL signal on MR imaging takes longer to normalize.[44,45]

In previous studies, PET/CT was superior to MR imaging, in fact, the latter gave more false-positive results after treatment due to residual scar or necrotic tissue.[44,45] However, these studies were limited by the lack of whole-body coverage and DWI sequences. The mp WB-MR imaging can provide not only a visual qualitative approach, but also

Table 1
Comparison of FDG-PET/CT and mp WB-MRI techniques as part of the baseline work-up

	FDG-PET/CT	Mp WB-MRI
Scanning Time	15–20 min (including radiopharmaceutical injection ~60 min)	40–60 min.
Radiation Exposure	6–15 mSv	None
Focal bone involvement	High sensitivity (more lesion detected in upper extremities, ribs and scapulae)	Highest sensitivity (more lesions detected in skull, spine and pelvis)
Diffuse Bone Marrow infiltration	Good sensitivity	Higher sensitivity (Gold standard)
EMD and PMD	Favored technique to assess EMD	Less documented (possible complementary role)
Impact on clinical decision	Less documented (need further investigations). No statistically significant difference in the clinical decision to treat. Patient acceptancy. (WB-MRI>PET/CT)	
Prognostic Value (no direct comparisons between the two techniques)	FL number, SUVmax value, presence/absence of EMD/PMD MTV and TLG	Less data are available. > 25FLs >3 large FLs (>5 cm^2) ADC value Diffuse pattern

Abbreviations: ADC, apparent diffusion coefficient; FDG PET/CT, fluorodeoxyglucose positron emission tomography–computed tomography; FL, focal lesion; mp WB-MRI, multiparametric whole-body MRI; MTV, metabolic tumor volume; SUVmax, maximum standardized uptake value; TLG, total lesion glycolysis.

a means for response assessment distinguishes the presence of active lesions from scar or necrotic inactive tissue.[14] Indeed, a comparison of ADC values and FF percentage between pretreatment and posttreatment mp WB-MR imaging may help to identify residual viable neoplasm.[46] ADC of FLs increases in patients with a biochemical response, and thus at least up to 21 weeks post-chemotherapy, whereas it is more uncertain in patients with diffuse bone disease.[47] An increase in ADC is thought to reflect tumor necrosis, tumor edema, and a decrease in cell density, whereas in late posttreatment fatty reconversion, a normalization of BM appearance and a decrease in ADC are seen.[48] However, ADC cut-off values may be influenced by the timing of measurement (in previous studies assessed early at 3 or 8 weeks or later between 13 and 21 weeks after chemotherapy), the study population (NDMM or treated MM), or the choice of b-values for diffusion sequences, and the optimal timing after treatment has not been established.[49]

Of note, a recent meta-analysis confirmed that a 35% increase in ADC from baseline values is found to classify response after induction chemotherapy.[50] Furthermore, treatment response evaluation and ADCmean value changes across different studies, based on a systematic literature review by Torkian and colleagues,[51] also showed that WB-MR imaging had a pooled sensitivity of 78% (95% CI: 72–83) and specificity of 73% (95% CI: 61–83) in distinguishing responders from nonresponders, highlighting the potential role of mp WB-MR imaging. When comparing PET/CT and mp WB-MR imaging, there are some key points that need to be validated and confirmed in future studies.

First, as with the PET-Impetus criteria, it is crucial to standardize and homogenize the interpretation of post-therapy WB-MR imaging and its integration in the assessment of minimal residual disease (MRD). To this end, the MY-RADS criteria have recently been published, providing a classification of the probability of response or progression.[14] These criteria differ from the IMPeTUs criteria, which provided a dichotomized classification of response. They are set on a 5 point scale of response assessment criteria (RAC) defining the probability of a response on imaging (RAC 1 and 2), stable disease (RAC 3), or progressive disease (RAC 4 and 5). These criteria need to be validated in further clinical trials, including assessment of repeatability and reproducibility. In this setting, few studies published so far provide promising data about both ADC and FF.[52,53] Belotti and colleagues[54] successfully applied the MY-RADS criteria to a population of 64 patients with consecutive MM undergoing first-line therapy. Notably, Heidemeier and colleagues recently proposed a multi-parametric assessment incorporating information from DWI, T2-weighted images, and FF. The study found substantial agreement between mp WB-MR imaging lesion classification and PET assessment based on a semiautomatically calculated 5 point scoring system analogous to the Deauville scores.[55]

Second, there is an enormous need for prospective data about the comparison between WB-MR imaging and PET/CT in the assessment of response to therapy, especially regarding the accuracy of both methods and their prognostic value.

A recent meta-analysis (n = 373) evaluating the diagnostic accuracy of WB-MR imaging and PET/CT suggested that PET/CT had a higher specificity, whereas WB-MR imaging had a higher sensitivity, although the latter was not statistically significant. Sensitivity and specificity were 93% and 57% for DWI versus 74% and 56% for WB-MR imaging without DWI, versus 66% and 81% for PET/CT.[56] However, the data were limited by the small numbers and the meta-analysis highlighted the need for larger prospective studies.

In Rasche and colleagues,[57] the predictive value of only WB-MR imaging positive at relapse was similar to that of PET/CT positive, with a non-statistically significant tendency of the latter to be superior (median PFS 3.4 vs 3.0 years, P = .2). By contrast, a prospective study of 30 patients with NDMM following induction-chemotherapy and ASCT found that PET/CT was significantly associated with PFS at both times, while mp WB-MR imaging showed no value as a prognostic factor.[58]

Third, the role of WB-MR imaging compared to PET/CT in the assessment of MRD. MRD negativity is a robust prognostic indicator in MM.[59] For this reason, the IMWG has introduced new response criteria with the addition of MRD in disease assessment both in the bone marrow (BM-MRD, by modern biological diagnostic tool) and in extramedullary sites (by functional imaging).[1] FDG-PET is considered a first-line imaging modality for its metabolic prognostic value and accuracy in assessing response to therapy. The creation of patient groups MRD-PET- (double negative), MRD +- PET+- (either positive), and MRD + PET+ (both positive) showed a more refined prognostic stratification in terms of PFS and OS.[60,61]

Fonseca and colleagues showed, in a retrospective study (n = 186), that MRD + PET + patients may represent a subcohort with more aggressive disease, while patients with MRD-PET disease at day 100 after treatment had a significantly longer time to next treatment.[62] A recent sub-analysis of the randomized phase II FORTE trial confirmed the prognostic role of double-negative patients, which showed significantly prolonged PFS in univariate and multivariate analysis. Notably, the BM-MRD negativity rate was higher in patients with negative PET (91%) than in patients with positive PET (50%).[43] Recently, an expert panel published recommendations to improve the quality of MRD research worldwide. PET-CT is the recommended functional imaging modality; however, it is noted that a possible WB-MR imaging complementary role in the future cannot be excluded.[63] Indeed, in Belotti and colleagues' retrospective study (n = 64), the 3 year post-ASCT survival rate was 92% versus 69% for RAC1 versus RAC of 2 or greater, confirming DW-MR imaging prognostic value. Combining DW-MR imaging and BM-MRD, 3 subgroups of patients were identified (RAC1 and MRD– vs RAC $\geq$2 and MRD + vs RAC1/MRD + or RAC $\geq$2/MRD–) with a significantly different outcome. In particular, a significantly better PFS was observed in patients with RAC1 and MRD negativity before maintenance compared to patients with RAC of 2 or greater and MRD-positive results.[54] The retrospective nature of the observations and the relatively small number of patients were limitations of the study. In parallel with PET/CT, the potential role of WB-MR imaging was investigated by Rasche and colleagues, who performed BM-MRD, PET/CT, and WB-MR imaging (without standardized reading criteria) in 168 patients who achieved CR after first-line or salvage treatment.[57] Fewer patients had residual FLs on FDG-PET/CT (21% of MR imaging vs 6% of PET/CT); however, there were 5 patients with FLs on PET alone, suggesting that the 2 techniques are complementary.

Bocke and colleagues included 102 patients with NDMM (n = 57) and relapsed/refractory MM (RRMM) (n = 45) in a single-center observation. PET/CT and WB-MR imaging were performed independently of BM-MRD results (in 78 patients, 39 PET/CT, 36 MR imaging, 3 PET/CT + MR imaging). Patients who did not achieve an optimal serologic response or MRD negativity by BM and imaging were offered an individualized consolidation approach. Functional imaging added to BMD-MRD assessment was helpful in tailoring treatment, with a greater impact on patients with RRMM compared to those with NDMM.[64] Indeed, even if PET/CT is the first choice; WB-MR imaging is a promising tool for the detection of MRD and seems to have a complementary role. Performing functional imaging in first-line therapy patients should be crucial for the detection of double-positive patients (BM-MRD + imaging+), who are associated with a particularly poor outcome, and for the detection of residual FLs/EMD in BM-MRD-negative patients (**Table 2**).

Table 2
Main characteristics of FDG PET/CT and mp WB-MRI for MM evaluation of response to treatment

	FDG-PET/CT	mp WB-MRI
Standardisation and reproducibility	Impetus criteria (CMR = disease uptake less than the liver uptake)	MY-RADS criteria (Probability of response or progression with morphologic images and "functional" information)
Diagnostic accuracy	Need of more comparative data. FDG-PET CT (Higher Specificity) mpWBMRI (probable higher sensitivity)	
FL signal change	Early changes (as soon as 7 d post-therapy)	Early changes (as soon as 21 d post-therapy)
Prognostic value (post-ASCT)	Gold Standard (reproduced in large prospective independent studies)	Lack of Data. Possibly less prognostic than FDG-PET/CT but need further investigations.
MRD evaluation	Gold Standard Defines the imaging MRD-negative/positive response category	Lack of Data. Initial promising results (Complementary role)

Abbreviations: ASCT, autologous stem cell transplant; CMR, complete metabolic response; FDG PET/CT, fluorodeoxyglucose positron emission tomography–computed tomography; FL, focal lesion; mpWB-MRI, multiparametric whole-body MRI.

SUMMARY

The precise future role and integration of the 2 imaging techniques are not so easy to predict.

While MR imaging is used for diagnosis due to its higher sensitivity and usefulness in detecting myeloma-defining events, FDG PET/CT is advised as the preferred modality for evaluating treatment response. The value of WB-MR imaging as a prognostic factor appears to be lower than that of FDG-PET/CT, although early results suggest a possible complementary role between the two techniques and larger studies are needed. The mp WB-MR imaging allows to obtain the maximum sensitivity of the MR imaging through DWI sequences and the maximum specificity of the modality by combining DWI data with morphologic sequences, ADC, and FF maps. On the PET/CT side, the importance of new and alternative radiotracers acting as potentially more sensitive and specific molecular imaging biomarkers than FDG, such as 11C-methionine or the CXCR4-targeting PET tracer, should be highlighted.[65] In addition, the recent advent of new PET/CT scanners, which allow dynamic studies collecting, will make dynamic PET/CT a possible tool to complement the information offered by conventional imaging.[66,67] Finally, new hybrid simultaneous PET/MR imaging has emerged recently; it might improve FLs detection and initial staging in patients with MM and might also help to guide treatment.[25,68] Nonetheless, further studies are needed to specify both the optimal imaging protocol in both staging and posttreatment evaluation and the standard hybrid interpretation, especially in case of discordance between MR imaging and PET.

CLINICS CARE POINTS

- Both PET/CT and WB-MR are able to identify focal lesion and diffuse pattern before osteolytic damage. In this context DWI and FF sequences should be part of WB-MR protocol, avoiding contrast media injection.

- Red marrow reconversion may occur in association with chemotherapy, anaemia, bone marrow stimulating factors or multiple factors. This may lead to false-positive results on WBMRI or FDG-PET/CT as it mimics diffuse infiltration.

- 18F-FDG can accumulate in coexisting infectious or inflammatory disorders, degenerative joints, recent benign fracture sites or other benign conditions, leading to false-positive results.

- Approximately 10% of the patients with NDMM revealed "false" negative findings on PET/CT in those who had the low expression of hexokinase-2. In such patients, FDG-PET/CT is not appropriate to evaluate metabolic response to therapy.

- Not all hyperintense bone lesions on high b-value images are malignant (e.g, artifacts around metal implants, bone infarcts, vertebral hemangiomas, chondromas, focal fat poor bone marrow...). To avoid misinterpretations it is essential to correlate high b-value DWI findings with morphological sequences, ADC and FF maps. Better standardisation of the technique by certifying MY-RADS, could further improve the accuracy.

- Bone marrow MRD (BM MRD) might lead to false negative results (spatial and heterogeneous infiltration of BM with false-negative results in the biopsy , extramedullary disease). For all these reasons, it has to be combined with functional imaging, however the future impact of functional imaging on clinical decisions has yet to be clarified.

DISCLOSURE

The authors have nothing to disclose.

REFERENCES

1. Kumar S, Paiva B, Anderson KC, et al. International myeloma working group consensus criteria for response and minimal residual disease assessment in multiple myeloma. Lancet Oncol 2016;17:e328–46.
2. Rajkumar SV, Dimopoulos MA, Palumbo A, et al. International Myeloma Working Group updated criteria for the diagnosis of multiple myeloma. Lancet Oncol 2014;15(12):e538–48.
3. Hillengass J, Usmani S, Rajkumar SV, et al. International myeloma working group consensus recommendations on imaging in monoclonal plasma cell disorders. Lancet Oncol 2019;20:e302–12.
4. Basha MAA, Hamed MAG, Refaat R, et al. Diagnostic performance of 18F-FDG-PET/CT and whole-body MRI before and early after treatment of multiple myeloma: a prospective comparative study. Jpn J Radiol 2018;36:382–93.
5. Summers P, Saia G, Colombo A, et al. Whole-body magnetic resonance imaging: technique, guidelines and key applications. Ecancermedicalscience 2021;15:1164.
6. Rossi A, Prochowski Iamurri A, Diano D, et al. Patient centered radiology: investigating 3 Tesla whole body MRI acceptance in cancer patients. Radiol Med 2023;128(8):960–9.
7. Barnes A, Alonzi R, Blackledge M, et al. UK quantitative WB-DWI technical workgroup: consensus meeting recommendations on optimisation, quality control, processing and analysis of quantitative whole-body diffusion-weighted imaging for cancer. Br J Radiol 2018;91(1081):20170577.
8. Cavo M, Terpos E, Nanni C, et al. Role of 18F-FDG-PET/CT in the diagnosis and management of multiple myeloma and other plasma cell disorders: a consensus statement by the International Myeloma Working Group. Lancet Oncol 2017;18:e206–17.
9. Fonti R, Salvatore B, Quarantelli M, et al. 18F-FDG PET/CT, 99mTc-MIBI, and MRI in evaluation of patients with multiple myeloma. J Nucl Med 2008;49:195–200.
10. Spinnato P, Bazzocchi A, Brioli A, et al. Contrast enhanced MRI and (1)(8)F-FDG PET-CT in the assessment of multiple myeloma: a comparison of results in different phases of the disease. Eur J Radiol 2012;81:4013–8.
11. Zamagni E, Nanni C, Patriarca F, et al. A prospective comparison of 18F-fluorodeoxyglucose positron emission tomography-computed tomography, magnetic resonance imaging and whole-body planar radiographs in the assessment of bone disease in newly diagnosed multiple myeloma. Haematologica 2007;92:50–5.
12. Moreau P, Attal M, Karlin L, et al. Prospective evaluation of MRI and PET-CT at diagnosis and before maintenance therapy in symptomatic patients with multiple myeloma included in the IFM/DFCI 2009 Trial. Blood 2015;126:395.
13. Bauerle T, Hillengass J, Fechtner K, et al. Multiple myeloma and monoclonal gammopathy of undetermined significance: importance of whole-body versus spinalMR imaging. Radiology 2009;252:477–85.
14. Messiou G, Hillengass J, Delorme S, et al. Guidelines for acquisition, interpretation, and reporcing of whole-body MRI in myeloma: myeloma response assessment and diagnosis system (MY-RADS). Radiology 2019;291(1):5–13.
15. Castagnoli F, Donners R, Tunariu N, et al. Relative fat fraction of malignant bone lesions from breast cancer, prostate cancer and myeloma are significantly lower than normal bone marrow and shows excellent interobserver agreement. Br J Radiol 2023;96(1152):20230240.
16. Messiou C, Porta N, Sharma B, et al. Prospective evaluation of whole-body MRI versus FDG PET/CT for lesion detection in participants with myeloma. Radiol Imaging Cancer 2021;3(5):e210048.
17. Mesguich C, Hulin C, Latrabe V, et al. Prospective comparison of 18-FDG PET/CT and whole-body diffusionweighted MRI in the assessment of multiple myeloma. Ann Hematol 2020;99:2869–80.
18. Westerland O, Amlani A, Kelly-Morland C, et al. Comparison of the diagnostic performance and impact on management of 18F-FDG PET/CT and whole-body MRI in multiple myeloma. Eur J Nucl Med Mol Imaging 2021;48:2558–65.
19. Bezzi D, Ambrosini V, Nanni C. Clinical value of FDG-PET/CT in multiple myeloma: an update. Semin Nucl Med 2023;53(3):352–70.
20. Rasche L, Angtuaco E, McDonald JE, et al. Low expression of hexokinase-2 is associated with false-negative FDG-positron emission tomography in multiple myeloma. Blood 2017;130(1):30–4.

21. Abe Y, Ikeda S, Kitadate A, et al. Low hexokinase-2 expression-associated false-negative (18)F-FDG-PET/CT as a potential prognostic predictor in patients with multiple myeloma. Eur J Nucl Med Mol Imaging 2019;46:1345–50.

22. Alberge JB, Kraeber-Bodere F, Jamet B, et al. Molecular signature of 18F-FDG-PET biomarkers in newly diagnosed multiple myeloma patients: a genome-wide transcriptome analysis from the CASSIOPET study. J Nucl Med 2022;63:1008–13.

23. Zamagni E, Nanni C, Mancuso K, et al. PET/CT improves the definition of complete response and allows to detect otherwise unidentifiable skeletal progression in multiple myeloma. Clin Cancer Res 2015;21(19):4384–90.

24. Lecouvet FE, Boyadzhiev D, Collette L, et al. MRI versus (18)F-FDG-PET/CT for detecting bone marrow involvement in multiple myeloma: diagnostic performance and clinical relevance. Eur Radiol 2020;30:1927–37.

25. Jamet B, Carlier T, Bailly C, et al. Hybrid simultaneous whole-body 2-[18F]FDG-PET/MRI imaging in newly diagnosed multiple myeloma: first diagnostic performance and clinical added value results. Eur Radiol 2023;33(9):6438–47.

26. Rosinol L, Beksac M, Zamagni E, et al. Expert review on soft-tissue plasmacytomas in multiple myeloma: definition, disease assessment and treatment considerations. Br J Haematol 2021;194:496–507.

27. Rasche L, Angtuaco EJ, Alpe TL, et al. The presence of large focal lesions is a strong independent prognostic factor in multiple myeloma. Blood 2018; 132(1):59–66.

28. Chen J, Li C, Tian Y, et al. Comparison of whole-body DWI and 18F-FDG PET/CT for detecting intramedullary and extramedullary lesions in multiple myeloma. AJR Am J Roentgenol 2019;213(3):514–23.

29. Gómez León N, Aguado BB, Herreros PM, et al. Agreement between 18F-FDG PET/CT and whole-body magnetic resonance compared with skeletal survey for initial staging and response at end-of-treatment evaluation of patients with multiple myeloma. Clin Nucl Med 2021;46(4):310–22.

30. Han S, Woo S, Kim YI, et al. Prognostic value of 18F-fluorodeoxyglucose positron emission tomography/computed tomography in newly diagnosed multiple myeloma: a systematic review and meta-analysis. Eur Radiol 2021;31:152–62.

31. Li Q, Hu L, Charwudzi A, et al. Prognostic value of ^{18}F-fluorodeoxyglucose positron emission tomography/computed tomography at diagnosis in untreated multiple myeloma patients: a systematic review and meta-analysis. Clin Exp Med 2023; 23(1):31–43.

32. Rasche L, Schinke C, Maura F, et al. The spatio-temporal evolution of multiple myeloma from baseline to relapse-refractory states. Nat Commun 2022;13:4517.

33. Walker R, Barlogie B, Haessler J, et al. Magnetic resonance imaging in multiple myeloma: diagnostic and clinical implications. J Clin Oncol 2007;25: 1121–8.

34. Mai EK, Hielscher T, Kloth JK, et al. A magnetic resonance imaging-based prognostic scoring system to predict outcome in transplant-eligible patients with multiple myeloma. Haematologica 2015; 100:818–25.

35. Zhang B, Bian B, Zhang Y, et al. The apparent diffusion coefficient of diffusion-weighted whole-body magnetic resonance imaging affects the survival of multiple myeloma independently. Front Oncol 2022; 12:780078.

36. Kim DK, Jung JY, Kim H, et al. Development of a semi-quantitative whole-body MRI scoring system for multiple myeloma. Radiology 2023;308(3):e230667.

37. Latifoltojar A, Boyd K, Riddell A, et al. Characterising spatial heterogeneity of multiple myeloma in high resolution by whole body magnetic resonance imaging: towards macro-phenotype driven patient management. Magn Reson Imaging 2021;75:60–4.

38. Charalampous C, Goel U, Broski SM, et al. Utility of PET/CT in assessing early treatment response in patients with newly diagnosed multiple myeloma. Blood Adv 2022;6:2763–72.

39. Davies FE, Rosenthal A, Rasche L, et al. Treatment to suppression of focal lesions on positron emission tomography-computed tomography is a therapeutic goal in newly diagnosed multiple myeloma. Haematologica 2018;103:1047–53.

40. Nanni C. PET-FDG: impetus. Cancers (Basel) 2020; 12:1030.

41. Sachpekidis C, Merz M, Raab MS, et al. The prognostic significance of [18F] FDG-PET/CT in multiple myeloma according to novel interpretation criteria (IMPeTUs). EJNMMI Res 2021;11:100.

42. Zamagni E, Nanni C, Dozza L, et al. Standardization of 18F-FDG-PET/CT according to deauville criteria for metabolic complete response definition in newly diagnosed multiple myeloma. J Clin Oncol 2021;39: 116–25.

43. Zamagni E, Oliva S, Gay F, et al. Impact of minimal residual disease standardised assessment by FDG-PET/CT in transplant-eligible patients with newly diagnosed multiple myeloma enrolled in the imaging sub-study of the FORTE trial. EClinicalMedicine 2023;60:102017.

44. Derlin T, Peldschus K, Munster S, et al. Comparative diagnostic performance of (1)(8)F-FDG PET/CT versus whole-body MRI for determination of remission status in multiple myeloma after stem cell transplantation. Eur Radiol 2013;23:570–8.

45. Moreau P, Attal M, Caillot D, et al. Prospective evaluation of magnetic resonance imaging and [(18)F] fluorodeoxyglucose positron emission tomography-computed tomography at diagnosis and before

maintenance therapy in symptomatic patients with multiple myeloma included in the IFM/DFCI 2009 Trial: results of the IMAJEM study. J Clin Oncol 2017;35:2911–8.

46. Koutoulidis V, Terpos E, Papanikolaou N, et al. Comparison of MRI features of fat fraction and ADC for early treatment response assessment in participants with multiple myeloma. Radiology 2022;304(1):137–44.

47. Mesguich C, Hulin C, Latrabe V, et al. 18F-FDG PET/CT and MRI in the management of multiple myeloma: a comparative review. Front. Nucl. Med 2022;1:808627.

48. Ormond Filho AG, Carneiro BC, Pastore D, et al. Whole-body imaging of multiple myeloma: diagnostic criteria. Radiographics 2019;39(4):1077–97.

49. Wu C, Huang J, Xu W-B, et al. Discriminating depth of response to therapy in multiple myeloma using whole-body diffusion-weighted MRI with apparent diffusion coefficient. Acad Radiol 2018;25:904–14.

50. Wang K, Lee E, Kenis S, et al. Application of diffusion-weighted whole-body MRI for response monitoring in multiple myeloma after chemotherapy: a systematic review and meta-analysis. Eur Radiol 2022;32:2135–48.

51. Torkian P, Mansoori B, Hillengass J, et al. Diffusion-weighted imaging (DWI) in diagnosis, staging, and treatment response assessment of multiple myeloma: a systematic review and meta-analysis. Skeletal Radiol 2023;52:565–83.

52. Barwick T, Orton M, Koh DM, et al. Repeatability and reproducibility of apparent diffusion coefficient and fat fraction measurement of focal myeloma lesions on whole body magnetic resonance imaging. Br J Radiol 2021;94(1120):20200682.

53. Michoux NF, Ceranka JW, Vandemeulebroucke J, et al. Repeatability and reproducibility of ADC measurements: a prospective multicenter whole-body-MRI study. Eur Radiol 2021;31(7):4514–27.

54. Belotti A, Ribolla R, Cancelli V, et al. Predictive role of diffusion-weighted whole-body MRI (DW-MRI) imaging response according to MY-RADS criteria after autologous stem cell transplantation in patients with multiple myeloma and combined evaluation with MRD assessment by flow cytometry. Cancer Med 2021;10(17):5859–65.

55. Heidemeier A, Schloetelburg W, Thurner A, et al. Multi-parametric whole-body MRI evaluation discerns vital from non-vital multiple myeloma lesions as validated by 18F-FDG and 11C-methionine PET/CT. Eur J Radiol 2022;155:110493.

56. Rama S, Suh CH, Kim KW, et al. Comparative performance of whole-body MRI and FDG PET/CT in evaluation of multiple myeloma treatment response: systematic review and meta-analysis. AJR Am J Roentgenol 2022;218(4):602–13.

57. Rasche L, Alapat D, Kumar M, et al. Combination of flow cytometry and functional imaging for monitoring of residual disease in myeloma. Leukemia 2019;33(7):1713–22.

58. Mesguich C, Latrabe V, Hulin C, et al. Prospective comparison of 18-FDG PET/CT and whole-body MRI with diffusion-weighted imaging in the evaluation of treatment response of multiple myeloma patients eligible for autologous stem cell transplant. Cancers (Basel) 2021;13:1938.

59. Bravo-Perez C, Sola M, Teruel-Montoya R, et al. Minimal residual disease in multiple myeloma: something old, something new. Cancers (Basel) 2021;13:4332.

60. Alonso R, Cedena MT, Gomez-Grande A, et al. Imaging and bone marrow assessments improve minimal residual disease prediction in multiple myeloma. Am J Hematol 2019;94:853–61.

61. Jamet B, Zamagni E, Nanni C, et al. Functional imaging for therapeutic assessment and minimal residual disease detection in multiple myeloma. Int J Mol Sci 2020;21:5406, 29.

62. Fonseca R, Arribas M, Wiedmeier-Nutor JE, et al. Integrated analysis of next generation sequencing minimal residual disease (MRD) and PET scan in transplant eligible myeloma patients. Blood Cancer J 2023;13(1):32.

63. Costa LJ, Derman BA, Bal S, et al. International harmonization in performing and reporting minimal residual disease assessment in multiple myeloma trials. Leukemia 2021;35:18–30.

64. Bockle D, Tabares P, Zhou X, et al. Minimal residual disease and imaging-guided consolidation strategies in newly diagnosed and relapsed refractory multiple myeloma. Br J Haematol 2022;198:515–22.

65. von Hinten J, Kircher M, Dierks A, et al. Molecular imaging in multiple myeloma—novel PET radiotracers improve patient management and guide therapy. Front. Nucl. Med 2022;2:801792.

66. Wu Y, Sun X, Zhang B, et al. Marriage of radiotracers and total-body PET/CT rapid imaging system: current status and clinical advances. Am J Nucl Med Mol Imaging 2023;13(5):195–207.

67. Sachpekidis C, Hillengass J, Goldschmidt H, et al. Treatment response evaluation with 18F-FDG PET/CT and 18F-NaF PET/CT in multiple myeloma patients undergoing high-dose chemotherapy and autologous stem cell transplantation. Eur J Nucl Med Mol Imaging 2017;44:50–62.

68. Burns R, Mule S, Blanc-Durand P, et al. Optimization of whole-body 2- [18F]FDG-PET/MRI imaging protocol for the initial staging of patients with myeloma. Eur Radiol 2022;32:3085–96.

Applications of 18F-Fluorodesoxyglucose PET Imaging in Leukemia

Francesco Dondi, MD[a],*, Francesco Bertagna, MD[a]

KEYWORDS

- PET • PET/CT • 18F FDG • Leukemia • Richter's transformation • Acute leukemia
- Chronic leukemia

KEY POINTS

- PET with 18F-Fluorodesoxyglucose (18F FDG-PET) imaging is able to evaluate leukemia, in particular those with high proliferating behavior such as acute leukemia.
- Chronic leukemia could be characterized by the presence of low 18F FDG uptake; however, PET imaging is able to drive the diagnosis and assess the presence of Richter's transformation.
- 18F FDG-PET imaging has a clear value in identifying the site of bone marrow involved in the disease that can be further analyzed with biopsy.
- 18F FDG-PET imaging can help in the diagnosis of leukemia in patients with unspecific symptoms, and also to assess the response to therapy and the presence of relapse.

INTRODUCTION

The term leukemia refers to a wide class of malignant clonal hematologic malignancies that arise from hematopoietic stem cells and infiltrate the bone marrow (BM), resulting in either focal or diffuse marrow replacing that can lead to an inhibition of its normal hematopoietic function. Moreover, other hemopoietic tissues and organs can be interested by neoplastic infiltration with specific symptoms that can arise. Leukemia is the third most common hematologic malignancy after lymphoma and multiple myeloma (MM) and it is the most frequent form of cancer in children, accounting roughly for 40% of all neoplasms.[1–4]

Different types of leukemia can be described and classified according to the differentiation, the speed of disease progression, and the maturity of the cells involved in the process. This classification has fundamental implications since every class of leukemia has different clinical course and prognosis. In general, leukemia can be divided into acute leukemia (AL) and chronic leukemia (CL) depending on the speed of cellular proliferation and therefore of their clinical onset. Generally speaking, the 4 main types of leukemia are acute lymphoblastic leukemia (ALL), acute myeloblastic leukemia (AML), chronic lymphoblastic leukemia (CLL) and chronic myeloblastic leukemia.[1] Interestingly, CLL is the most frequent form in elderly patients, while ALL is more frequent in the pediatric population. Nevertheless, there also other rare types of leukemia such as hairy cell leukemia, acute promyelocytic leukemia, and T-cell prolymphocytic leukemia.[5]

The correct diagnosis of leukemia is mandatory to start specific therapy and in the case of aggressive forms, such as AL or when Richter's transformation (RT) of CLL is present, the clear assessment of the disease needs to be quickly and early determined in order to have a prognostic impact on the patients. In this setting, blood

a Nuclear Medicine, Department of Medicine and Surgery, Università degli Studi di Brescia and ASST Spedali Civili di Brescia, Brescia, 25123, Italy
* Corresponding author.
E-mail address: francesco.dondi@unibs.it

PET Clin 19 (2024) 535–542
https://doi.org/10.1016/j.cpet.2024.05.007
1556-8598/24/© 2024 Elsevier Inc. All rights are reserved, including those for text and data mining, AI training, and similar technologies.

examinations searching for clonal neoplastic cells, the alteration of the value of different tumor markers, and biopsy are fundamental tools to reach the correct diagnosis.[6] Conventional imaging, in particular with MR imaging and computed tomography (CT), could offer specific information reflecting the presence of anatomic abnormalities in the tissues involved by the disease.[7] However, in the last decades, PET/CT imaging has experienced a relevant and constant increase in its indication. Different tracers that are able to image different metabolic pathways can be used to assess various conditions both benign and malignant. ^{18}F-Fluorodesoxyglucose (^{18}F FDG) is the most common PET tracer used worldwide and it has the ability to underline tissues with elevated glycolytic activity, a characteristic that is typical of some neoplasms but also of inflammatory diseases.[8,9] The role of this imaging modality for the assessment of some hematological malignancies has been proven, in particular for lymphomas and MM, where ^{18}F-FDG PET/CT has been widely used as a useful and noninvasive molecular imaging technique in diagnosing, staging, restaging, and response assessment after therapy. Despite that, the use of ^{18}F-FDG PET/CT in leukemia has no clear and established value, being proposed in particular for AL and aggressive forms of CLL.[4,10]

DISCUSSION

General Consideration on the Use of PET/Computed Tomography with ^{18}F-Fluorodesoxyglucose in Different Types of Leukemia

One of the main point that needs to be taken into account when evaluating the role of ^{18}F-FDG PET/CT in the assessment of different types of leukemia is that, depending on the fact that usually these neoplasms are not characterized by solid localizations, this imaging modality is not commonly used for their evaluation. However, in general, leukemia presents with increased tracer uptake in the BM that can be either focal or diffuse (**Fig. 1**). Different studies have revealed that patients with leukemia could have increased BM uptake in the vertebrae, pelvis, sternum, ribs, and extremities, reflecting the increased number and the elevated metabolic activity of leukemic cells in these tissues.[11,12] Interestingly, different distribution patterns of tracer uptake can be present when assessing BM involvement: some subjects can experience focal or inhomogeneous uptakes especially in the extremities and these findings may reflect the presence of focal bone sites of disease and the reduced activity of some leukemic cells due to BM necrosis.[12] In addition, it has also been reported that in patients with relapsed leukemia, increased focal bone uptakes of ^{18}F FDG could reflect focal localization of the disease and need to be therefore further investigated.[13]

^{18}F-FDG PET/CT may become a critical diagnostic tool for the early diagnosis in some specific cases such as in patients without remarkable abnormalities in peripheral blood analysis or in subjects presenting with nonspecific symptoms. In particular, in this specific setting, different case reports revealed its usefulness in diagnosing ALL in patients with fever of unknown origin and/or diffuse bone pain and negative conventional imaging such as CT and MR imaging. In addition, these insights were also confirmed in the pediatric population.[14,15]

Some significant limitations of ^{18}F-FDG PET/CT imaging, however, need to be taken into account when evaluating its role in leukemia assessment. First and most important of all, increased uptake of tracer in the BM is not a specific feature of these neoplasms and it can occur in many different benign or malignant conditions. As an example, in patients treated with granulocyte colony–stimulating factor or erythropoietin, which may be typical medications used in the treatment of hematological patients, diffuse increased BM uptake could be present.[16,17] In addition, the presence of infections can result in an increase of BM uptake and in this particular situation, it is difficult to differentiate whether this finding is related to disease infiltration or to an inflammatory response. However, some articles have reported the tendency of BM malignant infiltration from leukemia to present with markedly higher uptake as compared to benign conditions.[12,18]

The Role of PET/Computed Tomography with ^{18}F-Fluorodesoxyglucose in Acute Leukemia

AL is a general definition to indicate the presence of a type of leukemia that has rapid onset and development, resulting in a premature appearance of specific symptoms and a possible worst prognosis. In this setting, ALL presents with symptoms related to BM infiltration that could lead to pancytopenia and it is the most frequent form of leukemia in the pediatric population. As mentioned, ^{18}F-FDG PET/CT may be a beneficial noninvasive tool for assessing pediatric patients as well as adult subjects who present with nonspecific symptoms, including bone pain and fever.[14]

The potential role of ^{18}F-FDG PET/CT for the assessment of AL extent at staging and the evaluation of response to therapy has been underlined. Cunningham and colleagues[19] revealed

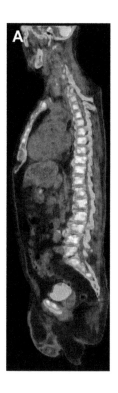
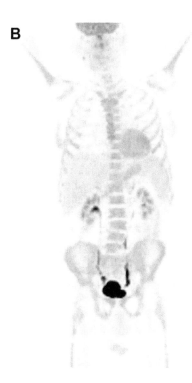

Fig. 1. Sagittal fused PET/computed tomography (*A*) and maximum intensity projection (*B*) images of a ^{18}F-Fluorodesoxyglucose scan performed in a patient with acute myeloblastic leukemia for staging purpose. The examination demonstrated intense and diffuse uptake of tracer in the BM. Subsequent biopsy confirmed the localization of the disease.

that the comparison between pretreatment and posttreatment imaging could evaluate the efficacy of therapy, suggesting that the use of PET imaging could increase the ability to eradicate all foci of leukemia, and divide responsible from refractory tumors, residual, and relapsed disease. Moreover, the use of PET imaging to assess response to therapy in extraosseous disease has also been reported.[20] These insights have also been translated in the setting of pediatric disease revealing that PET/CT could be a complementary modality to improve the detection of subtle leukemic infiltration in children with suspected leukemia progression or recurrence after chemotherapy or allogeneic hematopoietic stem cell transplantation (allo-HSCT). In particular, a study revealed that 4 patients who underwent allo-HSCT were characterized by increased multifocal BM uptake and extramedullary leukemia on ^{18}F-FDG PET/CT, while they showed negative BM biopsies. Therefore, PET-guided targeted biopsies may overcome the fact that focal BM involvement could be missed by BM biopsy alone.[21] Additionally, a case series has reported that in 2 children with AML who underwent PET/CT at diagnosis and in remission, 5 extramedullary disease lesions were demonstrated of which only 2 were detectable on clinical examination.[22]

In the presence of leukemia cells that appear within 2 years from complete remission after therapy, it is possible to define leukemia relapse that can occur intramedullary, extramedullary, or in both the sites together, although the first localization is the most frequent. Even though it is not a frequent finding, relapse is one of the major events able to drive the prognosis of the patients in particular in AL, despite the fact that high rates of complete remission are present after initial treatment.[23–26] Extramedullary AL is defined as the presence of lesions that occur in any anatomic site outside the BM and it is more common in monocytic and myelomonocytic leukemia. Typically, extramedullary manifestations are most frequent in the skin although they can affect almost all parts of the body.[27–30] The presence of extramedullary AL is, however, a rare finding with a prevalence that remains between 10% and 30%.[31,32] Symptoms and laboratory test changes related to extramedullary infiltration could not be specific or even present in the first stages of the disease. As a consequence, this manifestation is not easily diagnosed, in particular in recurrent form of AL, since the diagnosis is reached only in advanced stages with large or widespread lesions that can therefore result in poor prognosis.[4] Intramedullary relapse can often be easily diagnosed by BM biopsy and blood cell examination while it is difficult to detect extramedullary relapse. Traditional imaging with CT or MR imaging has limited sensitivities in particular in small and occult extramedullary lesions. In contrast, ^{18}F-FDG PET/CT may be a useful tool to detect and diagnose extramedullary AL since it has the ability to determine the location and the metabolic activity of the disease, demonstrating a high sensitivity of 93.3% and the ability to guide biopsy in particular for AML.[29] Most of these patients relapse within a short period of time after initiation of therapy or have refractory disease and therefore PET imaging could have an important impact on treatment decisions and outcomes.[31,33,34] In addition, it has been reported that PET/CT avoids false-positive or false-negative findings compared to PET and CT alone in patients with granulocytic sarcoma, that it can reveal more than twice as many patients with extramedullary AL than found by clinical examination and that the responses of extramedullary AL detected by ^{18}F-FDG PET/CT were concordant with the BM responses assessed by pathology examination.[29,32,35] Stölzel and colleagues[36] performed a study on 10 patients with de novo and relapsed AML, reporting that PET/CT was able to reveal the known site of extramedullary lesions in 90% of these subjects and to detect additional localization of the disease in 60% of the patients. Similar insights were obtained by Tan and colleagues[37] that reported a case of an ALL patient with a mass in the left eye 9 years from complete remission after allo-HSCT. ^{18}F-FDG PET/CT revealed increased tracer uptake with extramedullary relapse confirmed by biopsy, despite the BM aspiration biopsy was negative. Recently Li and colleagues[38] developed a machine learning model based on radiomics analysis of ^{18}F-FDG PET/CT images that, in patients with suspicious relapsed AL, can complement the visual analysis to derive a more comprehensive, confident, and accurate diagnosis.

The Value of PET with ^{18}F-Fluorodesoxyglucose Imaging in the Assessment of Chronic Leukemia

In contrast with acute forms of leukemia, chronic forms are characterized by a slower proliferation of the clonal neoplastic cells, resulting therefore in more slight symptoms. CLL is the most common type of leukemia in the Western communities and in elderly population and it is generally an indolent disease characterized by a low grade of proliferation.[39] As a consequence, the metabolic activity on ^{18}F-FDG-PET/CT in sites affected by the disease is typically low and therefore CT could safely replace PET/CT in the initial staging of this neoplasm.[1] Despite that, RT refers to the development of an aggressive form of CLL that switches to lymphoma, most commonly diffuse large B-cell

lymphoma (DLBCL), and could be experienced in roughly 8% to 10% of patients affected by CLL.[40,41] However, even if less frequently, transformations into prolymphocytic leukemia, Hodgkin lymphoma, and small non-cleaved cell lymphoma have also been documented.[42] RT is one of the main complications of CLL and, based on its rapid evolution, patients usually present with rapidly enlarging nodes and increasing size of hepatosplenomegaly, with a poor prognosis and a median survival that ranges between 5 and 8 months.[43] Moreover, the management of these subjects could be difficult and the ability to make a clear distinction between CLL and RT is crucial since they can benefit from different therapeutic regimens.[44,45]

The prompt diagnosis of RT is therefore crucial to set up a correct therapeutic approach; however, clinical symptoms (such as fever and the presence of enlarging lymph nodes) and serum laboratory findings (such as elevated lactate dehydrogenase and β-2 microglobulin levels) are not specific. As mentioned, conventional imaging and in particular CT could play a role for its assessment, highlighting the presence of lymphomatous lesions with compressive or infiltrative patterns. In addition, ^{18}F-FDG PET/CT is extremely beneficial in order to confirm the diagnosis, aiming for a clear definition of the metabolic behavior of such lesions. In this setting, it has been reported that this imaging modality has high sensitivity, specificity, and negative predictive value in the detection of RT from CLL to large cell lymphoma. In particular, evidence underlined that, depending on its low mitotic activity and therefore glucose consumption, low degree of ^{18}F FDG uptake could be present in patients affected by CLL or small lymphocytic lymphoma, while a high degree of tracer uptake is underlined in the case of RT (**Fig. 2**).[46] In fact, PET/CT has proven its usefulness to endorse the suspect of RT to lymphoma and to choose the best location to perform a biopsy aiming therefore for a definitive diagnosis.[41,45,47–50] In addition, fine needle aspiration is sometimes ineffective in the identification of disease transformation in CLL and therefore, the importance of using ^{18}F FDG-PET imaging for the assessment of these patients rises.[41] Interestingly, this fact was also underlined in the case of novel therapy for CLL, where it was suggested that patients receiving B-cell receptor pathway inhibitor therapy should undergo ^{18}F-FDG PET/CT for the evaluation of potential disease progression and that a biopsy should be considered in patients with suspected RT when a maximum standardized uptake value (SUVmax) greater than 5 is present.[45] In this scenario, it is important to underline

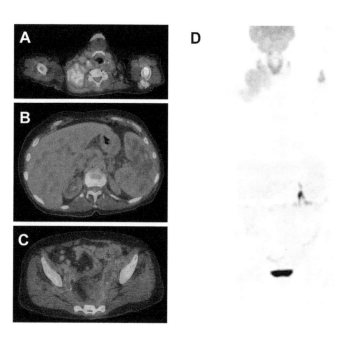

Fig. 2. Transaxial fused PET/computed tomography (*A–C*) and maximum intensity projection (*D*) images of a ^{18}F-Fluorodesoxyglucose scan performed in a patient with diagnosis of chronic lymphoblastic leukemia to assess the possible progression of disease to lymphoma. The examination demonstrated intense laterocervical nodal uptake, focal uptake in the parenchyma of the spleen, and focal uptake on the head of the left humerus. Furthermore, only moderate uptake was demonstrated on iliac lymph adenopathies.

that populations of untransformed CLL and transformed lymphoma may coexist in the same patient and, in the case of cytotoxic chemotherapy directed against the transformed tumor, little response is often seen in the sites of untransformed CLL. Again, the possibility to underline the presence of both these entities by metabolic imaging is a clear advantage of PET/CT.[4,51]

One of the main studies that investigated the role of ^{18}F-FDG PET/CT in RT was performed by Bruzzi and colleagues[47], revealing that in 37 patients with CLL and the suspicion of transformation to DLBCL, subjects with a histologically proven diagnosis had a higher SUVmax compared to those without a clear histologic evidence of transformation. A SUVmax greater than 5 was suggested by the investigators as a reliable threshold to distinguish RT with high diagnostic accuracy, with overall sensitivity, specificity, and positive and negative predictive values of 91%, 80%, 53%, and 97%, respectively. Similar values of SUVmax were subsequently validated as the limits to identify subjects with CLL who were clinically suspected of RT on PET/CT scans.[49] An SUVmax of 10 was demonstrated in another study as the strongest parameters able to predict the outcomes of the patients with a high discriminatory power, because it was independently linked to a reduction in overall survival (OS).[52] In addition, it was also suggested that patients with higher SUVmax values had a higher tendency to be characterized by negative prognostic factors, such as the presence of p17 deletion and/or ZAP-70 positivity.[50] An article reported that the median

SUVmax were 3.4 and 3.1 in newly diagnosed and relapsed CLL, respectively, while the median SUVmax observed in patients with either suspected or confirmed RT was 16.5 with a statistically significant difference between these values.[49] Falchi and colleagues[53] evaluated ^{18}F-FDG PET/CT in 322 patients with CLL, including 120 histologically indolent forms, 117 histologically aggressive forms, and 95 subjects with RT. The investigators underlined that subjects with aggressive forms or RT were characterized by comparable PET/CT patterns with higher SUVmax values and also shared characteristics typical for an aggressive disease, such as constitutional symptoms and an elevation of serum levels of lactate dehydrogenase. Despite that, subjects with aggressive forms of CLL had a longer median survival compared to patients with RT (17.6 and 7.7 months, respectively). In addition, age, performance status, bulky illness, and SUVmax 10 or higher were all individually linked to a shorter OS. Fine needle aspiration failed to provide a reliable diagnosis in 23%, 29%, and 53% of indolent, aggressive, and RT patients who underwent both aspiration and biopsy, respectively.[53]

Volumetric parameters are semiquantitative values that can be extracted from PET/CT imaging and that have a proven role for the assessment of many different hematological diseases, in particular for their prognostic value.[54] In this scenario, 2 different studies explored the role of metabolic tumor volume (MTV) and total lesion glycolysis (TLG) for the prognostic assessment of CLL, revealing, however, conflicting results.[55–57] In particular, an article reported that staging MTV in patients with RT was a prognostic factor at univariate analysis for OS even if not confirmed at multivariate analysis, while the other article did not confirm this insight. This finding is particularly interesting when taking into account the fact that all other PET/CT semiquantitative parameters were significantly higher in the group of patients with RT compared to those without RT, while MTV and TLG were the only parameters that did not demonstrate a correlation with the presence of transformation.[55,56]

SUMMARY

Even if ^{18}F FDG-PET imaging is not routinely performed for the assessment of leukemia, some evidence on its role has been reported. Generally speaking, the main finding that this imaging modality can reveal is the presence of BM infiltration, aiming therefore for the correct evaluation of disease extension in staging setting and also for known or suspected relapse assessment. Moreover, this ability can influence and guide the use of BM biopsy, in particular for focal infiltration aiding the formulation of a correct diagnosis even in the pediatric population. [18]F FDG-PET imaging has been reported as particularly useful for the diagnosis of leukemia in patients with nonspecific symptoms. Focusing on AL, this imaging modality revealed a role for the evaluation of therapy response and for the assessment of relapse, in particular for extramedullary forms. [18]F FDG uptake is generally low in CL; however, the usefulness of PET/CT has been underlined for the initial diagnosis and the evaluation of relapse of CLL with RT, given its ability to evaluate high metabolic lesion that had a transformation, underlining moreover the possible site of biopsy. Lastly, in the case of patients with RT, SUVmax revealed its value for the diagnosis of the disease and, with less evidence, some insights on its prognostic role have emerged.

CLINICS CARE POINTS

- ^{18}F-FDG PET imaging is able to evaluate leukemias and BM infiltration with different pattern can be demonstrated. The site of BM involved by the disease can be further analyzed with biopsy. Extramedullary forms can also be evaluated with this imaging modality.
- Other conditions that can lead to an increased tracer in the BM (eg, infection) need to be carefully considered.

- AL have higher tracer uptake compared to CL that could be characterized by the presence of low ^{18}F-FDG uptake, however PET imaging is able to drive the diagnosis and assess the presence of RT.
- ^{18}F-FDG PET imaging can help in the diagnosis of leukemias in patients with unspecific symptoms, but also to assess the response to therapy and the presence of relapse.

DISCLOSURE

The authors have nothing to disclose.

REFERENCES

1. Salem AE, Shah HR, Covington MF, et al. PET-CT in clinical adult oncology: I. Hematologic malignancies. Cancers (Basel) 2022;14(23):5941.
2. Méndez-Ferrer S, Bonnet D, Steensma DP, et al. Bone marrow niches in haematological malignancies. Nat Rev Cancer 2020;20(5):285–98.
3. Xu B, Hu R, Liang Z, et al. Metabolic regulation of the bone marrow microenvironment in leukemia. Blood Rev 2021;48:100786.
4. Zhao Z, Hu Y, Li J, et al. Applications of PET in diagnosis and prognosis of leukemia. Technol Cancer Res Treat 2020;19. 1533033820956993.
5. Mayerhoefer ME, Archibald SJ, Messiou C, et al. MRI and PET/MRI in hematologic malignancies. J Magn Reson Imaging 2020;51(5):1325–35.
6. Staber PB, Herling M, Bellido M, et al. Consensus criteria for diagnosis, staging, and treatment response assessment of T-cell prolymphocytic leukemia. Blood 2019;134(14):1132–43.
7. Averill LW, Acikgoz G, Miller RE, et al. Update on pediatric leukemia and lymphoma imaging. Semin Ultrasound CT MR 2013;34(6):578–99.
8. Dondi F, Albano D, Giubbini R, et al. 18F-FDG PET and PET/CT for the evaluation of gastric signet ring cell carcinoma: a systematic review. Nucl Med Commun 2021;42(12):1293–300.
9. Sammartino AM, Falco R, Drera A, et al. Vascular inflammation and cardiovascular disease: review about the role of PET imaging. Int J Cardiovasc Imaging 2023;39(2):433–40.
10. Buck AK, Bommer M, Juweid ME, et al. First demonstration of leukemia imaging with the proliferation marker 18F-fluorodeoxythymidine. J Nucl Med 2008;49(11):1756–62.
11. Arimoto MK, Nakamoto Y, Nakatani K, et al. Increased bone marrow uptake of 18F-FDG in leukemia patients: preliminary findings. Springerplus 2015;4:521.
12. Alam MS, Fu L, Ren YY, et al. 18F-FDG super bone marrow uptake: a highly potent indicator for the

malignant infiltration. Medicine (Baltimore) 2016; 95(52):e5579.

13. Endo T, Sato N, Koizumi K, et al. Localized relapse in bone marrow of extremities after allogeneic stem cell transplantation for acute lymphoblastic leukemia. Am J Hematol 2004;76(3):279–82.

14. Arslan F, Yilmaz M, Çakir T, et al. Significant contribution of fluorodeoxyglucose positron emission tomography/computed tomography (FDG PET/CT) in a case of acute lymphoblastic leukemia presenting with fever of unknown origin. Intern Med 2014; 53(7):789–91.

15. Ennishi D, Maeda Y, Niiya M, et al. Incidental detection of acute lymphoblastic leukemia on [18F]fluorodeoxyglucose positron emission tomography. J Clin Oncol 2009;27(36):e269–70.

16. Sugawara Y, Fisher SJ, Zasadny KR, et al. Preclinical and clinical studies of bone marrow uptake of fluorine-1-fluorodeoxyglucose with or without granulocyte colony-stimulating factor during chemotherapy. J Clin Oncol 1998;16(1):173–80.

17. Blodgett TM, Ames JT, Torok FS, et al. Diffuse bone marrow uptake on whole-body F-18 fluorodeoxyglucose positron emission tomography in a patient taking recombinant erythropoietin. Clin Nucl Med 2004; 29(3):161–3.

18. Zhou M, Chen Y, Liu J, et al. A predicting model of bone marrow malignant infiltration in 18F-FDG PET/CT images with increased diffuse bone marrow FDG uptake. J Cancer 2018;9(10):1737–44.

19. Cunningham I, Kohno B. 18 FDG-PET/CT: 21st century approach to leukemic tumors in 124 cases. Am J Hematol 2016;91(4):379–84.

20. Doma A, Škerget M, Žagar I. 18F-FDG PET/CT for staging and evaluation of therapy in a patient with unusual hairy cell leukemia presentation. Clin Nucl Med 2019;44(7):e458–60.

21. Kaya Z, Akdemir OU, Atay OL, et al. Utility of 18-fluorodeoxyglucose positron emission tomography in children with relapsed/refractory leukemia. Pediatr Hematol Oncol 2018;35(7–8):393–406.

22. Matsui M, Yamanaka J, Shichino H, et al. FDG-PET/CT for detection of extramedullary disease in 2 pediatric patients with AML. J Pediatr Hematol Oncol 2016;38(5):398–401.

23. de Lima M, Porter DL, Battiwalla M, et al. Proceedings from the National Cancer Institute's Second International Workshop on the biology, prevention, and treatment of relapse after hematopoietic stem cell transplantation: part III. Prevention and treatment of relapse after allogeneic transplantation. Biol Blood Marrow Transplant 2014;20(1):4–13.

24. Mortimer J, Blinder MA, Schulman S, et al. Relapse of acute leukemia after marrow transplantation: natural history and results of subsequent therapy. J Clin Oncol 1989;7(1):50–7.

25. Lee KH, Lee JH, Choi SJ, et al. Bone marrow vs extramedullary relapse of acute leukemia after allogeneic hematopoietic cell transplantation: risk factors and clinical course. Bone Marrow Transplant 2003; 32(8):835–42.

26. Lee KH, Lee JH, Kim S, et al. High frequency of extramedullary relapse of acute leukemia after allogeneic bone marrow transplantation. Bone Marrow Transplant 2000;26(2):147–52.

27. Chong G, Byrnes G, Szer J, et al. Extramedullary relapse after allogeneic bone marrow transplantation for haematological malignancy. Bone Marrow Transplant 2000;26(9):1011–5.

28. Tsimberidou AM, Kantarjian HM, Wen S, et al. Myeloid sarcoma is associated with superior event-free survival and overall survival compared with acute myeloid leukemia. Cancer 2008;113(6): 1370–8.

29. Zhou WL, Wu HB, Wang LJ, et al. Usefulness and pitfalls of F-18-FDG PET/CT for diagnosing extramedullary acute leukemia. Eur J Radiol 2016;85(1): 205–10.

30. Arrigan M, Smyth L, Harmon M, et al. Imaging findings in recurrent extramedullary leukaemias. Cancer Imag 2013;13(1):26–35.

31. Ciarallo A, Makis W, Novales-Diaz JA, et al. Extramedullary gastric relapse of acute lymphoblastic leukemia following allogeneic stem cell transplant: staging with F-18 FDG PET/CT. Clin Nucl Med 2011;36(8):e90–2.

32. Cribe AS, Steenhof M, Marcher CW, et al. Extramedullary disease in patients with acute myeloid leukemia assessed by 18F-FDG PET. Eur J Haematol 2013;90(4):273–8.

33. Elojeimy S, Luana Stanescu A, Parisi MT. Use of 18F-FDG PET-CT for detection of active disease in acute myeloid leukemia. Clin Nucl Med 2016;41(3): e137–40.

34. Cistaro A, Saglio F, Asaftei S, et al. The role of 18F-FDG PET/CT in pediatric lymph-node acute lymphoblastic leukemia involvement. Radiol Case Rep 2015;6(4):503.

35. Aschoff P, Häntschel M, Oksüz M, et al. Integrated FDG-PET/CT for detection, therapy monitoring and follow-up of granulocytic sarcoma. Initial results. Nuklearmedizin 2009;48(5):185–91.

36. Stölzel F, Röllig C, Radke J, et al. 18F-FDG-PET/CT for detection of extramedullary acute myeloid leukemia. Haematologica 2011;96(10):1552–6.

37. Tan G, Aslan A, Tazeler Z. FDG-PET/CT for detecting relapse in patients with acute lymphoblastic leukemia. Jpn J Clin Oncol 2016;46(1):96–7.

38. Li H, Xu C, Xin B, et al. 18F-FDG PET/CT radiomic analysis with machine learning for identifying bone marrow involvement in the patients with suspected relapsed acute leukemia. Theranostics 2019;9(16): 4730–9.

39. Shaikh F, Janjua A, Van Gestel F, et al. Richter transformation of chronic lymphocytic leukemia: a review of fluorodeoxyglucose positron emission tomography-computed tomography and molecular diagnostics. Cureus 2017;9(1):e968.

40. Robertson LE, Pugh W, O'Brien S, et al. Richter's syndrome: a report on 39 patients. J Clin Oncol 1993;11(10):1985–9.

41. Molica S. FDG/PET in CLL today. Blood 2014; 123(18):2749–50.

42. Brecher M, Banks PM. Hodgkin's disease variant of Richter's syndrome. Report of eight cases. Am J Clin Pathol 1990;93(3):333–9.

43. Tsimberidou AM, Keating MJ. Richter syndrome: biology, incidence, and therapeutic strategies. Cancer 2005;103(2):216–28.

44. Wang Y, Tschautscher MA, Rabe KG, et al. Clinical characteristics and outcomes of Richter transformation: experience of 204 patients from a single center. Haematologica 2020;105(3):765–73.

45. Wang Y, Rabe KG, Bold MS, et al. The role of 18F-FDG-PET in detecting Richter's transformation of chronic lymphocytic leukemia in patients receiving therapy with a B-cell receptor inhibitor. Haematologica 2020;105(11):2675–8.

46. Jerusalem G, Beguin Y, Najjar F, et al. Positron emission tomography (PET) with 18F-fluorodeoxyglucose (18F-FDG) for the staging of low-grade non-Hodgkin's lymphoma (NHL). Ann Oncol 2001;12(6):825–30.

47. Bruzzi JF, Macapinlac H, Tsimberidou AM, et al. Detection of Richter's transformation of chronic lymphocytic leukemia by PET/CT. J Nucl Med 2006; 47(8):1267–73.

48. Conte MJ, Bowen DA, Wiseman GA, et al. Use of positron emission tomography-computed tomography in the management of patients with chronic lymphocytic leukemia/small lymphocytic lymphoma. Leuk Lymphoma 2014;55(9):2079–84.

49. Papajík T, Mysliveček M, Urbanová R, et al. 2-[18F]fluoro-2-deoxy-D-glucose positron emission tomography/computed tomography examination in patients with chronic lymphocytic leukemia may reveal Richter transformation. Leuk Lymphoma 2014;55(2):314–9.

50. Parikh SA, Kay NE, Shanafelt TD. How we treat Richter syndrome. Blood 2014;123(11):1647–57.

51. Litz CE, Arthur DC, Gajl-Peczalska KJ, et al. Transformation of chronic lymphocytic leukemia to small non-cleaved cell lymphoma: a cytogenetic, immunological, and molecular study. Leukemia 1991;5(11): 972–8.

52. Michallet AS, Sesques P, Rabe KG, et al. An 18F-FDG-PET maximum standardized uptake value > 10 represents a novel valid marker for discerning Richter's Syndrome. Leuk Lymphoma 2016;57(6): 1474–7.

53. Falchi L, Keating MJ, Marom EM, et al. Correlation between FDG/PET, histology, characteristics, and survival in 332 patients with chronic lymphoid leukemia. Blood 2014;123(18):2783–90.

54. Albano D, Dondi F, Mazzoletti A, et al. Prognostic impact of pretreatment 2-[18F]-FDG PET/CT parameters in primary gastric DLBCL. Medicina (Kaunas) 2021;57(5):498.

55. Pontoizeau C, Girard A, Mesbah H, et al. Prognostic value of baseline total metabolic tumor volume measured on FDG PET in patients with richter syndrome. Clin Nucl Med 2020;45(2):118–22. PMID: 31876819.

56. Albano D, Camoni L, Rodella C, et al. 2-[18F]-FDG PET/CT role in detecting richter transformation of chronic lymphocytic leukemia and predicting overall survival. Clin Lymphoma, Myeloma & Leukemia 2021;21(3):e277–83.

57. Albano D, Bertagna F, Dondi F, et al. The role of 2-[18F]-FDG PET/CT in detecting richter transformation in chronic lymphocytic leukemia: a systematic review. Radiation 2021;1:65–76.

Role of Novel Quantitative Imaging Techniques in Hematological Malignancies

Rahul V. Parghane, MBBS, MD[a,b],
Sandip Basu, MBBS (Hons), DRM, DNB, MNAMS[a,b],*

KEYWORDS

- Hematological malignancies • PET/CT • Metabolic tumor volume (MTV)
- Total lesion glycolysis (TLG) • Total metabolic tumor volume (TMTV) • Dmax
- Artificial intelligence (AI) • Convolutional neural networks (CNNs)

KEY POINTS

- Hematological malignancies such as lymphoma and multiple myeloma affect various body parts and the entire skeletal system, requiring global disease assessment on PET/computed tomography imaging.
- In clinical practice, visual analysis using Deauville 5 point scoring system and semiquantitative parameters (SUVmax) is used commonly to assess ^{18}F-FDG -PET/CT response for hematological malignancies. But visual analysis is subjective in nature, and maximum SUV represents the highest level of metabolic activity within the region of interest and does not provide an indication of the global disease burden activity.
- Using novel quantitative metrices like metabolic tumor volume (MTV), total lesion glycolysis (TLG), and total MTV (TMTV), and maximum distance between 2 sites of disease (Dmax) can help assess the global disease burden in hematological malignancies and solve deficiencies associated with visual/SUVmax analysis.
- The measurement of these novel quantitative metrices is commonly done manually or semiautomatically. However, manual approach is time-consuming task with a high degree of intraobserver and interobserver variability.
- The artificial intelligence (AI) can determine novel PET/CT imaging quantitative parameters using convolutional neural networks algorithms with fully or semiautomated methods. AI determined TMTV can be beneficial in evaluating several aspects of hematological malignancies. It aids in characterizing tumors, quantifying their heterogeneity, predicting treatment response, determining survival rates, and assessing the risk of recurrence.

INTRODUCTION

PET imaging has revolutionized clinical oncology by enabling the visualization of cancer biology in its distinct manifestations. PET-based targeted radiotracers can serve as biomarkers to accurately characterize diseases, estimate prognosis, measure treatment response, and predict long-term response and survival. This is achieved through the usage of noninvasive measurements of tumor physiology by using PET imaging, which can be used to customize therapeutic regimens based on the tumor's biology. For the PET system, the process of image acquisition is based on the detection

[a] Radiation Medicine Centre (BARC), Tata Memorial Hospital Annexe, Parel, Mumbai, India; [b] Homi Bhabha National Institute, Mumbai, India
* Corresponding author. Radiation Medicine Centre, Bhabha Atomic Research Centre, Tata Memorial Hospital, Annexe Building, Jerbai Wadia Road, Parel, Mumbai 400 012, India.
E-mail address: drsanb@yahoo.com

PET Clin 19 (2024) 543–559
https://doi.org/10.1016/j.cpet.2024.05.008
1556-8598/24/© 2024 Elsevier Inc. All rights are reserved, including those for text and data mining, AI training, and similar technologies.

of photons that are produced by the annihilation of positrons that are emitted from positron-emitting radiopharmaceuticals that have been injected in patients. Fluorine-18 (^{18}F)-fluorodeoxyglucose (FDG) is a PET radiotracer that is extensively employed in clinical practice to assess glucose metabolism in tissues due to its wide range of clinical applications.[1–3] In terms of the clinical adoption of PET imaging, the introduction of hybrid PET/computed tomography (CT) was a significant step forward. Optimal localization and characterization of tissue metabolic activity (detected on PET images) can be achieved by the utilization of co-registered anatomic information, which is provided by the CT component of hybrid PET/CT. When CT and PET are used together, the number of false-positive and false-negative PET findings is reduced. Furthermore, PET/CT enables a reduction in the amount of time required for PET scanning. This is because the information on tissue densities that is obtained from CT is utilized for the purpose of attenuation correction of PET photons. A useful feature about PET/CT is that it can quantify the tracer uptake by comparing the measured tissue activity from PET images to the dose injected and the patient's body weight. This gives us a standardized uptake value (SUV). In clinical practice, the maximum level of activity within a region of interest (ROI) of tumor is usually used and recorded as maximum SUV (SUVmax). When compared to CT and ^{18}F-FDG-PET as independent imaging modalities, the 1 stop hybrid ^{18}F-FDG-PET/CT combines the functional and anatomic information as well as the quantification of tracer activity in tumor lesions. This hybrid imaging technique outperforms both options.[4–6] As a consequence of this, a number of cancer organizations, including the European Society for Medical Oncology, the American Society of Clinical Oncology, and the National Comprehensive Cancer Network, have made recommendations regarding the utilization of ^{18}F-FDG-PET/CT for staging, restaging, monitoring during therapy, and evaluating treatment response, in hematological malignancies.[7–10] This article will review hematological malignancies along with the clinical application of PET/CT imaging with standard response evaluation criteria for these malignancies. We will also discuss novel quantitative PET/CT imaging techniques for assessing global disease burden and how the use of artificial intelligence (AI) has helped to determine these parameters instantaneously in the evaluation of hematological malignancies.

HEMATOLOGICAL MALIGNANCIES

The term "hematological malignancies" refers to a broad collection of cancers that can be distinguished by their individual occurrences, prognoses, and underlying causes. These malignancies are caused by either cells that are responsible for producing blood (from bone marrow) or cells that are associated with the immune response. Lymphoma is a commonly seen hematological malignancy in clinical practices. Lymphomas are caused by the uncontrolled multiplication of lymphocytes or lymphocyte precursors. There are almost 50 distinct subtypes that vary greatly in terms of their histology, etiology, clinical behavior, and therapeutic response. The 2022 World Health Organization classification categorizes them into 2 main types: non-Hodgkin lymphoma (NHL) and Hodgkin lymphoma (HL).[11] Lymphomas are further classified based on their level of aggressiveness, which can be either indolent (low grade) or aggressive (high grade) kinds. The majority of the low-grade lymphomas are derived from NHL. Indolent lymphomas have lower levels of aggressiveness, yet pose greater challenges in terms of achieving a cure. Due to their reduced tumor proliferation, they exhibit a lower response to traditional chemotherapy regimens. Lymphoma has the potential to affect virtually any organ in the body. However, in the beginning, HL typically manifests as lymph node disease, with or without involvement of the spleen. NHL spreads randomly throughout various groups of lymph nodes and frequently affects multiple organs including the bone marrow and presents as extra-nodal disease.[12] The majority of lymphoma subtypes demonstrates increased glucose metabolic activity, leading to an increased FDG uptake on PET/CT imaging. HL and diffuse large B-cell lymphoma (DLBCL) are highly FDG-avid lymphomas. In HL, the cancerous Hodgkin and Reed–Sternberg cells make up a small portion of the cells that invade the affected tissue, occurring at a frequency between 0.1% and 10%. The main component of an HL lesion consists of a reactive infiltration composed of nonneoplastic small lymphocytes, eosinophilic and neutrophilic granulocytes, histiocytes, plasma cells, and fibroblasts in different proportions. The FDG uptake in activated lymphocytes, eosinophilic and neutrophilic granulocytes, histiocytes, and plasma cells is comparable to that observed in inflammatory lesions. ^{18}F-FDG-PET/CT imaging in HL reveals increased glucose metabolism throughout the tumor, indicating that noncancerous cells that are activated are responsible for a substantial percentage of the metabolic activity. DLBCL, follicular lymphoma (FL), and mantle cell lymphoma (MCL) as subtypes of NHL are often distinguished by a predominant population of cancerous lymphoid cells and a smaller proportion of noncancerous inflammatory cells. Unlike HL, the majority of the cellular infiltration in DLBCL consists of neoplastic lymphoid cells, and these subtypes of lymphomas exhibit a high FDG affinity on PET/CT imaging. Other lymphomas that exhibit high uptake of FDG include Burkitt lymphoma, as well as lymphomas originating from T cells, such as natural killer/T-cell lymphoma and anaplastic large cell lymphoma. Small lymphocytic lymphoma, extranodal marginal zone lymphoma, and cutaneous lymphomas have varying levels of glucose metabolic activity.[13–18]

Multiple myeloma (MM), which accounts for approximately 10% of all hematological malignancies, is the second most prevalent hematological cancer after lymphoma. Furthermore, it is the most prevalent primary malignancy of the bone. MM is caused by the uncontrolled proliferation of plasma cells in the bone marrow, which produces diffuse or focal osteolytic lesions. It is postulated that non-immunoglobulin M monoclonal gammopathy of undetermined significance (MGUS) serves as the progenitor cell for all cases of myeloma. MGUS typically transforms into smouldering MM (SMM), a transitional phase situated between MGUS and MM, over the course of time. MGUS advances to MM at a rate of approximately 1% annually. During the initial 5 years, SMM may progress to MM at a 10% annual rate, which may be rapid or gradual. Patients who have developed genuine MM typically exhibit the following CRAB symptoms: hypercalcemia, renal failure, anemia and bone lesions. The gold standard for diagnosing MM is a bone marrow biopsy; however, imaging is also crucial and can assist with guided bone marrow biopsy. In comparison to MR imaging and PET/CT, conventional radiography has a high false-negative rate of 30% to 70%, resulting in a substantial underestimation of the presence and extent of disease. In the imaging evaluation of MM, whole-body MR imaging or CT and ^{18}F-FDG-PET/CT have essentially replaced conventional radiography at present. ^{18}F-FDG-PET/CT provides a comprehensive evaluation of the entire body, surpassing the sensitivity of MR imaging in its ability to identify extramedullary sites of disease.[19–24]

Leukemia ranks as the third most prevalent hematological malignancy, following lymphoma and MM. It is the most prevalent malignancy in children, comprising around 40% of all malignancies. Leukemia originates from blood-forming cells, invading the bone marrow and other blood-forming tissues, causing either a localized or widespread replacement of the marrow. Additionally, it exhibits a minor preference for extra-osseous soft tissues. Leukemias are typically categorized based on their clinical characteristics and cellular development into 4 primary subgroups: acute lymphoblastic leukemia, acute myeloblastic leukemia (AML), chronic lymphoblastic leukemia (CLL), and chronic myeloblastic leukemia. Nevertheless, additional distinct classifications of precursor leukemia/lymphomas have been included. The category of precursor lymphoma/leukemia encompasses both B-cell-derived and T-cell-derived cases.[25–29] The utilization of ^{18}F-FDG-PET/CT in the evaluation of leukemia is infrequent. Nevertheless, numerous case studies have illustrated the capability of ^{18}F-FDG-PET/CT in diagnosing and monitoring leukemic bone marrow infiltration. The efficacy of ^{18}F-FDG-PET/CT in diagnosing extramedullary illness in individuals with newly diagnosed or relapsed AML has been demonstrated in several studies. ^{18}F-FDG-PET/CT can also be valuable in identifying Richter's syndrome, a condition with an unfavorable outlook that necessitates intensive treatment. Several groups have proposed using an SUV cutoff value of 5.0 or higher to accurately diagnose the progression of CLL into Richter syndrome. In addition, ^{18}F-FDG-PET/CT can assist in directing a diagnostic biopsy and may possibly offer prognostic insights in individuals with CLL.[30–40]

HYBRID PET/COMPUTED TOPOGRAPHY IMAGING

Various imaging techniques have been utilized for lymphoma, such as ultrasonography, CT, MR imaging, and ^{18}F-FDG-PET/CT. Ultrasound is utilized to evaluate superficial structures and aid in doing biopsies. In the past, CT imaging was regarded as the standard technique for lymphoma imaging. CT scans of the neck, chest, abdomen, and pelvis can be utilized as a standalone method for imaging low-grade lymphomas, particularly those who have a low affinity for FDG. MR imaging is primarily used for evaluating the neural axis, pelvic tissues, and identifying musculoskeletal involvement. Currently, ^{18}F-FDG-PET/CT is the modality of choice for staging and response evaluation of all high-grade lymphomas or those that are FDG-avid.[41–45] The ^{18}F-FDG-PET/CT can be performed with contrast or without contrast and can utilize either a diagnostic or low-dose CT. Contrast-enhanced CT, when combined with PET, provides a more comprehensive assessment of findings and a more detailed analysis of tissues compared to non-contrast CT scans. The optimal axial range of ^{18}F-FDG-PET/CT for lymphoma has not been determined; nevertheless, in general, a torso scan ("eyes-to-mid thighs") is sufficient for the majority of lymphoma types. For lymphomas that are prone to distal or cutaneous involvement, such as T-cell lymphomas, or in cases where specific bone lesions are recognized (in lymphoma or MM), a whole-body scan "top-of-head-to-feet" is often utilized.

QUANTITATIVE PARAMETERS ROUTINELY USED IN CLINICAL PRACTICES

Attenuation-corrected PET images are commonly used for determination of various semiquantitative parameters in PET/CT imaging. The SUV is most commonly used metric parameters. SUVs are frequently adapted to correspond with a particular measurement of patient sizes, including body weight, lean body mass, or body surface area. When the SUV is adjusted for lean body mass, it is referred to as standardized uptake value (SUL) (for lean body mass). The SUV can be measured in many ways to assess the metabolic activity of a lesion in a specific ROI. These measurements include the SUVmax, which represents the highest metabolic activity in the ROI, the mean SUV (SUV-mean), which represents the overall metabolic activity in ROI, and the SUVpeak, which represents the highest activity within a 1 cm^3 area surrounding the most metabolically active pixel. SUVpeak has more stability compared to other metrics in a significant area of metabolic activity that is reasonably uniform, such as the liver. However, in clinical practice, SUVpeak is not as commonly utilized as SUVmax. The stability and reproducibility of these parameters are influenced by various factors such as the size and heterogeneity of the target lesion, the time between uptake and imaging, patient preparation, acquisition, processing and reconstruction techniques, and the performance of the individual scanner. It is crucial in clinical practice to accurately replicate these characteristics between scans and to use the same equipment and protocol for each imaging session in oncological patients for response evaluation and monitoring therapy.

In ^{18}F-FDG-PET/CT evaluation for lymphomas, it is common to compare the SUV in the lesion being examined with that of a normal reference background tissue, such as the mediastinal blood pool or liver, using a ratio. The Deauville 5 point scoring (D5PS) system is developed and utilized to assess the response in lymphoma. The fourth International Workshop on Positron Emission Tomography in Lymphoma, which took place in Menton, France, in 2014, aimed to expand the scope of lymphomas studied, utilizes D5PS for end-of-treatment ^{18}F-FDG-PET/CT (ePET) and interim PET/CT (iPET) response evaluation, and introduced the concept of ΔSUVmax from baseline to

iPET. They recommended ^{18}F-FDG-PET/CT imaging for initial staging of any FDG-avid lymphomas with nodal involvement. The meeting also presented the concept of partial metabolic response for iPET. The utilization of the D5PS system is accompanied by many technological factors that add to confusion in response evaluation of lymphomas patients. The D5PS was first developed using visual assessments. The utilization of semiquantitative evaluations of SUVs introduced numerous points of ambiguity. Initially, metabolic activity in tumors tends to gradually grow over a period of up to 70 minutes, whereas activity in the blood pool diminishes. It is crucial to rigorously standardize the time between injection and imaging in order to prevent any potential errors. The second concern pertains to the selection of SUVmean, SUVmax, or SUVpeak for quantifying the activity levels in both background reference tissues and tumors. Partial volume effects lead to a reduction in assessments of metabolic activity for small lesions. One would anticipate that the SUVmean or SUVpeak readings will exhibit a higher value. Tumor heterogeneity would lead to decreased average SUV measurements. Thus, SUVmax could be regarded as a more accurate indicator of remaining incompletely treated disease, even if it encompasses just a small fraction of the remaining tumor mass. In D5PS, the point spread function and visually visible activity in tumor lesions may be altered by the reconstruction techniques and the type of scanner used. Thus, it may be safer to use SUVmax instead of SUVmean for both background tissues and tumors. It is crucial to guarantee that a particular patient undergoes imaging consistently across time using the same scanner, with the same time interval between injection and imaging, and with the use of identical processing and reconstruction techniques. In the event that standardization cannot be achieved, the Lugano consensus suggests that visual evaluation of therapy response using PET should be given priority. For quality assurance purposes, it is recommended to include visual assessment in all semiquantitative parameters analysis.[46–48]

PET imaging is frequently used in the management of MM. According to the updated diagnostic criteria from the International Myeloma Working Group, treatment should be considered when there are a number of focal bone lesions detected on MR imaging and one or more osteolytic lesions found on skeletal radiograph, CT, or ^{18}F-FDG-PET/CT. The Italian Myeloma Criteria for PET Use proposed the use of visual analysis of ^{18}F-FDG-PET/CT imaging, taking into account the metabolic activity of the bone marrow according to the D5PS, the number and location of FDG-avid focal lesions, the number of osteolytic lesions, and the presence of extramedullary disease (EMD).[49,50]

NOVEL QUANTITATIVE PARAMETERS

Hematological malignancies exhibit a widespread pattern of involvement. For instance, lymphomas and leukemia are characterized by the invasion of lymph nodes, liver, spleen, and bone marrow, resulting in the extensive involvement of several body regions. Hence, a modality that enables the images acquisition of the full body is crucial for a thorough evaluation of persons who are affected. The latest advancements in data-processing techniques that offer body part segmentation are highly compatible for analyzing data produced by hybrid PET/CT imaging. Unfortunately, commonly used PET-based parameters suffer from significant shortcomings and require clarification and revamping to achieve optimal utilization of PET/CT imaging in the treatment of hematological malignancies. Performing quantitative analysis with PET can be complex and tedious when analyzing each individual lesion. Efforts should be emphasized to provide easy, simple, efficient, and fast analysis of all lesions, allowing for their best utilization across various clinical situations of hematological malignancies. The assessment of SUVmax is of limited significance as it only represents findings from a constrained sample of disease sites and can potentially be deceptive. Therefore, it is not possible to generalize the interpretation of data based on SUVmax to encompass the tumor lesion or lesions found across the entire body and to view it as a reliable indicator of the global disease burden activity. As mentioned earlier, hematological malignancies are widespread and therefore it is necessary to evaluate the severity and extent of the disease activity throughout the entire body.[51]

GLOBAL DISEASE ASSESSMENT

In order to fix the shortcomings mentioned earlier, it is recommended that the evaluation of global assessment of disease activity should prioritize the use of SUVmean, the maximum distance between 2 lesions (Dmax), metabolic tumor volume (MTV), total lesion glycolysis (TLG), and total MTV (TMTV) as the preferred quantitative analysis in clinical settings. The Dmax is determined by calculating the maximum distance between 2 sites of disease. The MTV is a measure of the total volume of tumor lesion within a volume of interest (VOI).

The TLG is calculated by multiplying SUVmean for VOI by MTV. The TMTV is the sum of all the individual lesion volumes multiplied by the mean lesion SUV. It represents the total glycolytic burden of the disease, tumor heterogeneity, total tumor surface, and spatial dispersion on PET/CT imaging. The determination of these quantitative parameters is highly dependent on the precise specification of a VOI that uniquely defines the volume of the tumor. For calculation of MTV and TLG, process consists of 2 stages: (1) accurately defining the lesion by delineating the VOI and (2) segmenting each lesion to determine the boundaries of the VOI. In PET/CT imaging, various methods can be used to generate a segmented VOI and include manual delineation approach, thresholding, adaptive thresholding, region growth, gradient-based algorithms, and classifiers method.[52–54] The manual delineation method involves manually outlining a border around a metabolically active lesion to include the entire tumor lesion and avoid healthy tissues. This method is commonly used in clinical settings. Calculating the TMTV necessitates manually delineating several VOI over each lesion in hematological malignancy, a process that can be time-consuming and dependent on the operator's skills. Therefore, there is a need for a tool that utilizes semiautomatic, fully automatic, and AI techniques to efficiently extract quantitative parameters from PET/CT scans in cases of hematological malignancies.

THE USE OF ARTIFICIAL INTELLIGENCE IN ASSESSING QUANTITATIVE PARAMETERS IN PET/COMPUTED TOPOGRAPHY

AI is an expanding area of study that has had a significant impact on several aspects of our life. AI systems have the potential to further facilitate a wide range of features in the field of medical imaging. These include clinical decision-making, the enhancement of image acquisition, quality evaluation, post-processing procedures (including lesion delineation, registration, and quantification), and estimates of dose. Recent studies have shown that AI-assisted ^{18}F-FDG-PET/CT imaging can autonomously locate lymphoma, segment lesions, summarize features and heterogeneity, and track disease progression or response as shown in **Fig. 1**. They employ an AI-based industrial software prototype to delineate, segment, and quantify lymphoma lesions in the PET/CT. Machine learning is a subfield of AI that focuses on the development and implementation of computer algorithms. Machine learning algorithms construct a model using the provided training data in order to generate predictions or make decisions. Deep

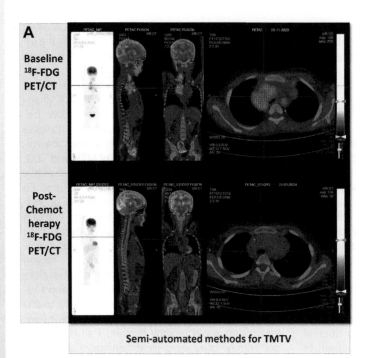

A

Baseline
¹⁸F-FDG
PET/CT

Post-
Chemot
herapy
¹⁸F-FDG
PET/CT

Semi-automated methods for TMTV

Fig. 1. A 11 year old male patient, known case of HL. The patient underwent baseline and post-chemotherapy ¹⁸F-FDG-PET/CT imaging. The baseline ¹⁸F-FDG-PET/CT showed (*A*) multiple enlarged FDG-avid cervical, supraclavicular, and mediastinal lymph nodes. Hence in this case, manual calculation of the newer quantitative metrices like MTV, TLG, and TMTV is time-consuming. Semiautomatic method using AI-aided software (Segami Oasis software) provides these values within few minutes as shown in panel *B*. Global disease activity was measured by using Segami Oasis software at thresholding of SUVmax 40% as shown in panels *A* and *B* with significant reduction of TMTV value from 408.8 to 18 after chemotherapy suggestive of favorable response to chemotherapy. (*With permission from* Segami Oasis Software.)

B

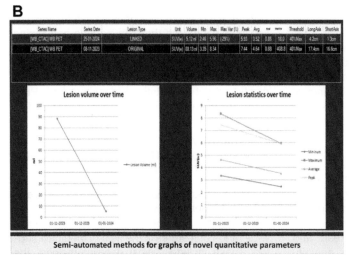

Semi-automated methods for graphs of novel quantitative parameters

learning is a machine learning approach that relies on artificial neural networks. Deep learning is a form of representation learning that encompasses a range of techniques enabling a machine to process raw data and automatically identify the relevant features for classification. Convolutional neural networks (CNNs) are a subset of machine learning that are currently being used to analyze medical images and have proven to be highly effective in visual tasks such as image recognition, object detection, and segmentation. AI carried out automated quantification, encompassing (1) the automatic identification of lesion locations, (2) the automatic segmentation of the lesion, and (3) the generation of a summary and total tumor burden. AI can provide registration at various intervals. This enables the assessment of hematological malignancies both prior to and following diagnosis or treatment as shown in **Fig. 2**. Therefore, the utilization of AI in PET/CT imaging for hematological malignancies is likely to be significant in the near future. As stated previously, novel quantitative parameters in hematological malignancies are assessed for global disease burden using MTV, TLG, and TMTV on PET/CT imaging as shown in **Fig. 3**. For quantification of these parameters, all lesions must be detected and segmented manually, which is time-consuming

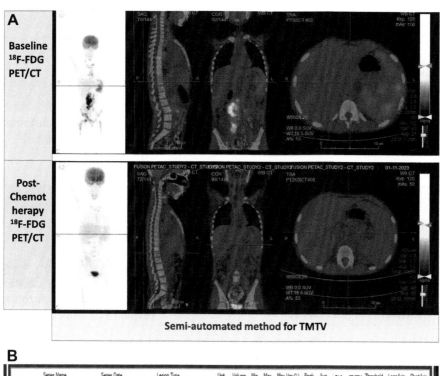

Semi-automated method for TMTV

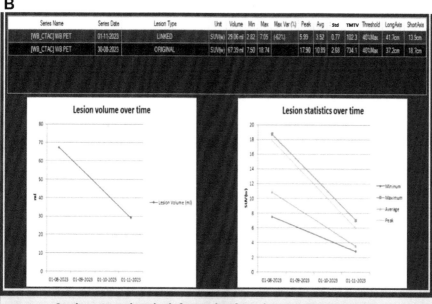

Series Name	Series Date	Lesion Type	Unit	Volume	Min	Max	Max Var (%)	Peak	Avg	Std	TMTV	Threshold	LongAxis	ShortAxis
[WB_CTAC] WB PET	01-11-2023	LINKED	SUV(w)	29.06 ml	2.82	7.05	(-62%)	5.99	3.52	0.77	102.3	40%Max	41.7cm	13.9cm
[WB_CTAC] WB PET	30-08-2023	ORIGINAL	SUV(w)	67.39 ml	7.50	18.74		17.90	10.89	2.68	734.1	40%Max	37.2cm	18.7cm

Semi-automated methods for graphs of novel quantitative parameters

Fig. 2. A 15 year old male patient of HL with extensive multi-organ disease involvement. Patient underwent baseline and post-chemotherapy ^{18}F-FDG-PET/CT imaging. Baseline ^{18}F-FDG-PET/CT showed (*A*) wide-spread involvement of lymph nodes all over body and extra-nodal disease involving multiple organs such as spleen and bone marrow. In this case, manual calculation of novel quantitative metrices is time-consuming task with a high degree of intra-observer and inter-observer variability. AI-aided software (Segami Oasis software) by using semiautomatic method (even in extensive disease with involvement of multiple organs) provided these values within few minutes as shown in panel *B*. Global disease activity was measured by using Segami Oasis software at thresholding of SUVmax 40%, showed (*A, B*) significant reduction of TMTV value from 734.1 to 102.3 after chemotherapy suggestive of favorable response to chemotherapy. (*With permission from* Segami Oasis Software.)

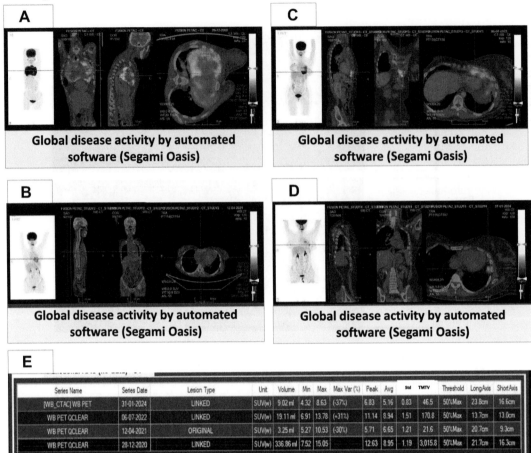

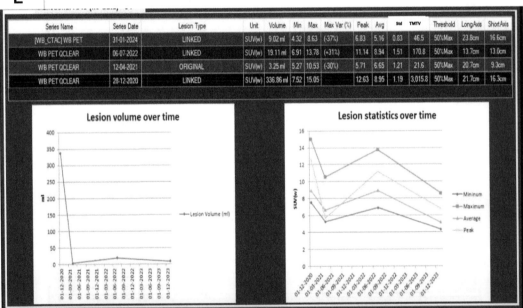

Semi-automated method used for graphs of novel quantitative parameters

Fig. 3. A 25 year old female patient known case of DLBCL involving mediastinal region. Patient underwent baseline, post-chemotherapy, and follow-up ^{18}F-FDG-PET/CT scans. Baseline ^{18}F-FDG-PET/CT scan (*A*) showed heterogeneous FDG uptake in the large mediastinal mass. Post-chemotherapy ^{18}F-FDG-PET/CT scan (*B*) showed complete metabolic response, but subsequent follow-up ^{18}F-FDG-PET/CT scans (*C, D*) showed FDG-avid lesions in mediastinal and left lung regions, suggestive of recurrence of disease. Use of novel quantitative metrices provided more accurate values of FDG uptake as compared to single pixel SUVmax measurement in evaluation of heterogenous tumor and also predicted response and recurrence appropriately in hematological malignancies. Global disease activity was measured by using Segami Oasis software at thresholding of SUVmax 50%, showed (*E*) high value (3015.8) of TMTV at baseline in heterogeneous tumor. This patient developed recurrence of disease within 14 months. Hence, novel quantitative analysis is useful for predicting prognosis in hematological malignancies. (*With permission from Segami Oasis Software.*)

and involves a significant amount of variability for intraobserver and interobserver. To quantify these novel parameters, AI can be employed using either of 2 approaches: (1) initially, a human (nuclear medicine physician) detects and selects the lesion, which is then followed by AI-based segmentation using a semiautomated approach as shown in **Fig. 4**. (2) In contrast, there is no involvement of a human (nuclear medicine physician) in identifying the lesion. AI will automatically detect and segment lesions in a fully automated manner. While fully automated models can eliminate the need for human to identify lesions, semiautomated models may offer advantages in terms of accuracy or precision. Human participation in semiautomatic methods is seen in 2 ways: (1) process involves using human input to detect and identify lesions before automatically segmenting the detected lesions. (2) Lesions with a high rate of false positives are automatically detected and segmented, but human are still needed to determine which lesions are true positive and dismiss the false positives.[55–57] Biodistribution of ^{18}F-FDG causes high normal activity (HiNA) zones with sites of FDG excretion and physiologic FDG uptake in the kidneys, bladder, brain, and heart, which can impair AI-based lesion recognition and segmentation in hematological malignancies. One may omit HiNA regions from the scene before lesion detection to improve AI model performance. This can be done manually or automatically preprocessing or postprocessing. Removing HiNA regions from training data improves automatic AI lesion detection and segmentation. Yu and colleagues employed a semiautomatic method to identify and delete HiNA regions, then used AI algorithm to detect lymphoma lesions in patients.[56] Therefore, an AI algorithm trained to identify and remove HiNA regions, while also quantifying tumor lesions in hematological malignancies will enhance workflow and facilitate integration into clinical practice. Currently, the absence of standardized, trustworthy, reproducible, generalizable, and precise approaches is hindering the broad application of AI-based models for quantifying novel parameters in clinical practice using PET/CT. However, the application of AI in PET/CT imaging offers extensive, optimistic, and promising possibilities. Nevertheless, there are challenges that must be immediately addressed, such as the requirement for high-quality and diverse PET/CT imaging datasets to construct AI algorithms. These databases can assist researchers in overcoming different challenges and expanding the diversity of the patient population and subtypes of hematological malignancies, hence improving generality of algorithms.

NOVEL QUANTITATIVE PARAMETERS: CLINICAL STUDIES IN HEMATOLOGICAL MALIGNANCIES

Novel quantitative parameters derived from ^{18}F-FDG-PET/CT imaging may have additional utility in lymphoma staging; for instance, it has been reported that TMTV defines risk more precisely than the Ann Arbor Staging.[58] The incorporation of TMTV as prognostic index into the management and treatment of patients with HL and DLBCL has better results.[59,60] In the analysis of the extensive REMARC trial involving older patients with DLBCL, Cottereau and colleagues found that the Dmax was a strong predictor of a worse prognosis.[61,62] In the analysis of the trial, Vercellino and colleagues found that a high TMTV value at the beginning of the study is a predictor of survival.[63] High baseline TLG and TMTV values independently predicted poor outcome in treatment-naive patients with DLBCL treated with chemoimmunotherapy in the GOYA trial.[64] High TMTV value predicts poor PFS and OS in FL. Similarly, in primary mediastinal B-cell and MCLs, metabolic heterogeneity observed by PET/CT imaging predicts a worse prognosis.[65,66]

In relapsed/refractory HL, TMTV predicts therapeutic success with autologous stem-cell transplantation (ASCT). Moskowicz and colleagues demonstrated that the TMTV enhanced the prognostic accuracy of pre-ASCT PET in comparison to PET positivity following initial treatment. They demonstrated baseline TMTV and pre-ASCT PET independently predicted three year event-free survival of 86% for low TMTV patients and 0% for high TMTV.[67] Mikhaeel and colleagues in DLBCL showed that TMTV could improve early PET response prediction, and a large prospective cohort of 510 patients with DLBCL treated in the PET-guided therapy optimization trial PETAL validated this.[68,69]

In MM, localized and diffuse bone lesions may coexist with varied FDG uptake; hence, ^{18}F-FDG-PET/CT interpretation may be difficult. In clinical routine, assessment of bone marrow involvement is mostly visual and subjective. Quantitative thus more objective assessments limited to the calculation of the semiquantitative parameter such as SUVmax, which is susceptible to several factors, such as reconstruction and acquisition parameters, partial-volume correction, blood glucose, and time between ^{18}F-FDG injection and image acquisition. ^{18}F-FDG-PET/CT imaging findings, including a SUVmax more than 4.2, the presence of more than 3 focal lesions, and the existence of EMD, are regarded as prognostic markers with inconsistent and nonreproducible measurement of tumor burden in MM. In this particular situation, MTV and TLG have

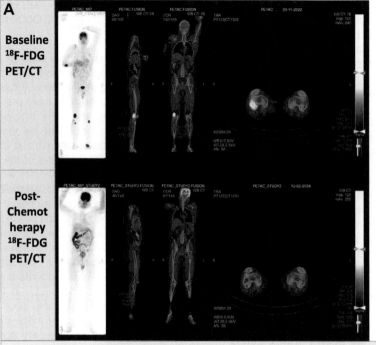

Semi-automated method by software (Segami Oasis) for calculating TMTV in patient of Multiple Myeloma with multi-site skeletal involvement

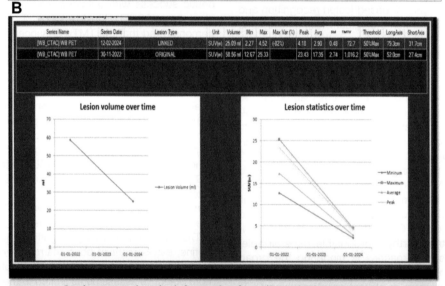

Semi-automated methods for graphs of novel quantitative parameters

Fig. 4. A 51 year old male patient known case of MM with multi-site bone involvement. The patient underwent baseline and post-chemotherapy ^{18}F-FDG-PET/CT imaging. Baseline ^{18}F-FDG-PET/CT showed (*A*) multiple bone involvement all over the body. Therefore, manual calculation of novel quantitative metrices was a time-consuming task. AI-aided software (Segami Oasis) by using semiautomatic method provided these values within few minutes as shown in (*B*). Global disease activity was measured by using Segami Oasis software at thresholding of SUVmax 50%, showed (*A, B*) significant reduction of TMTV values from 1016.2 to 72.7 after chemotherapy suggestive of favorable response to chemotherapy. (*With permission from* Segami Oasis Software.)

been suggested as potentially valuable metabolic indicators for measuring the extent of tumor burden and predicting the prognosis in patients with MM. In a retrospective study, Terao T and colleagues[70] examined and evaluated the prognostic significance of MTV, TLG, and high-risk PET/CT variables (a SUVmax >4.2, the presence of > 3 focal lesions, and the EMD) in 185 patients with newly diagnosed symptomatic MM. The authors found that high levels of MTV and TLG were independently associated with both poorer PFS and OS. Their findings indicate that pretreatment MTV and TLG can independently forecast survival outcomes in clinical settings, potentially surpassing the predictive value of high-risk PET/CT variables.

Studies mentioned earlier presented various threshold values for MTV, TLG, and TMTV in order to distinguish between high-risk and low-risk patients. However, the use of nonuniform quantification methodologies has resulted in confusion. Therefore, the implementation of standardized methods for measuring these parameters is anticipated to resolve this problem. Undoubtedly, the initial crucial phase involves integrating the measurement techniques and determining the optimal approach. Nevertheless, it is crucial to bear in mind that in these studies, the likelihood of events occurring rises as values for the global disease burden quantitative parameters increase.

ARTIFICIAL INTELLIGENCE APPLICATIONS IN CLINICAL STUDIES IN HEMATOLOGICAL MALIGNANCIES

Currently, there have been only a limited number of studies published on the utilization of AI in measurement of PET/CT-based quantitative parameters for hematological malignancies. The majority of the studies are retrospective in nature. Bi and colleagues applied AI through a deep CNN to classify areas of normal physiologic FDG uptake and FDG excretion on PET/CT images in a cohort of 40 lymphoma patients. The authors used multi-scale superpixel-based encoding to cluster several sections of normal FDG uptake into larger segments, enabling the CNN to extract the highly distinctive features.[71] The D5PS assesses the level of FDG uptake in a lesion by comparing it to the normal FDG uptake in the mediastinum (blood pool) and liver reference regions. Hence, assessment of FDG uptake in mediastinal blood pool and liver reference regions are essential for evaluation of lymphoma response to treatment. This information may be facilitated by AI-assisted technology in the near future.

Sadik and colleagues utilized an AI model to achieve automatic segmentation of the mediastinal blood pool and liver regions in CT images. Subsequently, transfer the ROI to the PET scans in order to compute the SUV of the reference regions. The authors employed this model on a cohort of 80 patients with lymphoma and observed that the automated quantification of the reference levels yielded results that were similar to those obtained through manual segmentation of the regions.[72]

Sibille L and colleagues assessed configurations of deep CNN for the purpose of identifying and classifying FDG uptake patterns on ^{18}F-FDG-PET/CT images in patients with lung cancer and lymphoma. A total of 629 patients were enrolled in their study, with 302 patients diagnosed with lung cancer and 327 patients diagnosed with lymphoma. Two nuclear medicine experts manually identified areas with increased FDG uptake, precisely determined their anatomic location, and classified these observations as either indicative of tumor lesion or metastasis, or non-tumor lesion. A CNN was developed to detect areas with positive FDG uptake, predict their anatomic location, and determine the expert classification, using these expert readings as the reference standard. The investigators found that a CNN demonstrated a high level of accuracy in automatically detecting and classifying areas with positive FDG uptake in patients with lung cancer and lymphoma, as observed in ^{18}F-FDG-PET/CT imaging. This accuracy was found to be comparable to that used by expert readers. For the most accurate FDG uptake pattern identification and classification, they recommended use of both ^{18}F-FDG-PET and CT data for analysis of PET/CT imaging.[73]

Blanc-Durand and colleagues utilized a 3 dimensional (3D) CNN to automatically segment TMTV in large datasets of patients with DLBCL, with the aim of evaluating the global disease burden. The dataset used in this study consists of pre-therapy ^{18}F-FDG-PET/CT scans obtained from 733 patients diagnosed with DLBCL who participated in 2 prospective trials conducted by the Lymphoma Study Association. The authors utilized the nnUNet Python library to train the model, which is an open-source deep learning framework that incorporates the latest domain knowledge and independently makes the necessary decisions to adapt a basic architecture. Their findings indicate that a CNN utilizing a U-Net architecture can yield remarkable outcomes in accurately segmenting lymphoma lesions. Therefore, this particular CNN conducted a fully automated evaluation of TMTV to assess the global disease burden. It accomplished this by utilizing both PET and CT image volumes as inputs, although there was a slight underestimation of TMTV.[74]

Capobianco and colleagues conducted a comparative analysis of the global disease burden measurement in patients with DLBCL using an AI-based technique to calculate TMTV, compared to manually measuring TMTV. The retrospective analysis of 301 patients with DLBCL from the REMARC study involved examining their baseline ^{18}F-FDG-PET/CT scans using prototype software called PET-assisted reporting system. The AI-based method was used to identify all 3D ROIs that showed increased FDG uptake. The obtained ROIs were subjected to analysis using a CNN. The ROIs were then classed as either showing non-suspicious or suspicious uptake. The AI-based measurement of TMTV was in agreement with that obtained by experts. Furthermore, the authors showed that AI-based measured TMTV as prognostic marker for PFS and OS in patients with DLBCL. They concluded that AI-based measurement of TMTV simplifies process of global disease burden estimation, reduces observer variability, and encourages the use of these parameters as a predictive factor in DLBCL patients.[75]

Girum and colleagues investigated the utilization of an AI method to assess the TMTV and Dmax in patients with DLBCL by analyzing 2 dimensional (2D) maximum-intensity projections (MIPs) of whole-body ^{18}F-FDG-PET images. The authors found that TMTV and Dmax computed from 2D PET MIP images can serve as predictive biomarkers in patients with DLBCL. These biomarkers can be automatically estimated from 2D images, rather than 3D images, enabling convenient and rapid assessment of TMTV and Dmax in clinical settings.[76]

Sachpekidis and colleagues investigated the performance of a new 3D deep learning technique on ^{18}F-FDG-PET/CT scans to automatically estimate the intensity of bone marrow metabolism in patients with MM. They compared the automatically estimated MTV and TLG with visual PET/CT imaging, as well as with histologic, cytogenetic, and clinical data of the patients. The authors found a significant and positive association between the values obtained from AI-based MTV and TLG calculations and the outcomes of the visual analysis of the PET/CT images. In addition, they showed a strong positive relationship between the infiltration of plasma cells in the bone marrow and the levels of β2-microglobulin in the plasma, with the automated quantitative PET/CT parameters MTV and TLG in patients with MM.[77]

FUTURE DIRECTIONS
PET/Computed Topography: Delta Quantitative Assessment

Currently, there is a limited comparison of quantitative analysis of PET/CT parameters between baseline PET and iPET/ePET images in both research and clinical settings. Temporal changes in a lesion can offer more valuable information in clinical practice than the imaging features of a lesion in a single examination. The Delta-quantitative assessment evaluates the changes in quantitative parameters before and after therapy to improve the extraction of information from PET/CT imaging analysis at multiple time-points, compared to a single time-point for analysis. Delta-quantitative assessment involves measuring the differences between baseline and interim/end parameters on PET/CT images, namely ΔSUV-mean, ΔMTV, ΔTLG, ΔTMTV, and ΔDmax.[78,79] Delta images can provide post-treatment tumor change, intra-lesion tumor heterogeneity, and prognosis prediction for oncological patients. Further studies should investigate the optimal methods of visualizing the Delta image to enhance its interpretability. Moreover, AI-based algorithms can focus on quantifying Delta images and identifying nonresponders at an early stage. This Delta-quantitative assessment allows the improvement of the treatment or guide biopsy of the unresponsive lesion for new mutations analysis.

Newer Radiopharmaceuticals for PET/ Computed Topography

Various new radiopharmaceuticals have been utilized for imaging hematological malignancies. For example, ^{18}F-labeled arginine-glycine-aspartic (RGD) specifically binds to the αvβ3 integrin, which is a biomarker for tumor neoangiogenesis. A preliminary examination of 18 patients with lymphoma who had RGD PET scans before treatment revealed high uptake of RGD in classical HL and gray zone lymphoma.[80] The chemokine C-X-C motif receptor 4 (CXCR4) molecules are present in hematopoietic cells, making it a potentially excellent choice for PET/CT imaging in hematological malignancies particularly in MM and lymphoma. ^{68}Ga-Pentixafor is a radiopharmaceutical that specifically targets CXCR4. It has demonstrated beneficial use in patients with MM and lymphoma. Recent research indicates that ^{68}Ga-Pentixafor is a highly promising substitute for ^{18}F-FDG in the staging of lymphoma patients, particularly in cases of lymphomas with low FDG uptake, such as marginal cell lymphoma and MALT lymphoma.[81–83] The fibroblast activation protein (FAP) is another promising target for imaging hematological malignancies, as it is specifically expressed by tumor-associated fibroblasts. The FAP inhibitor (FAPI) using ^{68}Ga-FAPI-04 PET/CT imaging has been investigated for its promise in different types of lymphoma and MM.[84] Hence, further research is necessary to explore the potential application of these newer radiopharmaceuticals in PET/CT imaging for quantitative analysis of hematological malignancies.

SUMMARY

Hematological malignancies exhibit diversity in terms of their incidence, prognosis, and causes. These diseases are induced by cells of the bone marrow or immune system. Hematological malignancies, such as lymphoma and MM, are known to be widespread and include the entire skeleton, contrary to the majority of solid tumors, which are confined to the bones and organs in the trunk. PET/CT is an essential and powerful diagnostic imaging technique used in oncology. It has a wide range of applications such as determining the initial stage of cancer, evaluating the effectiveness of treatment, restaging of cancer, and detecting suspected recurrence. This is especially beneficial in clinical settings for patients with FDG-avid lymphomas and MM, which frequently employ ^{18}F-FDG-PET/CT. Currently, routine clinical practice uses visual analysis utilizing D5PS and semiquantitative parameters (SUVmax) to assess response on ^{18}F-FDG-PET/CT in hematological malignancies. The significance of measuring SUVmax is notably restricted, as it solely represents measurements from a restricted sample of the disease sites and has the potential to be misleading. Therefore, the data derived from SUVmax cannot be extrapolated to the entire lesion and regarded as indicative of the global disease burden activity. Hence, the validity of the assertions made relying on SUVmax data is not ideal. Moreover, hematological malignancies exhibit a widespread distribution, necessitating the evaluation of disease activity over the entire body and/or skeletal system. The validity of relying just on the assessment of 3 or a few specific lesions for making clinical decisions is questionable, given that lymphoma affects many regions of the body and MM extensively infiltrates the bone marrow. An effective way to evaluate the global disease burden in hematological malignancies can be to utilize novel quantitative parameters such as MTV, TLG, TMTV, and Dmax, in addition to addressing the previous inadequacies. Currently, the measurement of these quantitative parameters is typically done using a manual or semiautomatic approach. However, this approach, particularly manual one is often time-consuming and demanding, as it necessitates substantial computing power and the creation of speedy and reproducible computer programs. The field of AI research is growing and has various applications in medical imaging, such as facilitating the ordering and protocoling of scans, screening, scheduling appointments, providing clinical decision support, managing image collections, assessing image quality, archiving image data, delineating tumors, registering images, and quantifying results. AI can utilize fully automated or semiautomated approaches and CNN algorithms to determine novel quantitative parameters on PET/CT imaging. This allows for the assessment of the global disease burden for hematological malignancies. AI-derived TMTV plays a crucial role in analyzing and assessing several aspects of hematological malignancies. It helps in characterizing tumors, measuring their heterogeneity, predicting treatment response, determining survival rates, and classifying the risk of recurrence. At present, clinical usage of AI-based models and ^{18}F-FDG-PET/CT-derived novel quantitative parameters are limited by the lack of standardized, reproducible, generalizable, and precise techniques. In the near future, we expect the integration of these novel quantitative parameters and AI algorithms into the routine clinical practices of hematological malignancies by using PET/CT imaging, as we enhance their reliability and validity.

CLINICS CARE POINTS

Pearls

- Hybrid 18F-FDG-PET/CT is considered as one-stop-shop imaging that provides both functional and anatomical information of tumor lesions, as well as crucial information regarding the quantification of tracer activity within the lesions.

- Hematological malignancies are characterized by a widespread distribution, which requires an assessment of disease activity throughout the entire body. PET/CT is an important imaging technique in this scenario, as it can provide a "top-of-head-to-feet" whole-body image.

- PET/CT imaging provides semiquantitative parameters such as SUVmax, which represents the highest metabolic activity in the region of interest (ROI), the mean SUV (SUVmean), which represents the overall metabolic activity in ROI, and the SUVpeak, which represents the highest activity within a 1 cm3 area surrounding the most metabolically active pixel. SUVpeak has more stability compared to other metrics. However, in clinical practice, SUVpeak is not as commonly utilized as SUVmax.

- The measurement of global disease burden activity in hematological malignancies by using SUVmax is of limited significance as it only represents findings from a limited sample of disease sites and can be at times deceptive. Therefore, it is not possible to generalize the interpretation of data based on SUVmax to encompass the tumor lesion or lesions found across the entire body. Therefore, the global assessment of disease in hematological malignancies should be performed using novel quantitative PET/CT-based parameters, including the maximum distance between two lesions (Dmax), metabolic tumor volume (MTV), total lesion glycolysis (TLG), and total MTV (TMTV).

- The TMTV is the sum of all the individual lesion volumes multiplied by the mean lesion SUV. The total glycolytic burden of the disease, tumor heterogeneity, total tumor surface, and spatial dispersion on PET/CT imaging are all represented by TMTV. Calculating the TMTV requires the manual delineation of multiple volume of interest (VOI) over each lesion in hematological malignancy, a procedure that is time-consuming and contingent upon the operator's abilities. Consequently, there is a requirement for a tool that employs artificial intelligence (AI), semiautomatic, and fully automatic techniques to effectively extract these quantitative parameters from PET/CT scans.

- Delta-quantitative assessment evaluates quantitative parameter changes before and after therapy to improve PET/CT imaging analysis at multiple time-points. Delta-quantitative assessment measures differences in baseline and interim/end parameters on PET/CT scans, including ΔSUVmean, ΔMTV, ΔTLG, ΔTMTV, and ΔDmax.

Pitfalls

- The Deauville 5 point scoring (D5PS) system is utilized to assess the response in lymphoma. In D5PS, the point spread function and visually visible activity in tumor lesions may be altered by the reconstruction techniques and the type of scanner used, which may lead to potential error in response evaluation. Thus, it is crucial to rigorously standardize the processing and reconstruction techniques between scans in order to prevent any potential errors.

- The stability and reproducibility of PET/CT based semiquantitative parameters are influenced by various factors such as the size (partial volume effects for small size lesion) and heterogeneity of the target lesion (lead to decreased average SUV measurements), the time between uptake and imaging, patient preparation, acquisition, processing and reconstruction techniques, and the performance of the individual scanner etc. It is crucial in clinical practice to accurately replicate these characteristics between scans and to use the same equipment and protocol for each imaging session for response evaluation and monitoring therapy in patients with hematological malignancies.

DISCLOSURE

No disclosure/conflict of interest declared by any of the authors.

REFERENCES

1. Kapoor V, McCook BM, Torok FS. An introduction to PET-CT imaging. Radiographics 2004;24:523–43.
2. Weber WA. Quantitative analysis of PET studies. Radiother Oncol 2010;96:308–10.
3. Almuhaideb A, Papathanasiou N, Bomanji J. 18F-FDG PET/CT imaging in oncology. Ann Saudi Med 2011;31:3–13.
4. Raynor WY, Al-Zaghal A, Zadeh MZ, et al. Metastatic seeding attacks bone marrow, not bone: rectifying ongoing misconceptions. Pet Clin 2019;14(1):135–44.
5. Houshmand S, Salavati A, Hess S, et al. An update on novel quantitative techniques in the context of evolving whole-body PET imaging. Pet Clin 2015;10(1):45–58.
6. Parghane RV, Basu S. PET/Computed tomography in treatment response assessment in cancer: an overview with emphasis on the evolving role in response evaluation to immunotherapy and radiation therapy. Pet Clin 2020 Jan;15(1):101–23.
7. Barrington SF, Mikhaeel NG, Kostakoglu L, et al. Role of imaging in the staging and response assessment of lymphoma: consensus of the international conference on malignant lymphomas imaging working group. J Clin Oncol 2014;32:3048–58.
8. Cheson BD, Fisher RI, Barrington SF, et al. Recommendations for initial evaluation, staging, and response assessment of Hodgkin and non-Hodgkin lymphoma: the Lugano classification. J Clin Oncol 2014;32:3059–68.
9. Dreyling M, Thieblemont C, Gallamini A, et al. ESMO Consensus conferences: guidelines on malignant lymphoma. part 2: marginal zone lymphoma, mantle cell lymphoma, peripheral T-cell lymphoma. Ann Oncol 2013;24:857–77.
10. Zelenetz AD, Wierda WG, Abramson JS, et al. Non-Hodgkin's Lymphomas, version 3.2012. J Natl Compr Cancer Netw 2012;10:1487–98.
11. Attygalle AD, Chan JKC, Coupland SE, et al. The 5th edition of the World Health Organization Classification

of mature lymphoid and stromal tumors - an overview and update. Leuk Lymphoma 2024;8:1–17.

12. Swerdlow SH, Campo E, Pileri SA, et al. The 2016 revision of the World Health Organization classification of lymphoid neoplasms. Blood 2016 May 19; 127(20):2375–90.

13. Weiler-Sagie M, Bushelev O, Epelbaum R, et al. (18)F-FDG avidity in lymphoma readdressed: a study of 766 patients. J Nucl Med 2010;51:25–30.

14. Swerdlow SH, Campo E, Harris NL, et al. WHO classification of tumours of haematopoietic and lymphoid tissues, In: Swerdlow SH, Campo E, Harris NL, et al. editors. WHO classification of tumours, 2008, IARC; Lyon (France). 10-15.

15. Armitage JO, Weisenburger DD. New approach to classifying non-Hodgkin's lymphomas: clinical features of the major histologic subtypes. Non-Hodgkin's Lymphoma Classification Project. J Clin Oncol 1998;16:2780–95.

16. Elstrom R, Guan L, Baker G, et al. Utility of FDG-PET scanning in lymphoma by WHO classification. Blood 2003;101:3875–6.

17. Tsukamoto N, Kojima M, Hasegawa M, et al. The usefulness of (18)F-fluorodeoxyglucose positron emission tomography ((18)F-FDG-PET) and a comparison of (18)F-FDG-pet with (67)gallium scintigraphy in the evaluation of lymphoma: relation to histologic subtypes based on the World Health Organization classification. Cancer 2007;110:652–9.

18. Lim MS, Beaty M, Sorbara L, et al. T-cell/histiocyte-rich large B-cell lymphoma: a heterogeneous entity with derivation from germinal center B cells. Am J Surg Pathol 2002;26:1458–66.

19. Dimopoulos M, Terpos E, Comenzo RL, et al, IMWG. International myeloma working group consensus statement and guidelines regarding the current role of imaging techniques in the diagnosis and monitoring of multiple Myeloma. Leukemia 2009;23(9):1545–56.

20. Collins CD. Multiple myeloma. Cancer Imag 2010; 10(1):20–31.

21. D'Agostino M, Cairns DA, Lahuerta JJ, et al. Second revision of the international staging system (R2-ISS) for overall survival in multiple myeloma: a European myeloma network (emn) report within the harmony project. J Clin Oncol 2022;40(29):3406–18.

22. Durie BG. The role of anatomic and functional staging in myeloma: description of Durie/Salmon plus staging system. Eur J Cancer 2006 Jul;42(11):1539–43.

23. Healy CF, Murray JG, Eustace SJ, et al. Multiple myeloma: a review of imaging features and radiological techniques. Bone Marrow Res 2011;2011: 583439.

24. Lütje S, de Rooy JW, Croockewit S, et al. Role of radiography, MRI and FDG-PET/CT in diagnosing, staging and therapeutical evaluation of patients with multiple myeloma. Ann Hematol 2009 Dec; 88(12):1161–8.

25. Salem AE, Zaki YH, El-Hussieny G, et al. Uncommon variants of mature T-cell lymphomas (MTCLs): imaging and histopathologic and clinical features with updates from the fourth edition of the world health organization (WHO) classification of lymphoid neoplasms. Cancers (Basel) 2021 Oct 18;13(20):5217.

26. Fox TA, Carpenter B, Taj M, et al. Utility of 18F-FDG-PET/CT in lymphoblastic lymphoma. Leuk Lymphoma 2021 Apr;62(4):1010–2.

27. Arslan F, Yilmaz M, Cakir T, et al. Significant contribution of Fluorodeoxyglucose positron emission tomography/computed tomography (FDG PET/CT) in a case of acute lymphoblastic leukemia presenting with fever of unknown origin. Intern Med 2014; 53(7):789–91.

28. Zhao Z, Hu Y, Li J, et al. Applications of PET in diagnosis and prognosis of leukemia. Technol Cancer Res Treat 2020 Jan-Dec;19. 1533033820956993.

29. Litz CE, Arthur DC, Gajl-Peczalska KJ, et al. Transformation of chronic lymphocytic leukemia to small non-cleaved cell lymphoma: a cytogenetic, immunological, and molecular study. Leukemia 1991 Nov; 5(11):972–8.

30. Endo T, Sato N, Koizumi K, et al. Localized relapse in bone marrow of extremities after allogeneic stem cell transplantation for acute lymphoblastic leukemia. Am J Hematol 2004;76:279–82.

31. Ennishi D, Maeda Y, Niiya M, et al. Incidental detection of acute lymphoblastic leukemia on [18F]fluorodeoxyglucose positron emission tomography. J Clin Oncol 2009;27:e269–70.

32. Kuenzle K, Taverna C, Steinert HC. Detection of extramedullary infiltrates in acute myelogenous leukemia with whole-body positron emission tomography and 2-deoxy-2-[18F]-fluoro-D-glucose. Mol Imag Biol 2002;4:179–83.

33. Stolzel F, Rollig C, Radke J, et al. (1)(8)F-FDG-PET/CT for detection of extramedullary acute myeloid leukemia. Haematologica 2011;96:1552–6.

34. Falchi L, Keating MJ, Marom EM, et al. Correlation between FDG/PET, histology, characteristics, and survival in 332 patients with chronic lymphoid leukemia. Blood 2014;123:2783–90.

35. Conte MJ, Bowen DA, Wiseman GA, et al. Use of positron emission tomography-computed tomography in the management of patients with chronic lymphocytic leukemia/small lymphocytic lymphoma. Leuk Lymphoma 2014;55:2079–84.

36. Papajik T, Myslivecek M, Urbanova R, et al. 2-[18F]fluoro-2-deoxy-D-glucose positron emission tomography/computed tomography examination in patients with chronic lymphocytic leukemia may reveal Richter transformation. Leuk Lymphoma 2014;55:314–9.

37. Bruzzi JF, Macapinlac H, Tsimberidou AM, et al. Detection of Richter's transformation of chronic lymphocytic leukemia by PET/CT. J Nucl Med 2006;47: 1267–73.

38. Parikh SA, Kay NE, Shanafelt TD. How we treat Richter syndrome. Blood 2014;123:1647–57.

39. Conconi A, Ponzio C, Lobetti-Bodoni C, et al. Incidence, risk factors and outcome of histological transformation in follicular lymphoma. Br J Haematol 2012;157:188–96.

40. Mauro FR, Chauvie S, Paoloni F, et al. Diagnostic and prognostic role of PET/CT in patients with chronic lymphocytic leukemia and progressive disease. Leukemia 2015;29:1360–5.

41. Barrington SF, Mikhaeel NG, Kostakoglu L, et al. Role of imaging in the staging and response assessment of lymphoma: consensus of the international conference on malignant lymphomas imaging working group. J Clin Oncol 2014 Sep 20;32(27): 3048–58.

42. Johnson SA, Kumar A, Matasar MJ, et al. Imaging for staging and response assessment in lymphoma. Radiology 2015 Aug;276(2):323–38.

43. Pinilla I, Gómez-León N, Del Campo-Del Val L, et al. Diagnostic value of CT, PET and combined PET/CT performed with low-dose unenhanced CT and full-dose enhanced CT in the initial staging of lymphoma. Q J Nucl Med Mol Imaging 2011 Oct; 55(5):567–75.

44. Albano D, Micci G, Patti C, et al. Whole-body magnetic resonance imaging: current role in patients with lymphoma. Diagnostics (Basel) 2021 May 31; 11(6):1007.

45. Cheson BD, Fisher RI, Barrington SF, et al. Recommendations for initial evaluation, staging, and response assessment of Hodgkin and non-Hodgkin lymphoma: the Lugano classification. J Clin Oncol 2014 Sep 20;32(27):3059–68.

46. Sher A, Lacoeuille F, Fosse P, et al. For avid glucose tumors, the SUV peak is the most reliable parameter for [(18)F]FDG-PET/CT quantification, regardless of acquisition time. EJNMMI Res 2016 Dec;6(1):21.

47. Adams MC, Turkington TG, Wilson JM, et al. A systematic review of the factors affecting accuracy of SUV measurements. AJR Am J Roentgenol 2010 Aug;195(2):310–20.

48. Parghane RV, Basu S. PET-CTBased quantitative parameters for assessment of treatment response and disease activity in cancer and noncancerous disorders. Pet Clin 2022 Jul;17(3):465–78.

49. Rajkumar SV, Dimopoulos MA, Palumbo A, et al. International Myeloma Working Group updated criteria for the diagnosis of multiple myeloma. Lancet Oncol 2014 Nov;15(12):e538–48.

50. Nanni C, Zamagni E, Versari A, et al. Image interpretation criteria for FDG PET/CT in multiple myeloma: a new proposal from an Italian expert panel. IMPeTUs (Italian Myeloma criteria for PET USe). Eur J Nucl Med Mol Imag 2016 Mar;43(3):414–21.

51. Kwee TC, Cheng G, Lam MG, et al. SUVmax of 2.5 should not be embraced as a magic threshold for separating benign from malignant lesions. Eur J Nucl Med Mol Imag 2013 Oct;40(10):1475–7.

52. Alavi A, Reivich M, Greenberg J, et al. Mapping of functional activity in brain with 18F-fluoro-deoxyglucose. Semin Nucl Med 1981;11:24–31.

53. Zaidi H, Ruest T, Schoenahl F, et al. Comparative evaluation of statistical brain MR image segmentation algorithms and their impact on partial volume effect correction in PET. Neuroimage 2006;32: 1591–607.

54. Soret M, Bacharach SL, Buvat I. Partial-volume effect in PET tumor imaging. J Nucl Med 2007;48: 932–45.

55. Guo R, Hu X, Song H, et al. Weakly supervised deep learning for determining the prognostic value of ^{18}F-FDG PET/CT in extranodal natural killer/T cell lymphoma, nasal type. Eur J Nucl Med Mol Imag 2021 Sep;48(10):3151–61.

56. Yu Y, Decazes P, Lapuyade-Lahorgue J, et al. Semiautomatic lymphoma detection and segmentation using fully conditional random fields. Comput Med Imag Graph 2018 Dec;70:1–7.

57. Lartizien C, Rogez M, Niaf E, et al. Computer-aided staging of lymphoma patients with FDG PET/CT imaging based on textural information. IEEE J Biomed Health Inform 2014 May;18(3):946–55.

58. Cheson BD, Meignan M. Current role of functional imaging in the management of lymphoma. Curr Oncol Rep 2021 Nov 4;23(12):144.

59. André MPE, Girinsky T, Federico M, et al. Early positron emission tomography response-adapted treatment in stage I and II Hodgkin lymphoma: final results of the randomized EORTC/LYSA/FIL H10 trial. J Clin Oncol 2017 Jun 1;35(16):1786–94.

60. Chang CC, Cho SF, Chuang YW, et al. Prognostic significance of total metabolic tumor volume on ^{18}F-fluorodeoxyglucose positron emission tomography/computed tomography in patients with diffuse large B-cell lymphoma receiving rituximab-containing chemotherapy. Oncotarget 2017 Aug 24;8(59):99587–600.

61. Cottereau AS, Meignan M, Nioche C, et al. Risk stratification in diffuse large B-cell lymphoma using lesion dissemination and metabolic tumor burden calculated from baseline PET/CT†. Ann Oncol 2021 Mar;32(3):404–11.

62. Bertolini V, Palmieri A, Bassi MC, et al. CT protocol optimisation in PET/CT: a systematic review. EJNMMI Phys 2020 Mar 16;7(1):17.

63. Vercellino L, Cottereau AS, Casasnovas O, et al. High total metabolic tumor volume at baseline predicts survival independent of response to therapy. Blood 2020 Apr 16;135(16):1396–405.

64. Kostakoglu L, Mattiello F, Martelli M, et al. Total metabolic tumor volume as a survival predictor for patients with diffuse large B-cell lymphoma in the GOYA study. Haematologica 2022 Jul 1;107(7):1633–42.

65. Ceriani L, Milan L, Martelli M, et al. Metabolic heterogeneity on baseline 18FDG-PET/CT scan is a predictor of outcome in primary mediastinal B-cell lymphoma. Blood 2018 Jul 12;132(2):179–86.

66. Liu F, Gu B, Li N, et al. Prognostic value of heterogeneity index derived from baseline ^{18}F-FDG PET/CT in mantle cell lymphoma. Front Oncol 2022 Apr 14;12: 862473.

67. Moskowitz AJ, Schoder H, Gavane S, et al. Prognostic significance of baseline metabolic tumor volume in relapsed and refractory Hodgkin lymphoma. Blood 2017;130:2196–203.

68. Mikhaeel NG, Smith D, Dunn JT, et al. Combination of baseline metabolic tumour volume and early response on PET/CT improves progression-free survival prediction in DLBCL. Eur J Nucl Med Mol Imag 2016 Jul;43(7):1209–19.

69. Schmitz C, Hüttmann A, Müller SP, et al. Dynamic risk assessment based on positron emission tomography scanning in diffuse large B-cell lymphoma: post-hoc analysis from the PETAL trial. Eur J Cancer 2020 Jan;124:25–36.

70. Terao T, Machida Y, Tsushima T, et al. Pre-treatment metabolic tumour volume and total lesion glycolysis are superior to conventional positron-emission tomography/computed tomography variables for outcome prediction in patients with newly diagnosed multiple myeloma in clinical practice. Br J Haematol 2020 Oct;191(2):223–30.

71. Bi L, Kim J, Kumar A, et al. Automatic detection and classification of regions of FDG uptake in whole-body PET-CT lymphoma studies. Comput Med Imag Graph 2017 Sep;60:3–10.

72. Sadik M, Lind E, Polymeri E, et al. Automated quantification of reference levels in liver and mediastinal blood pool for the Deauville therapy response classification using FDG-PET/CT in Hodgkin and non-Hodgkin lymphomas. Clin Physiol Funct Imag 2019 Jan;39(1):78–84.

73. Sibille L, Seifert R, Avramovic N, et al. ^{18}F-FDG PET/CT uptake classification in lymphoma and lung cancer by using deep convolutional neural networks. Radiology 2020 Feb;294(2):445–52.

74. Blanc-Durand P, Jégou S, Kanoun S, et al. Fully automatic segmentation of diffuse large B cell lymphoma lesions on 3D FDG-PET/CT for total metabolic tumour volume prediction using a convolutional neural network. Eur J Nucl Med Mol Imag 2021 May;48(5): 1362–70.

75. Capobianco N, Meignan M, Cottereau AS, et al. Deep-learning ^{18}F-FDG uptake classification enables total metabolic tumor volume estimation in diffuse large B-cell lymphoma. J Nucl Med 2021 Jan;62(1):30–6.

76. Girum KB, Rebaud L, Cottereau AS, et al. ^{18}F-FDG PET maximum-intensity projections and artificial intelligence: a win-win combination to easily measure prognostic biomarkers in DLBCL patients. J Nucl Med 2022 Dec;63(12):1925–32.

77. Sachpekidis C, Enqvist O, Ulén J, et al. Application of an artificial intelligence-based tool in [^{18}F]FDG PET/CT for the assessment of bone marrow involvement in multiple myeloma. Eur J Nucl Med Mol Imag 2023 Oct;50(12):3697–708.

78. Liu Y, Shi H, Huang S, et al. Early prediction of acute xerostomia during radiation therapy for nasopharyngeal cancer based on delta radiomics from CT images. Quant Imag Med Surg 2019 Jul;9(7):1288–302.

79. Nasief H, Zheng C, Schott D, et al. A machine learning based delta-radiomics process for early prediction of treatment response of pancreatic cancer. npj Precis Oncol 2019 Oct 4;3:25.

80. Tonnelet D, Bohn MDP, Becker S, et al. Angiogenesis imaging study using interim [^{18}F] RGD-K5 PET/CT in patients with lymphoma undergoing chemotherapy: preliminary evidence. EJNMMI Res 2021 Apr 12;11(1):37.

81. Albano D, Dondi F, Bertagna F, et al. The role of [^{68}Ga]Ga-pentixafor PET/CT or PET/MRI in lymphoma: a systematic review. Cancers (Basel) 2022 Aug 5;14(15):3814.

82. Mayerhoefer ME, Raderer M, Lamm W, et al. CXCR4 PET/MRI for follow-up of gastric mucosa-associated lymphoid tissue lymphoma after first-line Helicobacter pylori eradication. Blood 2022 Jan 13; 139(2):240–4.

83. Duell J, Krummenast F, Schirbel A, et al. Improved primary staging of marginal-zone lymphoma by addition of CXCR4-directed PET/CT. J Nucl Med 2021 Oct;62(10):1415–21.

84. Jin X, Wei M, Wang S, et al. Detecting fibroblast activation proteins in lymphoma using ^{68}Ga-FAPI PET/CT. J Nucl Med 2022 Feb;63(2):212–7.

Lymphoma
The Added Value of Radiomics, Volumes and Global Disease Assessment

Stéphane Chauvie, PhD[a],*, Alessia Castellino, MD[b], Fabrizio Bergesio, PhD[a],
Adriano De Maggi, PhD[a], Rexhep Durmo, MD[c]

KEYWORDS

- Positron emission tomography • Lymphoma • Total metabolic tumor volume • Radiomics
- Tumor dissemination

KEY POINTS

- Radiomics holds promise for making a significant clinical impact by offering a wealth of additional imaging information that can be quantified to monitor phenotypic changes during treatment. However, it is still in its early stages, and due to the limited number of patients enrolled in studies, the results remain controversial and inconclusive.
- Metabolic tumor volume, maximum tumor dissemination, and heterogeneity are all imaging biomarkers, and they face similar challenges encountered by other imaging biomarkers. Despite some biomarkers being extensively used and others showing great potential, only a limited number of them currently guide clinical decisions. For these biomarkers to be integrated into clinical practice, they must demonstrate reproducibility, relevance to clinical outcomes, and clinical utility.
- Clinical trials, prospective data collections, and retrospective studies are essential to test the reliability, accuracy, and precision of PET imaging biomarkers. Similar to the international effort made at Deauville, there is a need for a concerted global effort to advance the validation and standardization of these biomarkers. Such collaborative efforts are crucial to ensure the successful translation of PET imaging biomarkers into routine clinical practice.

INTRODUCTION

Outcomes of lymphomas, in general, have greatly improved in the last decades; however a percentage of patients did not respond to available treatments or ultimately relapse.

Identifying high risk patients, in each lymphoma subtype, at diagnosis and during treatment according to response achieved, remains one of the main challenging for clinicians, to be able to propose improving tailored strategies.

PET is a prevalent and frequently employed medical diagnostic technique in lymphoma. In particular, in Hodgkin's lymphoma (HL) and Non Hodgkin's aggressive and follicular lymphomas (FLs), PET represents the gold standard for staging disease and to guide the choice of the most appropriate site for biopsy at diagnosis or relapse, and the mile stone to assess the response after treatment.[1] PET reporting involves visually examining whole-body scans and describing the uptake areas using a binary scale, indicating either the presence or absence of uptake and their corresponding locations in the patient's body. However, recent advancements have prompted imaging specialists to transition from this binary scale to

[a] Department of Medical Physics, 'Santa Croce e Carle Hospital, Cuneo, Italy; [b] Department of Hematology, Santa Croce e Carle Hospital, Cuneo, Italy; [c] Nuclear Medicine Division, Department of Radiology, Azienda USL IRCCS of Reggio Emilia, Reggio Emilia, Italy
* Corresponding author.
E-mail address: chauvie.s@ospedale.cuneo.it

PET Clin 19 (2024) 561–568
https://doi.org/10.1016/j.cpet.2024.05.009

a quantitative approach. This involves analyzing PET scans on a discrete or continuous scale, where specific numerical values are assigned to the uptake areas, facilitating a tuned evaluation of the uptake.

Lugano classifications[2] for lymphoma staging and re-staging uses the discrete Deauville 5-point scale that defines the areas of uptake in the disease compared to physiologic districts.[3] The integration to it of a quantitative index has been a pursuit in PET imaging since its inception, yet its significance has only recently been amplified with the introduction of several metrics. These include the Total Metabolic Tumor Volume (TMTV), which offers a comprehensive evaluation of the volume of metabolically active tumor tissue within the patient's body. Additionally, dissemination features, such as the maximum distance between the 2 lesions that are the farthest apart (maximum tumor dissemination [Dmax]) in the whole body, have gained importance in assessing disease spread. Furthermore, on a per lesion basis, phenotyping through the analysis of heterogeneity features has become essential for characterizing the diversity within individual tumor lesions. These advancements underline the evolving role of quantitative metrics in enhancing the precision and effectiveness of PET imaging in oncology.

Thanks to the improving of quantitative analysis and precision of PET images, PET scan starting to show a role, not only in staging and response assessment in lymphoma, but also the possibility of a prognostic and predictive value, able to help in define higher risk patients.

It is well known[4] that a variety of physical, technical and biologic factors affect uptake repeatability,[5] but, recent advances in PET imaging, the use of common protocol for preparation and acquisition of the patient, and cross-calibration of the PET scanners,[6] reduced greatly the variability paving the way to a quantitative use of PET.

Semi-quantitative Metrics in PET/Computed Tomography: Metabolic Tumor Volume

Metabolic tumor volume (MTV) is a standardized uptake value (SUV)-based derived functional metrics, which measure metabolic activity in an entire tumor mass to reflect tumor biology. The MTV determines the total volume of the metabolically active tumor in an area of uptake, and is expressed in cm^3 or ml. When the volumes of the single lesions are summed up for the whole patient TMTV is defined.

Many publication demonstrated the usefulness of TMTV in different lymphoma subtypes in

particular for prognosis and several good reviews exists,[7,8] the last in particular.

For example, in Diffuse Large B-cell Lymphoma (DLBCL) setting, the prognostic and predictive role of PET has been investigated within the GOYA trial cohort.[9] One thousand three hundred and five of 1418 enrolled newly diagnosed DLBCL patients, treated with rituximab or obinutuzumab plus cyclophosphamide, doxorubicin, vincristine, and prednisone (CHOP), had a baseline PET with detectable lesions. High TMTV and total lesion glycolysis (TLG) predicted poorer progression free survival (PFS). TMTV maintained its prognostic role for PFS in subgroups with International Prognostic Index (IPI) scores 0 to 2 and 3 to 5, and those with different cell-of-origin (COO) subtypes. Moreover, high TMTV associated with high IPI risk or non-germinal center B-cell (non-GCB) COO subtype, identifying the highest-risk cohort for unfavorable outcome. Indeed, very high TMTV showed to be predictive of primary refractoriness to front-line treatment.

Also, the prognostic and predictive role of PET has been recently investigated in the setting of patients with aggressive lymphoma treated with Chimeric Antigen Receptor T-cells (CART-cells). Dean and colleagues,[10] showed that patients with baseline low MTV had significantly superior PFS and overall survival (OS), in a cohort of 96 relapse per refractory DLBCL cases treated with axicabtagene ciloleucel. These interesting results were successfully validated in a second cohort of 48 analogous patients.

Similar findings were showed by Iacoboni and colleagues,[11] who demonstrated that high baseline TMTV was associated with a lower PFS, with a trend toward shorter OS, in a population of 35 DLBCL patients treated with CART-cells therapy.

The prognostic role of semi-quantitative PET metrics has been investigated also in the setting of FL. In the phase III RELEVANCE trial,[12] newly diagnosed FL were randomly assigned to be treated with immunomodulatory combination of lenalidomide and rituximab versus R-chemotherapy, both followed by R maintenance. High TMTV and follicular lymphoma international prognostic index (FLIPI) were significantly associated with an inferior PFS, in both univariate and multivariate analyses. These 2 adverse factors combined were found able to stratify the overall population into 3 risk groups: patients with no risk factors (40%), with 1 factor (44%), or with both (16%), with a 6-year PFS of 67.7%, 54.5%, and 41.0%, respectively. No significant interaction between treatment arms and TMTV or FLIPI was observed. Moreover, baseline TMTV was predictive of PFS, independently of FLIPI, even in the context of rituximab maintenance.

In FL, Delfau-Larue and colleagues,[13] investigated the role of correlation between TMTV and circulating tumor cells (CTCs) and cell-free DNA (cfDNA), which may also reflect tumor burden, and its prognostic value on impact on lymphoma outcomes. They retrospectively analyzed 133 patients with previously untreated FL and a baseline PET from 2 cohorts with either a baseline plasma sample or a bcl2-JH informative peripheral blood sample. Quantification of circulating bcl2-JH1 cells and cfDNA was performed by droplet digital polymerase chain reaction. A significant correlation was found between TMTV and both CTCs ($P<.0001$) and cfDNA ($P<.0001$). With a median 48-month follow-up, 4-year PFS was lower in patients with TMTV greater than 510 cm^3 ($P = .0004$), CTCs greater than .0.0018 peripheral blood cells ($P = .03$), or cfDNA greater than .2550 equivalent-genome per mL ($P = .04$). In a Cox multivariate analysis, both cfDNA and TMTV remained predictive of outcome, showing that PFS was shorter for patients with high cfDNA and TMTV, suggesting that these parameters provide relevant information for tumor-tailored therapy.

In the setting of HL, many studies have investigated the prognostic role of PET. Within the population of the multicenter phase III HD16 trial,[14] including early stage favorable hemodialysis (HL) patients, MTV and TLG demonstrated to positively correlate with response and to have a predictive value after 2 standard chemotherapy cycles, particularly when using the fixed threshold of SUV4.0 for MTV and TLG calculation.

Similar findings were showed, in the setting of Advanced Stage HL, within the COG AHOD0031 trial,[15] conducted in children and adolescent patients. In this analysis, MTV and TLG were associated with Event Free Survival (EFS). MTV, in particular, was highly associated with EFS when controlling for disease bulk and response to chemotherapy, suggesting that incorporation of baseline MTV into risk-based treatment algorithms may improve outcomes in intermediate-risk HL.

Therefore, while numerous studies have unequivocally demonstrated the prognostic significance of TMTV, further clinical trials involving patients with various types of lymphoma are imperative. These trials will help determine whether these novel findings can be effectively integrated into diverse prognostic models, ultimately leading to enhanced risk stratification and more tailored treatment selection strategies. Currently, there is only 1 ongoing trial, RAFTING (NCT04866654), which utilizes MTV as a stratification tool for patient allocation into different treatment arms for early

HL. A clear demonstration of the possible prospective use of TMTV is clearly represented by the work of Mickaeles and colleagues

One of the reasons why this useful clinical parameter has not been yet integrated in clinical applications is because of its lack of validation.[16] One of the major hurdles is that the segmentation process, that is the act of defining where the metabolic activity of the tumor is higher than the surrounding tissue, is challenging to define. A flavor of methods have been defined in the past, among them the most commonly used in lymphoma where the fixed threshold of MTV = 2.5 or MTV = 4 and the percentage threshold, for example, 41% or 26% of SUV$_{max}$. Since in the last 30 years no method has been demonstrated to be more precise than other, an initiative to standardize the use of MTV was launched within the Menton meeting,[17] to at least definite an accurate method to be used in clinical practice. The primary objective was to conduct a technical validation of MTV measurement, aimed at establishing benchmark reference ranges for delineation approaches utilized in various software platforms. Following 3 years of dedicated effort, the findings of this initiative were unveiled during the Menton 2023 meeting. A consensus emerged among experts, advocating for the adoption of a fixed SUV threshold of 4 for segmenting lymphoma lesions. This methodology yielded remarkably consistent results and boasted the advantage of being readily applicable in clinical settings, as it is supported by the majority of software viewers available on the market. Moreover, it requires minimal human intervention compared to alternative methods, thereby enhancing efficiency and ease of implementation.

In conclusion, MTV emerges as a robust prognosticator, and since the method of segmentation is now standardized, the authors do expect that investigations into the dependence of MTV on risk can be pursued, facilitating the development of optimized treatment strategies.

Lesion dissemination: maximum distance between 2 lesions

Recently, there has been a focus on studying lesion dissemination as a surrogate marker for tumor burden and Ann Arbor Staging. Lesion dissemination, which can be assessed in various ways, serves as an indicator of the extent of the tumor spread throughout the body. The underlying hypothesis is that a wider dissemination of the tumor correlates with a poorer prognosis, in the context of radio-chemotherapy treatment. One straightforward metric used to quantify lesion dissemination is the D$_{max}$ between 2 lesions (d$_{max}$), or between a lesion and the bulky mass, or between a lesion and the spleen.[18] This metric offers several advantages, notably its simplicity and the avoidance of many technical complexities. Indeed, measuring the distance between 2 active lesions in the body can be easily accomplished using a ruler, making it a practical and accessible tool for clinical assessment.

The French group was the first to introduce this metrics and to prove its significance in DLBCL. Cotterau and colleagues[19] studied 4 dissemination features on 95 DLBCL patients with Ann Stage 3 to 4 (90% stage 4) and at least 2 lesions on baseline PET/computed tomography (CT) from the population of patients aaIPI 2 to 3 enrolled in the LNH073 B trial randomly assigned to R-CHOP14 or R-ACVP (rituximab, doxorubicin, cyclophosphamide, vindesine, bleomycin, prednisone). Among the 4 dissemination features D_{max}, the maximum distance among lesions, create 2 groups with better PFS and OS separation respect to MTV. MTV (>394 cm3) or D_{max} (>58 cm) create 3 groups of high, intermediate, and low-risk patients with 4-year PFS rates of 94%, 73%, and 50%, respectively and 4-year OS rates of 97%, 88%, and 53%, respectively. The same group performed the same analysis in 290 patients aged 60 to 80 years included in the REMARC study.[20] 91% had an advanced stage and 71% IPI greater than or equal to 3. High versus low Dmax significantly impacted PFS ($P<.0001$) and OS ($P=.0027$). Patients with SDmax greater than 0.32 m^{-1} ($n = 82$) had a 4-year PFS and OS of 46% and 71%, respectively, versus 77% and 87%, respectively, for patients with low SDmax. high SDmax and high MTV were independent prognostic factors of PFS ($P=.0001$ and $P=.0010$, respectively) and OS ($P=.0028$ and $P=.0004$, respectively). Combining MTV and SDmax yielded 3 risk groups with no ($n = 109$), 1 ($n = 122$) or 2 ($n = 59$) factors ($P<.0001$ for both PFS and OS). The 4-year PFS were 90%, 63%, 41%, respectively and the 4-year OS were 95%, 79%, 66%, respectively. In addition, patients with at least 2 of the 3 factors including high SDmax, high MTV, Eastern Cooperative Oncology Group greater than or equal to 2 had a higher number of central nervous system relapse ($P=.017$). Respect to the previous analysis, they normalized the Dmax to the patient body surface area (SDmax).

D_{max} was also tested in HOVON-84 trial,[21] 317 newly diagnosed DLBCL patients were included. The optimal radiomics model comprised the natural logarithms of MTV and of SUV_{peak} and the maximal distance between the largest lesion and any other lesion ($Dmax_{bulk}$) yielded an area under the curve (AUC = 0.76) with more accurate selection of high-risk patients compared to the IPI model

(progression at 2-year TTP, 44% vs 28%, respectively).In HL setting, Durmo and colleagues.[22] studied 155 HL patients performing ABVD (doxorubicin hydrochloride [Adriamycin], bleomycin sulphate, vinblastine suphate, dacarbazine). Using a median value of 20 cm for Dmax, they showed that it was the only variable independently associated with PFS (heart rate [HR] = 2.70, 95% CI 1.1–6.63, probability Value = .03) in multivariate analysis of PFS for all patients and for those with early complete metabolic response (iPET-). Among patients with iPET-low Dmax was associated with a 4-year PFS of 90% (95% CI 82.0–98.9) significantly better compared to high Dmax (4-year PFS 72.4%, 95% CI 61.9–84.6). Regarding FL setting, the Italian research group has recently presented the preliminary data on FL, indicating that TMTV and tumor dissemination, calculated from PET/CT scans conducted before first-line therapy, serve as predictors of patient outcomes. The 5-year PFS rates were significantly lower for patients with high TMTV (60% vs 70%; HR = 1.87 [95%CI: 1.41–2.49], $P<.001$) and D_{max} greater than 0.4 m (56% vs 69%; HR = 1.67 [95%CI: 1.24–2.25], $P = .001$). Moreover, combining D_{max} with TMTV, D_{max} identified varying levels of risk of progression among high TMTV cases: patients with TMTV greater than 200 mL and D_{max} less than 0.4 m had an HR of 1.59 (95% CI: 1.16–2.17) compared to 2.53 (95% CI: 1.73–3.61) for TMTV greater than 200 and Dmax greater than 0.4 m. [Luminari, EANM 2022 & ASH 2022]. Despite lesion dissemination, expressed as Dmax, is emerging as a promising prognostic factor, not all the studies were concord on its independent value.

In FL, Rodier and colleagues,[23] evaluated 201 patients with grade 1-3a low-tumor burden FL, diagnosed in 4 French centers between 2010 and 2020 and managed by a watch and wait strategy in real-life settings. On multivariate analysis, elevated lactate dehydrogenase, more than 4 nodal areas involved and more than 1 extranodal involvement were identified as independent predictors of Time to Lymphoma Treatment (TLT). In a subanalysis of 75 patients staged with PET-CT, TMTV greater than or equal to 14 cm3 and standardized Dmax greater than 0.32 m-1 were also associated with shorter TLT (HR = 3.4; $P=.004$ and HR = 2.4; $P=.007$, respectively). However, when analyzed in multivariate models combining PET-CT parameters and clinical variables, only TMTV, but no Dmax, remained independent predictor of shorter TLT.

Also in the multicenter phase III trial RELEVANCE,[12] both SUVmax and SDmax were not predictive of worse PFS ($P=.08$ and $P=.12$, respectively), while TMTV was.

In conclusion, lesion dissemination emerges as a promising prognostic factor in lymphoma, even if results from some trials are controversy. While its potential has been recognized, it has not undergone extensive testing. However, when combined with other prognostic indexes, it enhances risk stratification, indicating its value as a complementary tool in predicting patient outcomes and guiding treatment decisions.

Radiomics Indexes

Radiomics refers to the extraction of quantitative features that result in the conversion of images into mineable data and the subsequent analysis of these data for decision support.[24] The radiomics process culminates when radiomics features are correlated with clinical variables and patient outcomes. The underlying hypothesis driving radiomics is that these quantitative features, which encompass characteristics such as shape, morphology, and heterogeneity of the lesion, mirror the physio-pathologic properties of the tumor. Pioneering work by Aerts and colleagues demonstrated that radiomics untraveled a broad prognostic phenotype present across multiple cancer types, elucidating associations with underlying gene-expression patterns. This innovative research highlights the potential of radiomics to provide deeper insights into tumor biology and prognosis, paving the way for more personalized and effective cancer management strategies.[25]

Similarly, the pattern of F-18 flurodeoxyglucose FDG uptake within a lymphoma lesion could reflect a multitude of biologic characteristics, including vascularization, cellularity, hypoxia, metabolism, cell density, and necrosis, but, on the basis of results published to date on FDG PET, it is still unclear which features should be used and what they represent.

Preliminary studies showed that radiomics could discriminate lymphoma versus physiologic organ or tissue,[26] lymphomatous versus non-lymphomatous lesions,[27] and lymphomatous versus gastro-intestinal lesion.[28]

One of the first works of prognostic value of radiomics in a small mixed population of 57 Hodgkin and Non-Hodgkin lymphoma patients is that of Ben Boallegue and colleagues[29] showing that adding radiomics features to MTV and histology increased AUC in the early response evaluation. Among the features selected by multi-variate analysis contrast, granularity and AUC-cumulative SUV-volume histograms (CSH), this latter was also shown by Ceriani and colleagues[30] to discriminate 2 groups of patients with different prognosis in a population of 103 patients with Primary Mediastinal B-cell

Lymphoma (PMBCL) enrolled in a prospective multi-centre clinical trial (IELSG26).

In DLBCL some experience with few patients and in retrospective studies were carried out showing that radiomics correlates with objective response at end-of-treatment PET evaluated with Lugano classification,[31] correlates with bone marrow biopsy (BMB),[32] and increase predictive power of MTV.[33] All this studies have important limitations, being conducted on a small population,[32,33] with mixed treatment and performing only a Cox-analysis[31] and using only 1 feature.[33]

Ceriani and colleagues[34] analyzed baseline PET/CT of 141 patients with DLBCL treated with R-CHOP14 in the prospective SAKK38/07 study demonstrating that elevated metabolic heterogeneity (MH) significantly predicted poorer outcomes in the subgroups of patients with elevated MTV. A model integrating MTV and MH identified high-risk patients with shorter PFS (testing set: HR, 5.6; 95% CI, 1.8–17; $P= .0001$; validation set: HR, 5.6; 95% CI, 1.7–18; $P =.0002$) and shorter OS (testing set: HR, 9.5; 95% CI, 1.7–52; $P= .0001$; validation set: HR, 7.6; 95% CI, 2.0–28 $P =.0003$). The same authors also demonstrated AUC-CSH discriminates 2 risk groups with high and low metabolic heterogeneity in 144 DLBCL[35] and in 103 PMBCL[30] patients that performed baseline PET.

Kostakoglu and colleagues.[36] developed a radiomics prediction model using data from 1263 DLBCL patients in the GOYA trial. They combined PET/CT texture features and clinical risk factors into a random forest model, which outperformed the traditional IPI in PFS OS. Notably, the random forest model with cell-of-origin subgroups delineated a more distinct high-risk population (2-year PFS: 45% [95% CI 40%-52%]; 2-year OS: 65% [95% CI 59%-71%]) compared to the IPI (2-year PFS: 58% [95% CI 50%-67%]; 2-year OS: 69% [95% CI 62%-77%]).

Aide N. and colleagues studied the diagnostic and prognostic value of skeletal textural features on baseline FDG PET in DLBCL patients. Eighty-two patients with DLBCL who underwent a BMB and a PET scan were evaluated. Authors identified Skewness as independent prognostic factor of PFS in 82 patients with DLBCL but not for OS. Moreover they showed that Skewness was the best parameter for identifying bone marrow involvement with sensitivity and specificity of 81.8% and 81.7%, respectively.[32]

Similarly few works exist on HL, Milgrom and colleagues retrospectively analyzed [18F]FDG-PET scan of 251 patients with classical HL stage I-II to predict refractory or relapsed disease.[37] The analysis comprised histogram features, Gray Level Cooccurence Matrix features, and basic shape features, extracted from the mediastinal tumor volume on the one hand, and the total tumor volume on the other hand, segmented by a combination of manual and threshold-based delineation. Based on the 5 most predictive features of the mediastinal tumor volume, AUCs of 0.95 for the radiomic approach versus 0.78 for MTV and TLG, and just 0.65 for SUVmax were achieved; whereas total tumor volume PET features were not predictive of outcome. Lue and colleagues retrospectively analyzed single-scanner pre-therapeutic [18F] FDG-PET scans of 42 HL patients that subsequently underwent chemo- or radiochemotherapy.[38] This study also focused on survival prognostication by means of overall 450 3-dimensional radiomic features extracted from original/ normalized and wavelet-decomposed images. In their multivariate Cox regression analysis, only a single gray level run lenght matrix feature (intensity non-uniformity) remained prognostic for both OS and PFS, and a single histogram features (SUV kurtosis) was prognostic for PFS alone. Of note, MTV, a metric that has shown prognostic value in several studies in HL patients, was neither prognostic for OS or PFS. Similar results were obtained in an update of the paper.[39]

In FL, Tatsumi and colleagues conducted a study involving 51 FL patients, revealing that only low gray-level zone emphasis among all the texture features exhibited statistical significance in predicting complete response.

Montes de Jesus and colleagues.[40] presented a novel approach using radiomics to identify individuals with FL who progressed to DLBCL. They utilized radiomic features extracted from PET/CT scans and analyzed them with machine learning algorithms to differentiate between FL and DLBCL lesions. In a retrospective study involving 44 FL and 76 DLBCL cases, their machine learning classifier demonstrated superior discrimination performance using 136 radiomic features, achieving an AUC of 0.86 and an accuracy of 80%. Remarkably, it significantly outperformed SUVmax-based logistic regression ($P \leq .01$).

The challenges in this domain are manifold. Firstly, heterogeneity features encompass a wide array of characteristics, complicating analysis and interpretation. Secondly, the scarcity of patients and events further complicates statistical analysis and the generalizability of findings. To address these issues, some studies employ feature selection methods and Cox models to identify relevant predictors amidst the limited data. However, despite these efforts, many studies utilizing PET/CT with texture features encounter significant challenges. These include high false discovery rates (Type I error) and the identification of different statistically significant texture features across studies, even when they appear conceptually similar. These discrepancies highlight the need for standardized methodologies and rigorous validation in the utilization of texture features in lymphoma research.

In conclusion, while there exists some "proof of concept" regarding the potential utility of texture features in lymphoma research, it is important to acknowledge certain realities. Studies aiming for reliability and robustness often require the inclusion of thousands of patients, which can be challenging in the context of rare diseases like certain lymphoma subtypes. Moreover, these studies face inherent limitations, such as the complexity of translating findings into actionable and visible outcomes. However, addressing these challenges is inherent to the scientific process, and researchers continually strive to overcome them in their quest to improve patient care and outcomes.

SUMMARY

In summary, radiomics holds promise for making a significant clinical impact by offering a wealth of additional imaging information that can be quantified to monitor phenotypic changes during treatment. However, it is still in its early stages, and due to the limited number of patients enrolled in studies, the results remain controversial and inconclusive.

MTV, Dmax, and heterogeneity are all imaging biomarkers, and they face similar challenges encountered by other imaging biomarkers. Despite some biomarkers being extensively used and others showing great potential, only a limited number of them currently guide clinical decisions. For these biomarkers to be integrated into clinical practice, they must demonstrate reproducibility, relevance to clinical outcomes, and clinical utility.

Clinical trials, prospective data collections, and retrospective studies are essential to test the reliability, accuracy, and precision of PET imaging biomarkers. Similar to the international effort made at Deauville, there is a need for a concerted global effort to advance the validation and standardization of these biomarkers. Such collaborative efforts are crucial to ensure the successful translation of PET imaging biomarkers into routine clinical practice.

CLINICS CARE POINTS

- We do expect that an increasing evidence in the field concomitant to a new generation of PET-CT scanner could lead to a use of radiomics as a prognostic and stratification tool managing and guiding the therapy.

DISCLOSURE

The authors have no conflicts of interest to disclose related to the subjects, matter or materials discussed in this article.

REFERENCES

1. Cheson BD, Fisher RI, Barrington SF, et al. Recommendations for initial evaluation, staging, and response assessment of Hodgkin and non-Hodgkin lymphoma: the Lugano classification. J Clin Oncol 2014;32(27):1–10.
2. Cheson B, Fisher R, Barrington S. Recommendations for initial evaluation, staging, and response assessment of Hodgkin and Non-Hodgkin lymphoma: the Lugano classification. J Clin Oncol 2014;32(27):3059–68.
3. Ardeshna K, Smith P, Norton A, et al. Report on the Second International Workshop on interim positron emission tomography in lymphoma held in Menton, France, 8-9 April 2010. J Clin Oncol 2013;99(3): 946–53.
4. Chauvie S, Bergesio F. The strategies to Homogenize PET/CT metrics: the case of onco-haematological clinical trials. Biomedicine 2016;4(4):2124–30.
5. Biggi A, Bergesio F, Chauvie S, et al. Concomitant semi-quantitative and visual analysis improves the predictive value on treatment outcome of interim 18F-fluorodeoxyglucose/Positron Emission Tomography in advanced Hodgkin lymphoma. Q J Nucl Med Mol Imaging 2017. https://doi.org/10.23736/S1824-4785.17.02993-4.
6. Chauvie S, Bergesio F, Fioroni F, et al. The 68Ge phantom-based FDG-PET site qualification program for clinical trials adopted by FIL (Italian Foundation on Lymphoma). Phys Med 2016;32(5): 651–6.
7. Kostakoglu L, Chauvie S. PET-derived quantitative metrics for response and prognosis in lymphoma. Pet Clin 2019;14(3). https://doi.org/10.1016/j.cpet.2019.03.002.
8. Alderuccio JP, Kuker RA, Yang F, et al. Quantitative PET-based biomarkers in lymphoma: getting ready for primetime. Nat Rev Clin Oncol 2023;20(9):640–57.
9. Kostakoglu L, Mattiello F, Martelli M, et al. Total metabolic tumor volume as a survival predictor for patients with diffuse large B-cell lymphoma in the GOYA study. Haematologica 2022;107(7). https://doi.org/10.3324/haematol.2021.278663.
10. Dean EA, Mhaskar RS, Lu H, et al. High metabolic tumor volume is associated with decreased efficacy of axicabtagene ciloleucel in large B-cell lymphoma. Blood Adv 2020;4(14). https://doi.org/10.1182/bloodadvances.2020001900.
11. Iacoboni G, Simó M, Villacampa G, et al. Prognostic impact of total metabolic tumor volume in large

B-cell lymphoma patients receiving CAR T-cell therapy. Ann Hematol 2021;100(9). https://doi.org/10.1007/s00277-021-04560-6.
12. Cottereau AS, Rebaud L, Trotman J, et al. Metabolic tumor volume predicts outcome in patients with advanced stage follicular lymphoma from the RELEVANCE trial. Ann Oncol 2023;35(1):130–7.
13. Delfau-Larue MH, Van Der Gucht A, Dupuis J, et al. Total metabolic tumor volume, circulating tumor cells, cell-free DNA: distinct prognostic value in follicular lymphoma. Blood Adv 2018;2(7):807–16.
14. van Heek L, Stuka C, Kaul H, et al. Predictive value of baseline metabolic tumor volume in early-stage favorable Hodgkin Lymphoma – data from the prospective, multicenter phase III HD16 trial. BMC Cancer 2022;22(1):1–8.
15. Milgrom SA, Kim J, Pei Q, et al. Baseline metabolic tumour burden improves risk stratification in Hodgkin lymphoma: a Children's Oncology Group study. Br J Haematol 2023;201(6):1192–9.
16. Kostakoglu L, Chauvie S. Metabolic tumor volume metrics in lymphoma. Semin Nucl Med 2017;48(1): 50–66.
17. Barrington SF, Meignan M. Time to prepare for risk adaptation in lymphoma by standardizing measurement of metabolic tumor burden. J Nucl Med 2019; 60(8):1096–102.
18. Girum KB, Cottereau A-S, Vercellino L, et al. Tumor location relative to the spleen is a prognostic factor in lymphoma patients: a demonstration from the REMARC trial. J Nucl Med 2023;123:266322.
19. Cottereau A-S, Nioche C, Dirand A-S, et al. 18 F-FDG-PET dissemination features in diffuse large B cell lymphoma are prognostic of outcome. J Nucl Med 2019;119:229450.
20. Cottereau AS, Meignan M, Nioche C, et al. Risk stratification in diffuse large B-cell lymphoma using lesion dissemination and metabolic tumor burden calculated from baseline PET/CT. Ann Oncol 2021; 32(3):404–11.
21. Eertink JJ, Zwezerijnen GJC, Heymans MW, et al. Baseline PET radiomics outperforms the IPI risk score for prediction of outcome in diffuse large B-cell lymphoma. Blood 2023;141(25):3055–64.
22. Durmo R, Donati B, Rebaud L, et al. Prognostic value of lesion dissemination in doxorubicin, bleomycin, vinblastine, and dacarbazine-treated, interimPET-negative classical Hodgkin Lymphoma patients: a radiogenomic study. Hematol Oncol 2022;40(4):645–57.
23. Rodier C, Kanagaratnam L, Morland D, et al. Risk factors of progression in low-tumor burden follicular lymphoma initially managed by watch and wait in the era of PET and rituximab. Hemasphere 2023;7(5). https://doi.org/10.1097/HS9.0000000000000861.
24. Gillies RJ, Kinahan PE, Hricak H. Radiomics: images are more than pictures, they are data. Radiology 2016;278(2):563–77.

25. Aerts HJWL, Velazquez ER, Leijenaar RTH, et al. Decoding tumour phenotype by noninvasive imaging using a quantitative radiomics approach. Nat Commun 2014;5. https://doi.org/10.1038/ncomms5006.

26. Hsu CY, Doubrovin M, Hua CH, et al. Radiomics features differentiate between normal and tumoral high-fdg uptake. Sci Rep 2018;8(1):1–10.

27. Lartizien C, Rogez M, Niaf E, et al. Computer-aided staging of lymphoma patients with FDG PET/CT imaging based on textural information. IEEE J Biomed Health Inform 2014;18(3):946–55.

28. Watabe T, Tatsumi M, Watabe H, et al. Intratumoral heterogeneity of F-18 FDG uptake differentiates between gastrointestinal stromal tumors and abdominal malignant lymphomas on PET/CT. Ann Nucl Med 2012;26(3):222–7.

29. Ben Bouallegue F, Al Tabaa Y, Kafrouni M, et al. Association between textural and morphological tumor indices on baseline PET-CT and early metabolic response on interim PET-CT in bulky malignant lymphomas. Med Phys 2017;44(9):4608–19.

30. Ceriani L, Milan L, Martelli M, et al. Metabolic heterogeneity on baseline 18FDG-PET/CT scan is a predictor of outcome in primary mediastinal B-cell lymphoma. Blood 2018;132(2):179–86.

31. Parvez A, Tau N, Hussey D, et al. 18F-FDG PET/CT metabolic tumor parameters and radiomics features in aggressive non-Hodgkin's lymphoma as predictors of treatment outcome and survival. Ann Nucl Med 2018;32(6):410–6.

32. Aide N, Talbot M, Fruchart C, et al. Diagnostic and prognostic value of baseline FDG PET/CT skeletal textural features in diffuse large B cell lymphoma. Eur J Nucl Med Mol Imaging 2018;45(5):699–711.

33. Decazes P, Becker S, Toledano MN, et al. Tumor fragmentation estimated by volume surface ratio of tumors measured on 18F-FDG PET/CT is an independent prognostic factor of diffuse large B-cell lymphoma. Eur J Nucl Med Mol Imaging 2018;45(10):1672–9.

34. Ceriani L, Gritti G, Cascione L, et al. SAKK38/07 study: integration of baseline metabolic heterogeneity and metabolic tumor volume in DLBCL prognostic model. Blood Adv 2020;4(6):1082–92.

35. Zucca E, Cascione L, Ruberto T, et al. Prognostic models integrating quantitative parameters from baseline and interim positron emission computed tomography in patients with diffuse large B-cell lymphoma: post-hoc analysis from the SAKK38/07 clinical trial. Hematol Oncol 2020;38(5):715–25.

36. Kostakoglu L, Dalmasso F, Berchialla P, et al. A prognostic model integrating PET-derived metrics and image texture analyses with clinical risk factors from GOYA. eJHaem 2022;3(2):406–14.

37. Milgrom SA, Elhalawani H, Lee J, et al. A PET radiomics model to predict refractory mediastinal Hodgkin lymphoma. Sci Rep 2019;9(1):1–8.

38. Lue KH, Wu YF, Liu SH, et al. Prognostic value of pretreatment radiomic features of 18F-FDG PET in patients with Hodgkin lymphoma. Clin Nucl Med 2019;44(10):e559–65.

39. Lue KH, Wu YF, Liu SH, et al. Intratumor heterogeneity assessed by 18F-FDG PET/CT predicts treatment response and survival outcomes in patients with Hodgkin lymphoma. Acad Radiol 2020;27(8):e183–92.

40. de Jesus FM, Yin Y, Mantzorou-Kyriaki E, et al. Machine learning in the differentiation of follicular lymphoma from diffuse large B-cell lymphoma with radiomic [18F]FDG PET/CT features. Eur J Nucl Med Mol Imaging 2022;49(5). https://doi.org/10.1007/s00259-021-05626-3.

PET Imaging in Chimeric Antigen Receptor T-Cell Trafficking

Patrick Glennan, BA[a], Vanessa Shehu, BA[b], Shashi B. Singh, MBBS[c],
Thomas J. Werner, MSE[d], Abass Alavi, MD[d],
Mona-Elisabeth Revheim, MD, PhD, MHA[e,f,*]

KEYWORDS

- Chimeric antigen receptor T-cell (CAR T-cell) • Trafficking • Positron Emission Tomography • PET
- [18F]fluorodeoxyglucose ([18F]FDG)

KEY POINTS

- The high sensitivity of PET and the wide array of possible cell labeling methods make it an excellent imaging method to track CAR T-cell trafficking.
- PET reporter genes have potential to accurately track cell migration, which is the key to early detection of off-target activity.
- The ideal radiotracer for PET imaging of CAR T-cell trafficking eludes consensus, requiring high cell viability, patient safety, and practical half-life.

INTRODUCTION

Chimeric antigen receptor (CAR) T-cell therapy is a form of autologous immunotherapy that involves the modification of genes to specifically target tumor antigens (**Fig. 1**).[1] The efficacy of these treatments has been demonstrated in the management of relapsed leukemias and lymphomas following hematopoietic cell transplantation.[2] Due to their impressive outcomes, the US Food and Drug Administration (FDA) has approved autologous T cells that have been modified to express a CAR targeting the CD19 B-lymphocyte molecules for the treatment of resistant pre-B-cell acute lymphoblastic leukemia (ALL), diffuse large B-cell lymphoma, and multiple myeloma, the second most common hematological cancer, that has relapsed after or is refractory to at least 4 prior treatments.[2,3] Examples of FDA-approved CAR T-cell therapies include tisagenlecleucel/Kymriah for ALL; axicabtagene ciloleucel/Yescarta, lisocabtagene maraleucel/Breyanzi, and idecabtagene vicleucel/Abecma for multiple myeloma. Additionally, the recent FDA approval of ciltacabtagene autoleucel/Carvykti in February 2022 marks a significant advancement in multiple myeloma treatment, underscoring the promising role of CAR T-cell therapy in this disease.[4,5] Ongoing research is exploring the potential applications of CAR T cells in the treatment of other

[a] Rutgers Robert Wood Johnson Medical School, 675 Hoes Lane West, Piscataway, NJ 08854, USA; [b] University of Pittsburgh School of Medicine, 3550 Terrace Street, Pittsburgh, PA 15261, USA; [c] Molecular Imaging Program at Stanford (MIPS), Stanford University School of Medicine, The Richard M. Lucas Center for Imaging, 1201 Welch Road, Stanford, CA 94305, USA; [d] Department of Radiology, Hospital of the University of Pennsylvania, 3400 Spruce Street, Philadelphia, PA 19104, USA; [e] Division for Technology and Innovation, The Intervention Center, Oslo University Hospital, Rikshospitalet, Post Box 4950 Nydalen, Oslo 0424, Norway; [f] Institute of Clinical Medicine, Faculty of Medicine, University of Oslo, Postbox 1078, Blindern, Oslo 0316, Norway

* Corresponding author. Division for Technology and Innovation, The Intervention Center, Oslo University Hospital, Rikshospitalet, Post Box 4950 Nydalen, Oslo 0424, Norway.
E-mail addresses: mona.elisabeth.revheim@ous-hf.no; m.e.rootwelt-revheim@medisin.uio.no

PET Clin 19 (2024) 569–576
https://doi.org/10.1016/j.cpet.2024.06.002
1556-8598/24/© 2024 Elsevier Inc. All rights are reserved, including those for text and data mining, AI training, and similar technologies.

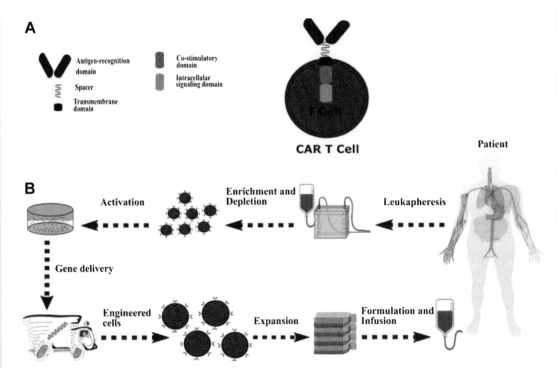

Fig. 1. An example of CAR T-cell construction. (*A*) A representation of one CAR composition with five labeled categories of protein domains, vary in CAR construction. (*B*) The simplified steps of autologous CAR-T cell manufacture and infusion including leukocyte collection, subset selection, CAR gene introduction, clonal expansion, and infusion. (*From* Ref.[11])

malignancies, such as chronic lymphocytic leukemia[6] and solid tumors,[7,8] as well as systemic rheumatic diseases[9] and autoimmune diseases.[10,11] Cell-based therapies hold significant potential in various medical fields; however, at present, there is a substantial lack of understanding regarding the homing pattern and migratory behaviors of CAR T cells in vivo and ex vivo, as well as their location within the body over extended periods of time.[12]

CAR T-cell trafficking refers to the movement and distribution of CAR T cells within the body after they have been administered to a patient. After infusion, the CAR T cells travel through the patient's body. The process of these cells moving to and accumulating in the appropriate anatomic sites (such as the tumor site) is known as trafficking. Effective trafficking is crucial for the success of the therapy, as it determines the ability of CAR T cells to reach and engage with cancer cells as opposed to depositing in healthy tissues and the central nervous system.[13,14] As new cell-based therapies are developed, there is a critical need for the advancement of imaging techniques that provide rapid assessment of these novel therapies, their molecular targets, and how effectively they traffic into tumor environments.[15]

PET imaging with [18F]fluorodeoxyglucose and other radiotracers has been crucial in the clinical management of patients with cancer undergoing CAR T-cell therapy.[16] It has also been instrumental in evaluating the systemic effects of CAR T-cell therapy in various organs.[17–19] However, the potential of PET imaging in CAR T-cell trafficking remains largely unknown.[13] In this article, the authors aim to explore the potential of PET imaging in the visualization of the distribution and movement of genetically engineered CAR T cells within the human body, as well as ex vivo.

PET AS A MODALITY FOR IMAGING CHIMERIC ANTIGEN RECEPTOR T-CELL TRAFFICKING

The scope for PET as an imaging modality for CAR T-cell trafficking is wide. Chief usages include the preclinical development of CAR T cells and evaluating their action on designed targets, development of adequate radiotracers and labeling for usage in human patients, identification of off-target activity including invasion of CAR T cells into the central nervous system (CNS), and use in conjunction with inducible signals that can use PET to potentially identify a tumor's antigen landscape (and thus CAR targets) without the need of a biopsy.[20]

PET benefits from being a noninvasive quantification method with very high sensitivity, with studies able to detect as few as 10,000 CAR T cells.[21] Laboratory techniques, including micropattern tumor array analysis and flow cytometry, have been used in an attempt to evaluate solid tumor infiltration and trafficking[22] but are not suitable for evaluating whole-body trafficking and are better suited as laboratory and preclinical tools. Fluorescence staining using lipophilic, near-infrared fluorescent cyanine dye (DiR) on natural killer (NK) cells has been proven in a small animal model,[23] which in itself is a variation of bioluminescence techniques that involve editing and inclusion of a "luciferase" gene for trafficking. The latter technique suffered from a key issue in that the bioluminescent factor's intensity depended on adenosine triphosphate, which was hindered by a decrease in T-cell mitochondrial function.[24] Many PET techniques, on the other hand, have been developed that have little-to-no effect on cell function and viability and maintain signal intensity.[13,21,25–27]

Novel CAR T-cell treatment development with varied gene expression to improve trafficking into solid tumors and decrease off-target activity can effectively use PET preclinically. CAR T-cell activity extraneous to the tumor can lead to the presentation of pseudoprogression or inflammation, both of which can be detected using PET.[28] In addition, off-target activity, especially in the CNS, is an important metric in the development of novel CAR T cells and targets. Inhibition of integrin

α4β1 and vascular cell adhesion molecule 1 interaction at the blood–brain barrier eliminates CAR T-cell extravasation.[29] This can be confirmed and used in conjunction with radionuclide labeling.

The ideal label of therapeutic cells is nontoxic, noninvasive, and will be retained by target cells for the desired monitoring period without compromising the viability and function of the cells.[30] Across the literature, efforts to label CAR T cells have employed 3 predominant methods: direct labeling of cells with a radioactive isotope in complex with a chelating molecule; indirect labeling via the expression of reporter genes by target cells; and, recently, nanoparticle tagging.[31]

DIRECT CELL LABELING

The first method by which CAR T cells can be labeled is direct labeling after the production of the CAR T cells and prior to reinfusion. Traditionally, cells have been labeled with a radiotracer by 2 means: passive diffusion of the tracer into the cells and binding of the tracer to targeted cell surface protein via a chelating molecule (**Fig. 2**).[30] One risk of cellular internalization of the tracer is that the tracer molecule disrupts the cell membrane of the CAR T cell, causing concerns for the viability and function of these therapeutic cells. Another issue with direct cellular labeling, broadly, is that cell death and cell division can lead to dilution of the radiotracer signal.[30,32] Efflux of the radioactive probe from the cells is also an issue associated with direct cell labeling,[31,32] albeit

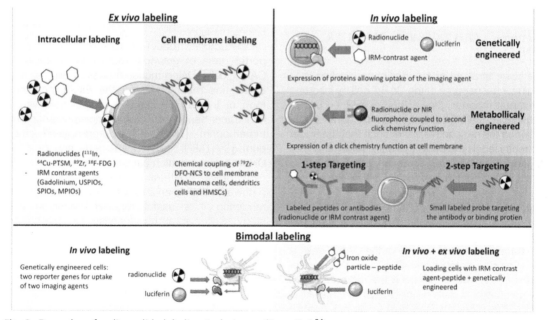

Fig. 2. Examples of radionuclide labeling techniques. (*From* Ref.[34])

efflux has also been observed with reporter gene-labeled cells.[33]

One development in immune cell imaging is the use of nanoparticles complexed to radioactive isotopes as a tracer of choice. In 2013, Bhatnagar and colleagues set a strong foundation for nano-tagging with their design of gold nanoparticles (GNPs) chelated to copper-64 ([^{64}Cu]) for PET imaging.[35] They used electroporation to directly label the CAR T cells in vitro. The half-life of [^{64}Cu] is 12.7 hours.[36] This group found that the size of the nanoparticles affected the efficiency by which the tracer crosses the cell membrane to enter the cell, noting that smaller particles were preferable for use. They reported no significant difference in the viability of the GNP-labeled CAR T cells upon electroporation in comparison to control CAR T cells.

Harmsen and colleagues published methods and findings for their dual-modal PET/near-infrared fluorescent tracer consisting of silica nanoparticles tagged to zirconium-89 ([^{89}Zr]) oxalate.[31] The nanoparticles were directly labeled with [^{89}Zr] in the presence of heparin and protamine ex vivo. The heparin and protamine enable the nano-tracer to bind to T cells. Given [^{89}Zr]'s half-life of 78.4 hours, this team was able to track CAR T-cell movement and migration in tumor-bearing immunodeficient mice for 7 days, after which the tracer was observed to dissociate. Another study used [^{89}Zr] desferrioxamine (DFO)-labeled CAR T cells that were found to have better stability compared to [^{89}Zr]oxine.[25] The long half-life of [^{89}Zr] makes it a useful radionuclide for direct labeling.

"Genomic LABELING" WITH REPORTER GENES

The basic strategy of reporter gene labeling is to engineer the genome of the CAR T cell by inserting the target reporter gene. When expressed by the transduced CAR T cells, the reporter gene should act upon the radioactive tracer such that the tracer indirectly labels the cells. Typically, reporter genes encode transporters, proteins with enzymatic functions, and receptors; in all 3 of these methods, the reporter protein will interact with the radiotracer to label the cells.[33,34] One goal for the usage of reporter genes is elucidating interactions between the protein gene products and the radioactive tracers such that activity of the CAR T cells is not altered. A notable benefit of reporter gene labeling is that the signal from the radiotracer will not be diluted as cells divide and/or die post-infusion.[32] This is because the CAR T cells need not be labeled in vitro with the radiotracer. Rather, the radiotracer can be injected into the patient immediately prior to the PET scan, and the genomic modification of the CAR T cells, which is retained by daughter cells upon proliferation, ensures that the CAR T cells will continue to be labeled by the radiotracer. This establishes the utility of reporter gene labeling for longitudinal tracking of the CAR T cells in vivo.

One type of reporter gene used to label cells is kinases, which will phosphorylate the target radiotracer, leading to its internalization by the cell. For example, herpes simplex virus type 1–thymidine kinase (HSV1-TK) has been employed in both preclinical and clinical studies for PET imaging.[13,37,38] Techniques to edit CAR T cells with HSV1-TK include the sleeping beauty transposon system, which has been verified through identification with 2'-deoxy-2'-[18F]fluoro-5-ethyl-1-β-D-arabinofuranosyl-uracil PET.[39] A benefit of nonhuman, viral reporter genes is that no tissues of the body will express the reporter gene, ensuring only the targeted CAR T cells are labeled. However, this benefit must be weighed against the reported immunogenicity of HSV1-TK in humans due to its viral origin.[13] The risk of a nonhuman reporter gene is that the foreign protein would trigger the immune system to attack the labeled CAR T cells.[40] An additional usefulness of a viral gene was shown with the HSV1-sr39tk gene, which provided a "kill-switch" for CAR T cells, whereby ganciclovir administration kills the cells due to the inclusion of the gene. It also has an increased sensitivity to the 9-[4-[18F]fluoro-3-(hydroxymethyl)butyl]guanine radionuclide.[38,41] Sakemura and colleagues contend that an additional drawback is the high background present with HSV1-TK, limiting the accuracy of cell trafficking measures.[26]

Dihydrofolate reductase (DHFR) is another reporter gene of growing interest for imaging of CAR T cells. Using mouse models, Sellmyer and colleagues recently tested the *Escherichia coli* form of the eDHFR gene in conjunction with a PET tracer based on the small molecule antibiotic trimethoprim (TMP), [18F]fluoropropyl-trimethoprim ([18F]TMP).[13] The DHFR gene encodes the DHFR enzyme, which catalyzes the conversion of dihydrofolate to tetrahydrofolate in biosynthetic pathways. TMP is an antibiotic inhibitor of eDHFR, rendering it a useful reporter tracer in this study. Sellmyer and colleagues designed anti-disialoganglioside 2 (GD2) CAR T cells that coexpressed eDHFR in addition to yellow fluorescent protein and Renilla luciferase, the latter 2 reporter genes being used for bioluminescent imaging to supplement the eDHFR-[18F]TMP PET.

During in vitro imaging tests, the CAR T cells demonstrated a 10 fold higher uptake of the PET tracer and a 50 fold higher signal intensity during bioluminescent imaging in comparison to control T cells. This successful result prompted the researchers to test this reporter gene tracking system in vivo with mice engrafted with GD2+ tumors, with PET scans being taken on day 7 and day 13, post-infusion of CAR T cells. The researchers report that the eDHFR reporter gene did not negatively impact the function of the CAR T cells. In addition, they found a pattern of initial uptake in the spleen followed by homing in the GD2+ tumors. While the pairing of eDHFR and [18F]TMP has yet to be studied in patients, this animal study demonstrates the longitudinal utility of reporter gene labeling. Furthermore, Sellmyer and colleagues claim that the eDHFR reporter system may be less immunogenic than the HSV1-TK, potentiating it to be more accessible for human use.

Human sodium iodide symporter (NIS) is another target that has been tested in preclinical models using [18F]tetrafluoroborate (TFB) PET and other radioisotopes, including technetium-99m and iodide-123. TFB, an iodide analog, has mild uptake in thyroid tissue and a shorter half-life compared to the other 2, at around 109.8 minutes. TFB, however, does not cross the blood–brain barrier. Thus, any attempts to use this imaging method to assess for neurotoxicity and errant trafficking into the CNS will be impossible using PET for NIS.[42] NIS has been used for CAR T-cell trafficking in triple-negative breast cancer models.[43] This reporter gene may be superior to HSV1-TK because of its reduced immunogenicity compared to the viral gene.[26]

Prostate-specific membrane antigen (PSMA), a type-II transmembrane glycoprotein, is a target that has been used for CAR T-cell trafficking since T cells rarely express the protein and thus provide a low background signal. [68Ga]Ga-PSMA-11, [177Lu]Lu-PSMA I&T, [18F]F-PSMA-1007, [18F]F-DCFPyL, and [68Ga]Ga-PSMA-617 have all been characterized for this purpose. A recent study reported being able to detect as few as 10,000 cells using [68Ga]Ga-PSMA-617.[21] Using [18F]F-DCFPyL requires at least 1 hour for complete uptake of the cells, which is perhaps a downside to this tracer.[26,44] However, PSMA tracers are highly available and in clinical use.

POTENTIAL RADIONUCLIDES FOR CHIMERIC ANTIGEN RECEPTOR T-CELL TRACKING

PET has been selected by many researchers as the imaging modality of choice to monitor adoptive cell therapy, or the immunotherapy method whereby either tumor-infiltrating lymphocytes or genetically modified T cells are used to treat cancers.[45,46]

However, trafficking in vivo using the ideal radio-tracer eludes consensus.

Lee and colleagues directly labeled CAR T cells with radioactive [89Zr]-DFO in an attempt at imaging in vivo cell trafficking. The marker was tested in mice only but highlights the interface of PET with the development of methods to monitor CAR T-cell activity. Overall, 95.2% of the CAR T cells were viable upon radiolabeling. The animal model used is adequate for [89Zr]-DFO testing given the noted comparable T-cell movement in the animal model to human patients.[25] In this study, there was no significant infiltration of tumors by the labeled cells. Nevertheless, [89Zr]'s half-life of approximately 78 hours allows a generous amount of time for the labeled cells to migrate to the tumor locations, provided that the cells assume regular migration patterns.[47]

[68Ga] labeling has been used for the last 20 years for the imaging of neuroendocrine tumors labeled to DOTATOC, the last 10 years for prostate cancer labeled with PSMA, and lately for labeling fibroblast-activation-protein inhibitors.[48] Its ability to act as an effective radionuclide for the imaging of cell trafficking has been assessed recently and has had promising results. [68Ga] has been compared to [89Zr] despite the large difference of the 2 radionuclides in half-life. The benefit of [89Zr] is the multiple-day half-life, giving time for the cells to migrate to the tumors. [68Ga] has a much shorter half-life, slightly more than 1 hour (68 minutes). One benefit of these radionuclides is that the absorbed dose of radiation is at least one order of magnitude lower than that of [89Zr].[49] In comparison with [89Zr], the 2 cell-attached radionuclides show similar migration to tumor microenvironments. Wang and colleagues employed mice and concluded that if cell trafficking in the first hours upon being labeled with [68Ga] is consistent with normal movement as compared to [89Zr]-labeled CAR T cells, future migration will be comparably normal. Additional investigation of [68Ga] labeling and cell migration is necessary to determine its long-term and predictive abilities to track cell trafficking.

[64Cu] is another radionuclide that has been the subject of a range of PET imaging studies for various cancers. Its versatility has been a highlight of its usefulness as a diagnostic tool, for example, its chelation abilities to be linked to peptides and other molecules.[50,51] One study showed that [64Cu] could be used to label daratumumab, a CD38 antibody. CD38 is a plasma cell receptor that is expressed in almost all patients with multiple myeloma and, therefore, a useful target for this cancer.[52] More recently, a human study has shown success with ex vivo [64Cu] labeling of CAR T cells using superparamagnetic iron oxide nanoparticles, which were then tracked in vivo. This PET/MR imaging study found high cell viability (>80%) after labeling and an ability to detect the cells at the tumor sites for several days.[53]

FUTURE PET APPLICATIONS

More investigation is necessary in the imaging of cell trafficking as a method for mitigation of damage caused by conditions such as cytokine release syndrome (CRS). The in vivo proliferation of CAR T cells introduced to patients is correlated with an increased presentation of CRS and neurotoxicity. Neurotoxicity effects have been associated with the migration of CAR T cells into the cerebrospinal fluid, releasing cytokines that could then cause damage to the central nervous system. Imaging of cell trafficking could allow physicians to more carefully administer safe doses that account for cell proliferation and subsequent damage.[54] The incorporation of PET for early tracking of immunotherapy cells can detect off-target activity and migration by the cells to counter detrimental effects such as CRS.

Regenerative medicine could benefit from in vivo imaging of cells. Transplanted stem cells require evaluation to determine whether they reach the target tissue, remain viable, and function properly in the transplanted patient.[55] PET is a possible imaging modality that could facilitate this evaluation.

As more cell immunotherapies are developed, especially the promising CAR NK therapy,[56] new methods will be required to allow for in vivo imaging of the therapeutic cells. The discovery of new radiotracers, reporter genes, and nanotags will provide a foundation for the translation of PET imaging and its application to other cell immunotherapies. A framework for therapy assessment via PET imaging could lead to future arbitration on immunotherapeutic effectiveness.

SUMMARY

The ability to monitor and track CAR T-cell trafficking is imperative for enhancing the effectiveness of immunotherapies in cancer treatment. Among various imaging modalities, PET imaging demonstrates significant promise due to its real-time and comprehensive tracking abilities. The use of reporter genes such as eDHFR, which have been shown to not negatively impact the function of CAR T cells, facilitates this imaging process. Furthermore, the incorporation of PET reporter genes holds potential in accurately tracking cell migration, thereby aiding in early detection of off-

target activity and controlling detrimental effects. However, despite these promising developments, further research and trials are necessary to standardize the PET imaging process for CAR T-cell tracking and to establish the ideal radiotracer suited for this task. These advancements are expected to ensure safe and optimal dosages for patients, leading to targeted and effective treatments.

CLINICS CARE POINTS

- A substantial lack of understanding of CAR T-cell homing patterns and migratory behaviors can lead to suboptimal therapy outcomes.
- Inadequate imaging and monitoring may result in CAR T-cells accumulating in non-target tissues, potentially causing off-target effects and adverse effects such as neurotoxicity and cytokine release syndrome.
- Effective CAR T-cell trafficking is essential for the success of CAR T-cell therapy, as it ensures that the engineered cells reach and engage with cancer cells rather than depositing in healthy tissues and causing adverse effects.
- PET has the potential to assess the distribution and movement of CAR T cells within the body, potentially enabling better evaluation and modification of therapeutic strategies.
- Incorporating PET imaging early in the therapy process can help detect off-target activity and migration of CAR T-cells, possibly allowing for timely intervention and modification of treatment. This approach can mitigate adverse effects like cytokine release syndrome and neurotoxicity by enabling physicians to administer safer doses and monitor cell proliferation closely.
- Modif.

DISCLOSURE

The authors have nothing to disclose. The authors declare that they have no conflicts of interest.

REFERENCES

1. UpToDate. Available at: https://www.uptodate.com/contents/immunotherapy-for-the-prevention-and-treatment-of-relapse-following-allogeneic-hematopoietic-cell-transplantation. [Accessed 30 March 2024].
2. June CH, O'Connor RS, Kawalekar OU, et al. CAR T cell immunotherapy for human cancer. Science 2018;359(6382):1361–5.

3. Sheykhhasan M, Ahmadieh-Yazdi A, Vicidomini R, et al. CAR T therapies in multiple myeloma: unleashing the future. Cancer Gene Ther 2024. https://doi.org/10.1038/s41417-024-00750-2.

4. Sheykhhasan M, Manoochehri H, Dama P. Use of CAR T-cell for acute lymphoblastic leukemia (ALL) treatment: a review study. Cancer Gene Ther 2022; 29(8–9):1080–96.

5. Turtle CJ, Hanafi LA, Berger C, et al. CD19 CAR–T cells of defined CD4+:CD8+ composition in adult B cell ALL patients. J Clin Invest 2016;126(6):2123–38.

6. Iovino L, Shadman M. CAR T-cell therapy for CLL: a new addition to our treatment toolbox? Clin Adv Hematol Oncol 2023;21(3):134–41. Available at: https://www.ncbi.nlm.nih.gov/pubmed/36867557.

7. Newick K, O'Brien S, Moon E, et al. CAR T cell therapy for solid tumors. Annu Rev Med 2017;68: 139–52.

8. Newick K, Moon E, Albelda SM. Chimeric antigen receptor T-cell therapy for solid tumors. Mol Ther Oncolytics 2016;3:16006.

9. Bhandari S, Bhandari S, Bhandari S. Chimeric antigen receptor T cell therapy for the treatment of systemic rheumatic diseases: a comprehensive review of recent literature. Ann Med Surg (Lond) 2023; 85(7):3512–8.

10. Su M, Zhao C, Luo S. Therapeutic potential of chimeric antigen receptor based therapies in autoimmune diseases. Autoimmun Rev 2022;21(1):102931.

11. Sadeqi Nezhad M, Seifalian A, Bagheri N, et al. Chimeric antigen receptor based therapy as a potential approach in autoimmune diseases: how close are we to the treatment? Front Immunol 2020;11: 603237.

12. Donnadieu E, Dupré L, Pinho LG, et al. Surmounting the obstacles that impede effective CAR T cell trafficking to solid tumors. J Leukoc Biol 2020;108(4): 1067–79.

13. Sellmyer MA, Richman SA, Lohith K, et al. Imaging CAR T cell trafficking with eDHFR as a PET reporter gene. Mol Ther 2020;28(1):42–51.

14. Slaney CY, Kershaw MH, Darcy PK. Trafficking of T cells into tumors. Cancer Res 2014;74(24):7168–74.

15. June CH, Sadelain M. Chimeric antigen receptor therapy. N Engl J Med 2018;379(1):64–73.

16. Sesques P, Tordo J, Ferrant E, et al. Prognostic impact of 18F-FDG PET/CT in patients with aggressive B-cell lymphoma treated with anti-CD19 chimeric antigen receptor T cells. Clin Nucl Med 2021;46(8):627–34.

17. Shrestha B, Singh S, Raynor W, et al. Role of 18F-FDG PET/CT to evaluate the effects of chimeric antigen receptor T-cell therapy on lymph node involvement in patients with non-Hodgkin lymphoma. J Nucl Med 2023;64(supplement 1):P1159. Available at: https://jnm.snmjournals.org/content/64/supplement_1/P1159.abstract. [Accessed 30 March 2024].

18. Shrestha B, Singh S, Raynor W, et al. Effects of chimeric antigen receptor T-cell therapy on pulmonary and hepatic FDG uptake in patients with non-Hodgkin lymphoma. J Nucl Med 2023;64(supplement 1):P1076. Available at: https://jnm.snmjournals.org/content/64/supplement_1/P1076.abstract. [Accessed 30 March 2024].

19. Shrestha B, Singh S, Ismoilov M, et al. Chimeric antigen receptor T-cell treatment for non-Hodgkin lymphoma: a comprehensive bone marrow evaluation with FDG PET/CT. J Nucl Med 2023;64(supplement 1):P1342. Available at: https://jnm.snmjournals.org/content/64/supplement_1/P1342.abstract. [Accessed 30 March 2024].

20. Shin J, Parker MFL, Zhu I, et al. Antigen-dependent inducible T-cell reporter system for PET imaging of breast cancer and glioblastoma. J Nucl Med 2023; 64(1):137–44.

21. Zhang Y, Song X, Xu Z, et al. Construction of truncated PSMA as a PET reporter gene for CAR T cell trafficking. J Leukoc Biol 2024;115(3):476–82.

22. Tokarew NJA, Gosálvez JS, Nottebrock A, et al. Flow cytometry detection and quantification of CAR T cells into solid tumors. Methods Cell Biol 2022;167: 99–122.

23. de Souza Fernandes Pereira M, Thakkar A, Lee DA. Non-invasive fluorescence imaging for tracking immune cells in preclinical models of immunotherapy. Methods Cell Biol 2022;167:163–70.

24. Serganova I, Moroz E, Cohen I, et al. Enhancement of PSMA-directed CAR adoptive immunotherapy by PD-1/PD-L1 blockade. Mol Ther Oncolytics 2017;4: 41–54.

25. Lee SH, Soh H, Chung JH, et al. Feasibility of real-time in vivo 89Zr-DFO-labeled CAR T-cell trafficking using PET imaging. PLoS One 2020;15(1): e0223814.

26. Sakemura R, Bansal A, Siegler EL, et al. Development of a clinically relevant reporter for chimeric antigen receptor T-cell expansion, trafficking, and toxicity. Cancer Immunol Res 2021;9(9):1035–46.

27. Leland P, Kumar D, Nimmagadda S, et al. Characterization of chimeric antigen receptor modified T cells expressing scFv-IL-13Rα2 after radiolabeling with 89Zirconium oxine for PET imaging. J Transl Med 2023;21(1):367.

28. Huang J, Rong L, Wang E, et al. Pseudoprogression of extramedullary disease in relapsed acute lymphoblastic leukemia after CAR T-cell therapy. Immunotherapy 2021;13(1):5–10.

29. Morales EA, Dietze KA, Baker JM, et al. Restricting CAR T cell trafficking expands targetable antigen space. bioRxiv 2024. https://doi.org/10.1101/2024.02.08.579002.

30. Xiao Z, Puré E. Imaging of T-cell responses in the context of cancer immunotherapy. Cancer Immunol Res 2021;9(5):490–502.

31. Harmsen S, Medine EI, Moroz M, et al. A dual-modal PET/near infrared fluorescent nanotag for long-term immune cell tracking. Biomaterials 2021;269:120630.

32. Wei W, Jiang D, Ehlerding EB, et al. Noninvasive PET imaging of T cells. Trends Cancer Res 2018;4(5):359–73.

33. Jurgielewicz P, Harmsen S, Wei E, et al. New imaging probes to track cell fate: reporter genes in stem cell research. Cell Mol Life Sci 2017;74(24):4455–69.

34. Perrin J, Capitao M, Mougin-Degraef M, et al. Cell tracking in cancer immunotherapy. Front Med 2020;7:34.

35. Bhatnagar P, Li Z, Choi Y, et al. Imaging of genetically engineered T cells by PET using gold nanoparticles complexed to Copper-64. Integr Biol 2013;5(1):231–8.

36. Zhou Y, Li J, Xu X, et al. 64Cu-based radiopharmaceuticals in molecular imaging. Technol Cancer Res Treat 2019;18. 1533033819830758.

37. Emami-Shahri N, Papa S. Dynamic imaging for CAR-T-cell therapy. Biochem Soc Trans 2016;44(2):386–90.

38. Keu KV, Witney TH, Yaghoubi S, et al. Reporter gene imaging of targeted T cell immunotherapy in recurrent glioma. Sci Transl Med 2017;9(373). https://doi.org/10.1126/scitranslmed.aag2196.

39. Najjar AM, Manuri PR, Olivares S, et al. Imaging of Sleeping Beauty-modified CD19-specific T cells expressing HSV1-thymidine kinase by positron emission tomography. Mol Imaging Biol 2016;18(6):838–48.

40. Mohseni YR, Tung SL, Dudreuilh C, et al. The future of regulatory T cell therapy: promises and challenges of implementing CAR technology. Front Immunol 2020;11:1608.

41. Murty S, Labanieh L, Murty T, et al. PET reporter gene imaging and ganciclovir-mediated ablation of chimeric antigen receptor T cells in solid tumors. Cancer Res 2020;80(21):4731–40.

42. Chen CH, Cheng MC, Hu TM, et al. Identification of rare mutations of the vasoactive intestinal peptide receptor 2 gene in schizophrenia. Psychiatr Genet 2022;32(3):125–30.

43. Volpe A, Lang C, Lim L, et al. Spatiotemporal PET imaging reveals differences in CAR-T tumor retention in triple-negative breast cancer models. Mol Ther 2020;28(10):2271–85.

44. Minn I, Huss DJ, Ahn HH, et al. Imaging CAR T cell therapy with PSMA-targeted positron emission tomography. Sci Adv 2019;5(7):eaaw5096.

45. Rosenberg SA, Packard BS, Aebersold PM, et al. Use of tumor-infiltrating lymphocytes and interleukin-2 in the immunotherapy of patients with metastatic melanoma. A preliminary report. N Engl J Med 1988;319(25):1676–80.

46. Wang Z, Cao YJ. Adoptive cell therapy targeting neoantigens: a frontier for cancer research. Front Immunol 2020;11:176.

47. García-Toraño E, Peyrés V, Roteta M, et al. Standardisation and half-life of 89Zr. Appl Radiat Isot 2018;134:421–5.

48. Kratochwil C, Flechsig P, Lindner T, et al. 68Ga-FAPI PET/CT: tracer uptake in 28 different kinds of cancer. J Nucl Med 2019;60(6):801–5.

49. Wang XY, Wang Y, Wu Q, et al. Feasibility study of 68Ga-labeled CAR T cells for in vivo tracking using micro-positron emission tomography imaging. Acta Pharmacol Sin 2021;42(5):824–31.

50. Wu N, Kang CS, Sin I, et al. Promising bifunctional chelators for copper 64-PET imaging: practical (64)Cu radiolabeling and high in vitro and in vivo complex stability. J Biol Inorg Chem 2016;21(2):177–84.

51. Anderson CJ, Ferdani R. Copper-64 radiopharmaceuticals for PET imaging of cancer: advances in preclinical and clinical research. Cancer Biother Radiopharm 2009;24(4):379–93.

52. Caserta E, Chea J, Minnix M, et al. Copper 64-labeled daratumumab as a PET/CT imaging tracer for multiple myeloma. Blood 2018;131(7):741–5.

53. Singla R, Wall DM, Anderson S, et al. First in-human study of in vivo imaging of ex vivo labeled CAR T cells with dual PET-MR. J Clin Orthod 2020;38(15_suppl):3557.

54. Brudno JN, Kochenderfer JN. Recent advances in CAR T-cell toxicity: mechanisms, manifestations and management. Blood Rev 2019;34:45–55.

55. Acton PD, Zhou R. Imaging reporter genes for cell tracking with PET and SPECT. Q J Nucl Med Mol Imaging 2005;49(4):349–60. Available at: https://www.ncbi.nlm.nih.gov/pubmed/16407818.

56. Sato N, Stringaris K, Davidson-Moncada JK, et al. In vivo tracking of adoptively transferred natural killer cells in rhesus macaques using 89Zirconium-oxine cell labeling and PET imaging. Clin Cancer Res 2020;26(11):2573–81.

Printed and bound by CPI Group (UK) Ltd, Croydon, CR0 4YY

08/05/2025

01864750-0014